JN443963

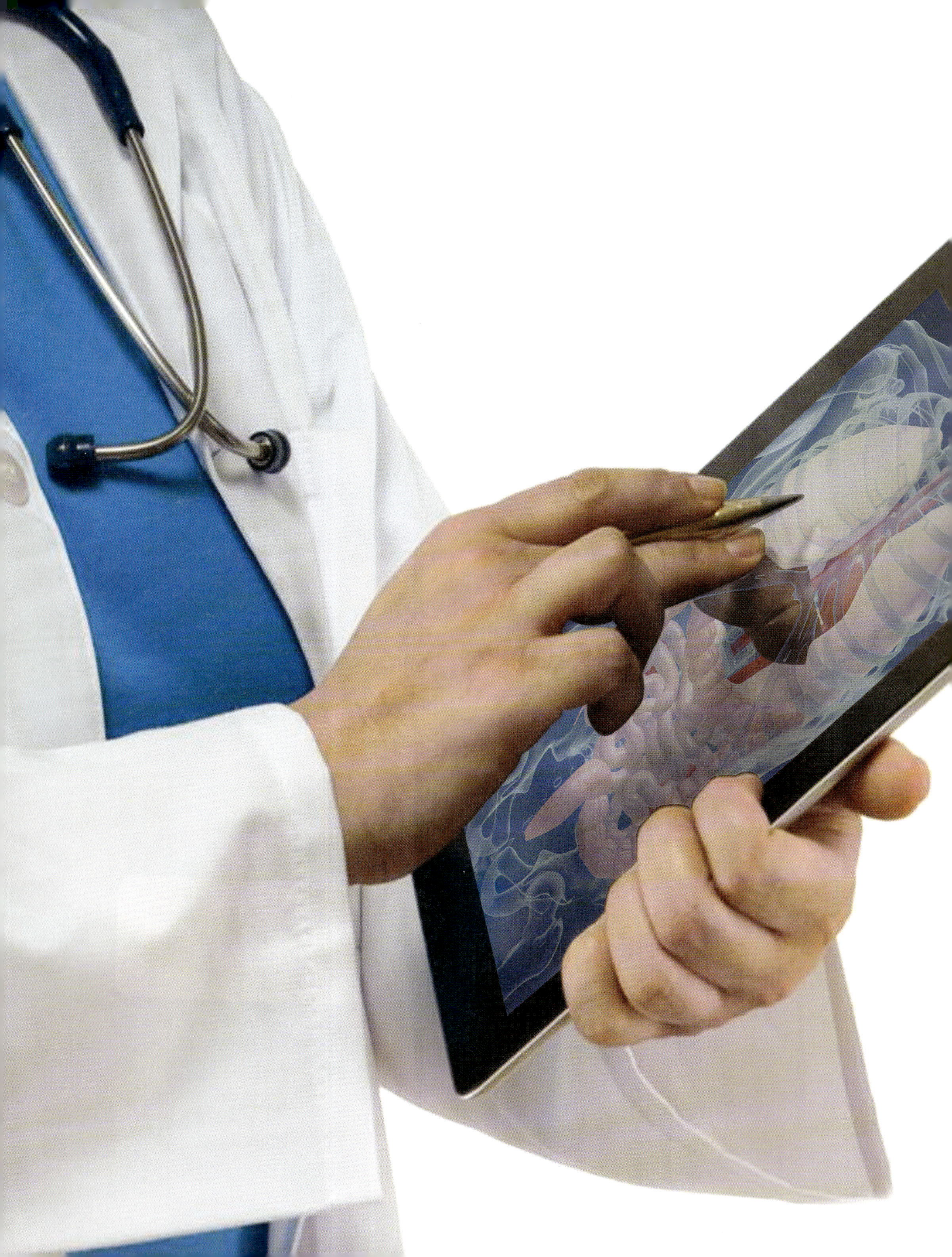

ESSENCE MEDICAL TERMINOLOGY

Kuk Hwan Lim, Eun Ha Kim, Hyun Sook Kim
Young Chul Kim, Hyun Ju Kwon, Byung Ki Lee
Kyu Hwa Lee, Kyung Sook Lee, Geun Hee Sul
Young Hui Nam, Ji Yeon Um, Sang man Hahn

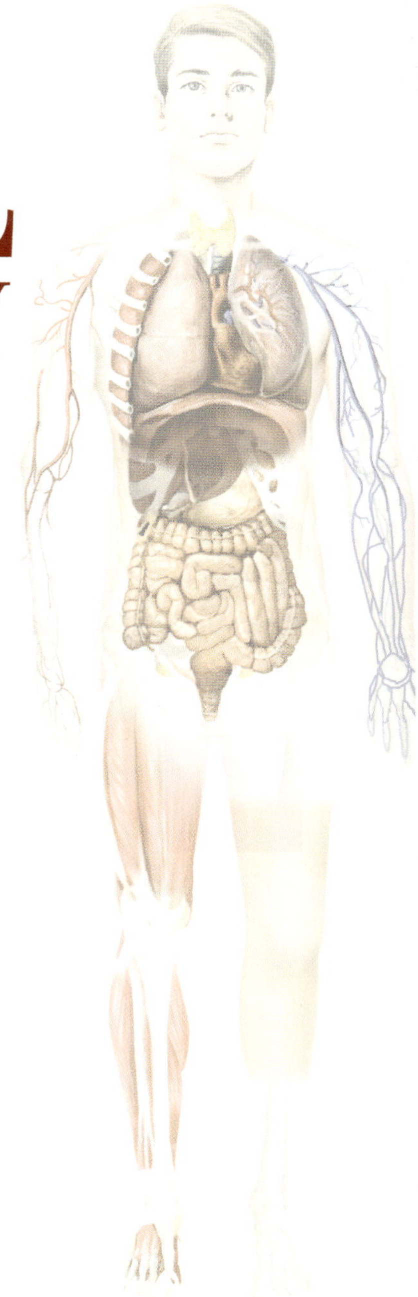

MEDI CEAN

Authors

Kuk Hwan Lim Korea University

Eun Ha Kim Catholic University of Pusan

Hyun Sook Kim Shinhan University

Young Chul Kim Keimyung University

Hyun Ju Kwon Namseoul University

Byung Ki Lee Daewon University

Kyu Hwa Lee Tongwon University

Kyung Sook Lee Soonchunhyang University

Geun Hee Sul Korea University

Young Hui Nam Namseoul University

Ji Yeon Um Kyungil University

Sang man Hahn Seoul National University
University of Texas at Austin.

Copyright © 2015 by MEDICEAN, Inc., Paju Book City, 209 Hoedong-gil Paju-si, Gyeonggi-do KOREA.

Tel : +82-31-955-7577 // Fax : +82-31-955-7730

Jigu Publishing Co., All rights reserved. Printed in the Korea. This publication is protected by Copyright and permission should be obtained from the publisher prior to any prohibited reproduction, storage in a retrieval system, or transmission in any form or by any means, electronic, mechanical, photocopying, recording, or likewise. For information regarding permission(s), writh to: Rights and Permissions Department.

MEDICEAN is a trademark of Jigu Publishing Inc., Paju Book City, KOREA.

MEDICEAN

ISBN 978-89-93033-92-2

Preface

Medical terminology is essential to describe such things as parts of the body, their locations, functions, diseases, surgical and clinical procedures, measurements, medical instruments, etc. It follows that physicians, nurses, medical technicians, medical recorders and administrative staff must use accurate medical terminology.

This book is built with chapters in which a rich mixture of human body illustrations and pictures are presented so that students of medicine, nursing, medical technology, healthcare informatics, public health science can easily understand.

Each chapter starts with study objectives and chapter composition. In Chapters 1 through 5, makeup of medical terminology, roots, prefixes, suffixes relating to human body and body organization are examined. Chapters 6 through 18 deal with human body systems in detail, by presenting anatomical terms, terms used for symptoms and diseases, analysis and meaning of key terms and abbreviations. "Memory Keys" are inserted and exercise questions are added in each chapter.

The book was coauthored by domestic professors and a scholar from the USA, with the contents deliberately co-examined for accuracy and easy reading. Thus it can be put to practical use not only in the USA and other English-speaking countries, but also in other countries such as China.

We will make a continuing effort to improve this book and seek advice and support from the teachers and the readers. We cordially extend our gratitude to President Joo, the editing staff and design team of Medicean publishing company. Lastly, we wish this book to be born as a favorite one loved by the readers.

In the spring of 2015,

One of the writers of this book

Structure and Features of this Book

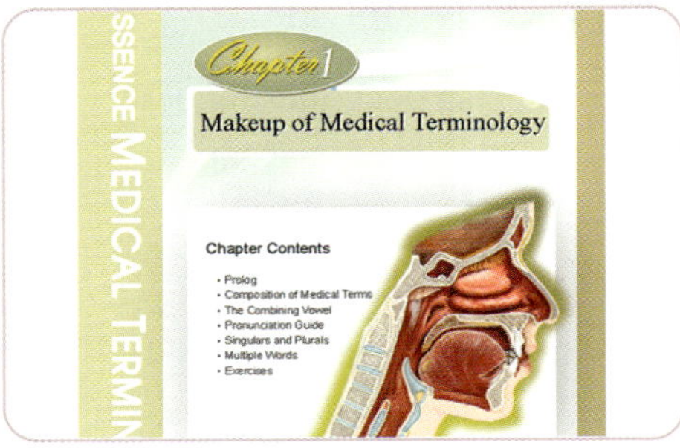

Chapter Contents

How the contents of the chapter are arranged is shown.

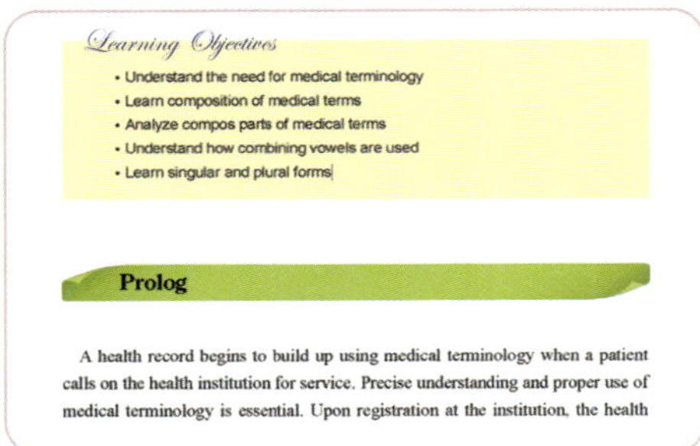

Learning Objectives

Core contents that readers must understand and strategy to learning are presented in each chapter.

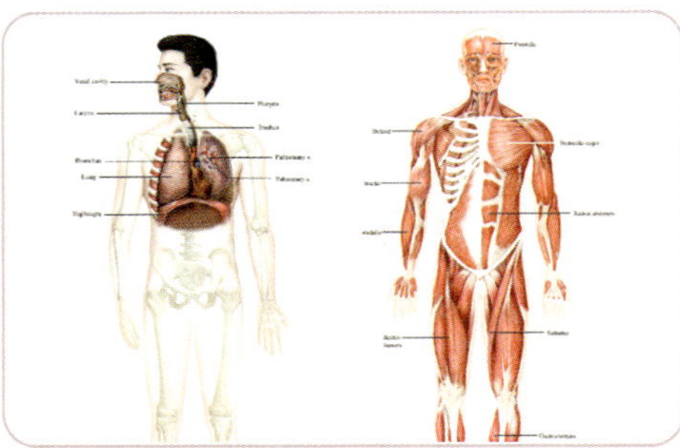

Anatomical Terms

Physiologically divided body systems in each chapter and frequently used terms for the anatomical location of the body are introduced along with illustrations.

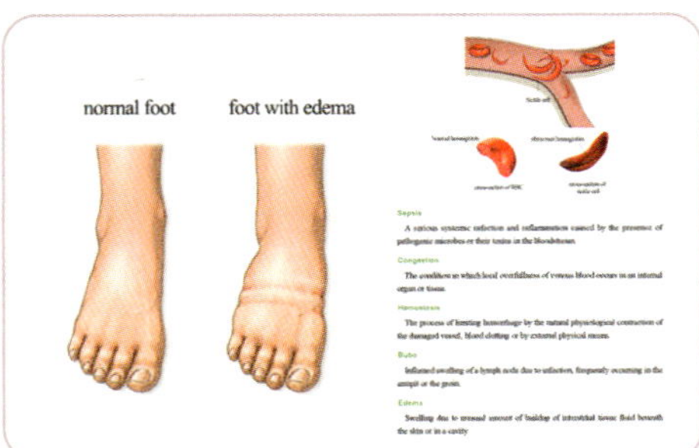

Terms for Symptoms and Diseases

Terminology for each part of the body related to symptoms and diseases are presented along with pictures, to help communicate with patients and other health professionals.

Struture & Feature

Terms for Surgery, Treatment and Diagnosis/Intervention

Terminologies used in various methods for diagnoses, surgery, treatment and intervention to help communicate in the medical field.

Terms for Surgery and Treatment

Angioplasty

Surgical reconstruction of the blood vessel by widening the narrowed portion using a balloon catheter or a stent.

Atherectomy

Surgical procedure to remove fatty plaque from an artery.

Atrial fibrillation ablation

The process of removing rapid, irregular or unsynchronized contractions of the atrium, typically by radiofrequency ablation.

Analysis and Meaning of Key Terms*

Key terms in each chapter are listed and analyzed to aid in understanding the meaning.

Analysis and Meaning of Key Terms

blood

Term	Term Analysis	Meaning
hemat/o, hem/o: blood		
hemolysis [himálәsis]	-lysis = breakdown, destruction, separation	breakdown of blood cells, esp. RBC
hematologist [hiːmәtaːlәdʒust]	-logist = specialist	scientist or doctor specializing in blood
hematology [hèmәtálәdʒi]	-logy = study of	study of blood and related organs and diseases

Abbreviations

Important multiple-word terms are listed as abbreviations and fully spelled terms.

Abbreviations

abbreviation	full term	meaning
AE	above elbow	above the elbow toward the attachment of the arm
AP	anterior-posterior	from front to back
BE	below elbow	below the elbow
BK	below knee	below the knee toward the feet
LE	lower extremity	leg
LLQ	left lower quadrant	lef lower quadrant of the abdominopelvic cavity
Lt.	left	

Momory Key

Some of the important items are encapsulated in the text to help the reader learn them by heart.

Memory Key

- There are several types of amblyopia: congenital amblyopia with no known cause; strabismic amblyopia, amblyopia due to severe refractive anomaly (near- or farsightedness, astigmatism); anisometropia (unequal refractive error between the two eyes), among others.

Exercises

Many terms are condensed at the end of each chapter as a test for the reader to practice with.

Exercises

1. Analyze the following terms into prefix, root, suffix and write the meaning.

① blepharoplasty — blephar/o + -plasty
plastic surgery of the eyelid

② keratomycosis — kerat/o + myc/o + -sis
inflammation of the cornea due to fungal infection

③ presbyopia — presby/o + -opia
inability of the eye to focus due to old age

④ ossiculoplasty — ossicul/o + -plasty

* Note : The word "term" in this book refers to a medical vocabulary, while "terminology" is a collective word for a group of terms as a study subject.

Contents

Preface / 03
Structure and features of this Book / 04
contents / 06

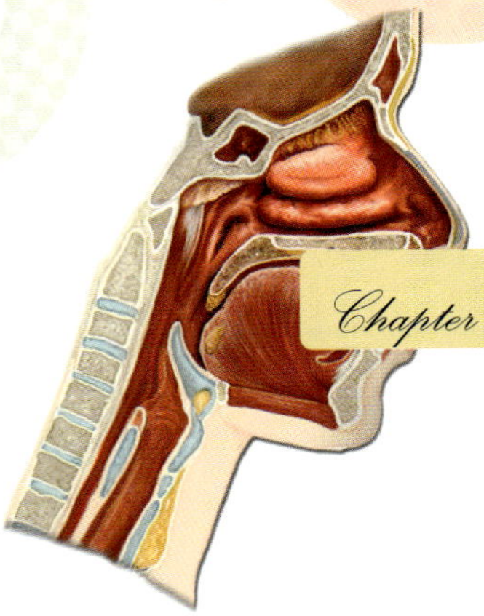

Chapter 1 Makeup of Medical Terminology

- Prolog 16
- Composition of medical terms 17
- The Combining Vowel 19
- Pronunciation Guide 20
- Singulars and Plurals 21
- Multiple Word Terms 24
- Exercises 25
- Medical Specialties 27
- Abbreviations for Diagnostic Procedures 28

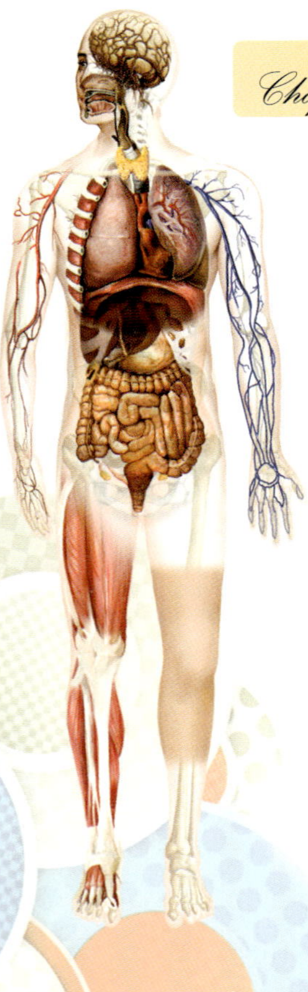

Chapter 2 Roots of Body Systems

- Prolog 30
- Anatomy and Physiology 30
- Organization of Human Body 31
- Anatomical Roots 32
    - Skeletal System / 32
    - Muscular System / 33
    - Integumentary System / 34
    - Respiratory System / 35
    - Digestive System / 36
    - Endocrine System / 37
    - Nervous System / 38
    - Circulatory System / 39
    - Lymphatic and Immune Systems / 40
    - Urinary System / 41
    - Male Reproductive System / 42
    - Female Reproductive System / 43
- Exercises 44

Contents

Chapter 3 Suffixes

- Prolog ···· 48
- General Suffixes ···· 48
- Adjectival Suffixes ···· 50
- Suffixes used to Indicate Pathological Conditions ···· 51
- Suffixes used to Indicate Diagnostic Procedures ···· 54
- Suffixes used to Indicate Surgical Procedures ···· 55
- Exercises ···· 57

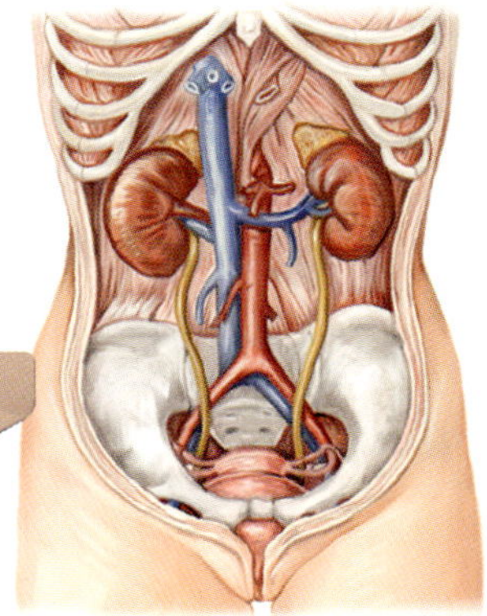

Chapter 4 Prefixes

- Prolog ···· 60
- Negative Prefixes ···· 60
- Prefixes Referring to Direction, Position, Posture, etc. ···· 61
- Prefixes Related to Time ···· 64
- Prefixes Referring to Numbers and Measurements ···· 65
- Miscellaneous Prefixes ···· 67
- Prefixes with Similar or Opposite Meaning ···· 69
- Exercises ···· 70

Chapter 5 Body Organization

- Prolog ···· 74
- Terms for Cavities in the Body ···· 75
  - Body Cavities / 75
  - Abdominopelvic Regions and Quadrants / 77
  - Anatomical Planes / 78
- Terms for Direction and Motion of the Body ···· 80
- Analysis and Meaning of Key Terms ···· 84
- Abbreviations ···· 85
- Exercises ···· 86

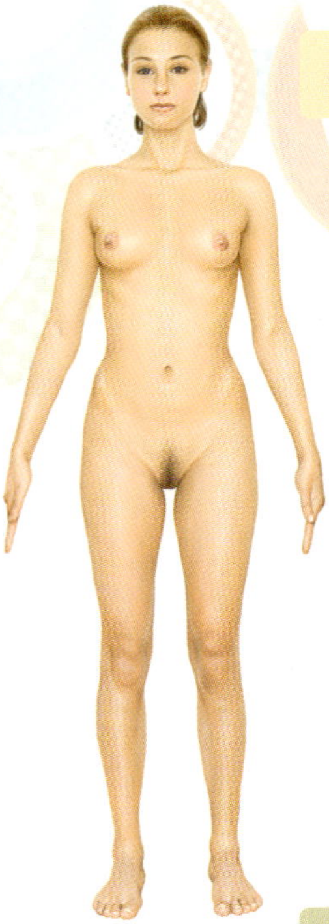

Chapter 6 Integumentary System

- Prolog 88
- Anatomical Terms 89
  - Epidermis / 89
  - Dermis / 90
  - Subcutaneous Tissue / 91
  - Skin Appendage / 91
- Terms for Symptoms and Diseases 94
- Terms for Surgery and Treatment 103
- Terms for Test and Intervention 105
- Analysis and Meaning of Key Terms 106
- Abbreviations 109
- Exercises 110

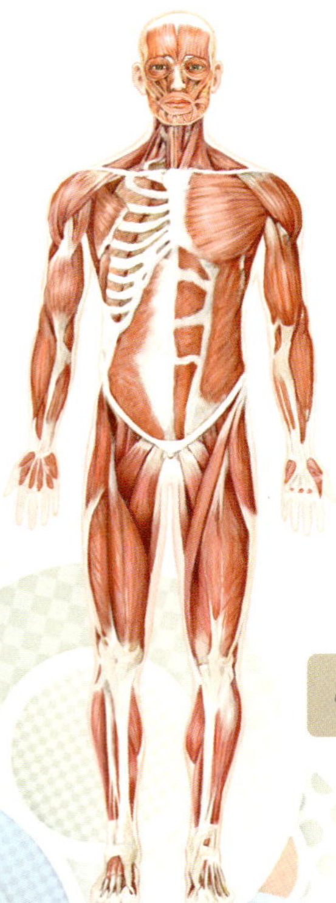

Chapter 7 Skeletal System

- Prolog 114
- Anatomical Terms 114
  - Bone Types / 114
  - Osteocytes / 116
  - Bone Structure / 116
  - Construction of the Skeleton / 118
- Terms for Symptoms and Diseases 125
- Terms for Test and Surgery 127
- Analysis and Meaning of Key Terms 128
- Abbreviations 133
- Exercises 134

Chapter 8 Muscular System

- Prolog 140
- Anatomical Terms 140
  - Attachment of Muscle / 140
  - Types of Muscles / 141
  - Structure of Muscles / 141

Contents

Motions by Skeletal Muscles / 143

- Terms for Symptoms and Diseases 145
- Terms for Test and Surgery 147
- Analysis and Meaning of Key Terms 147
- Abbreviations 150
- Exercises 151

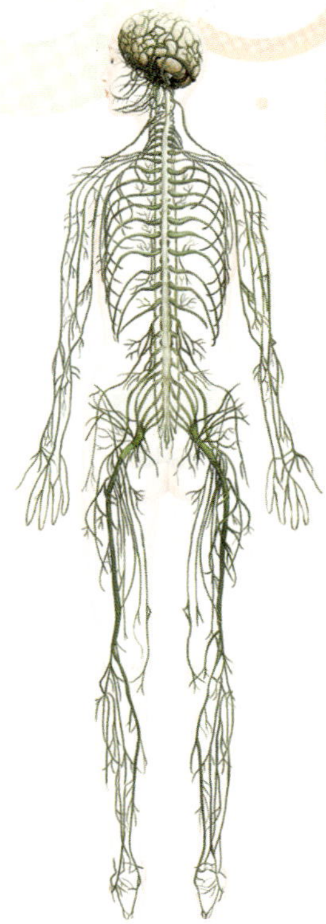

Chapter 9 Nervous System

- Prolog 154
- Anatomical Terms 155

  Central Nervous System / 155

  Peripheral Nervous System / 157
- Terms for Symptoms and Diseases 159
- Terms for Surgery and Treatment 160
- Terms for Test and Intervention 161
- Analysis and Meaning of Key Terms 162
- Abbreviations 165
- Exercises 166

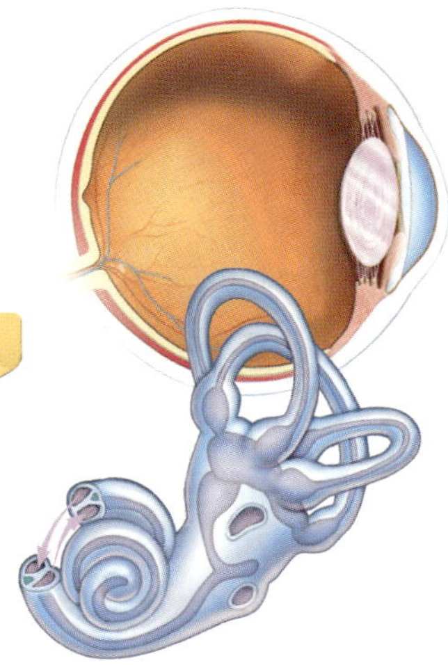

Chapter 10 Eye and Ear

- Understanding the Eye 170
- Anatomical Terms 171

  Outer Eye / 171

  Inner Eye / 171
- Terms for Symptoms and Diseases 176
- Terms for Surgery and Treatment 183
- Terms for Test and Intervention 185
- Analysis and Meaning of Key Terms 186
- Understanding the Ear 190
- Anatomical Terms 191

  Outer Ear / 191

  Middle Ear / 191

  Inner Ear / 193

- Terms for Symptoms and Diseases 195
- Terms for Surgery and Treatment 198
- Terms for Test and Intervention 199
- Analysis and Meaning of Key Terms 199
- Abbreviations 202
- Exercises 203

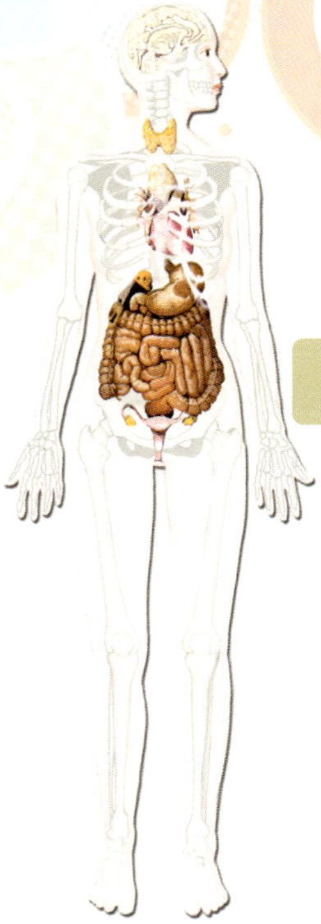

Chapter 11 Endocrine System

- Prolog 208
- Anatomical Terms 210
- Terms for Symptoms and Diseases 214
- Terms for Surgery and Treatment 217
- Terms for Test and Intervention 218
- Analysis and Meaning of Key Terms 219
- Abbreviations 223
- Exercises 224

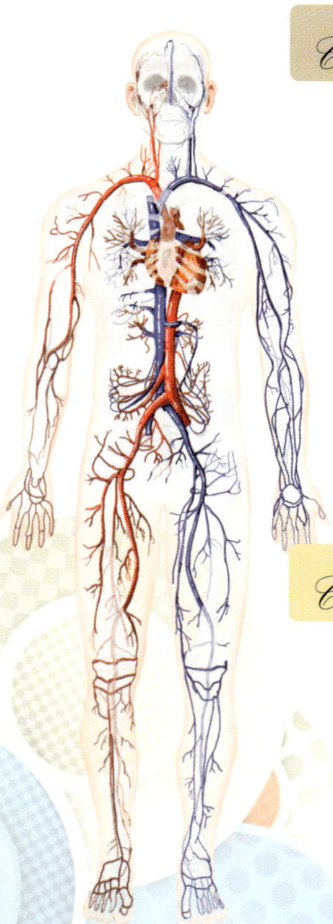

Chapter 12 Circulatory, Cardiovascular System

- Prolog 228
- Anatomical Terms 228
- Terms for Symptoms and Diseases 237
- Terms for Surgery and Treatment 241
- Terms for Test and Intervention 242
- Analysis and Meaning of Key Terms 245
- Abbreviations 247
- Exercises 250

Chapter 13 Blood and Immune/Lymphatic System

- Prolog 256
- Anatomical Terms 259
- Terms for Symptoms and Diseases 262
- Terms for Surgery and Treatment 264

Contents

- Terms for Test and Intervention ········ 265
- Analysis and Meaning of Key Terms ········ 266
- Abbreviations ········ 270
- Exercises ········ 271

Chapter 14 Respiratory System

- Prolog ········ 274
- Anatomical Terms ········ 275
    - Nose, Nasal Cavity and Paranasal Sinuses / 275
    - Pharynx, Larynx and Trachea / 276
    - Bronchus and Lung / 278
    - Pleural and Mediastinal Cavities / 281
- Terms for Symptoms and Diseases ········ 282
- Terms for Surgery and Treatment ········ 289
- Terms for Test and Intervention ········ 292
- Analysis and Meaning of Key Terms ········ 294
- Abbreviations ········ 299
- Exercises ········ 301

Chapter 15 Digestive System

- Prolog ········ 306
    - Oral Cavity / 307
    - Gastrointestinal Tract Activities / 308
- Anatomical Terms ········ 309
    - Oral Cavity / 309
    - Pharynx, Esophagus and Stomach / 313
    - Small and Large Intestines, Peritoneum / 316
    - Liver, Biliary system and Pancreas / 318
- Terms for Symptoms and Diseases ········ 320
    - Oral Cavity / 320
    - Pharynx, Esophagus and Stomach / 323
    - Small and Large Intestines, Peritoneum / 326
    - Liver, Biliary system and Pancreas / 330
- Terms for Surgery and Treatment ········ 332
    - Oral Cavity / 332
    - Pharynx, Esophagus and Stomach / 332

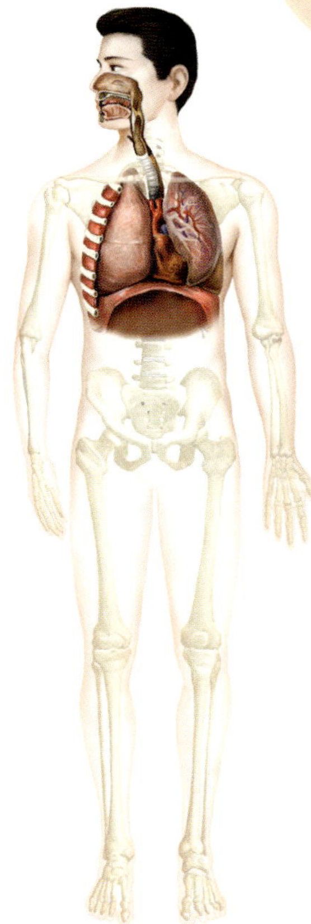

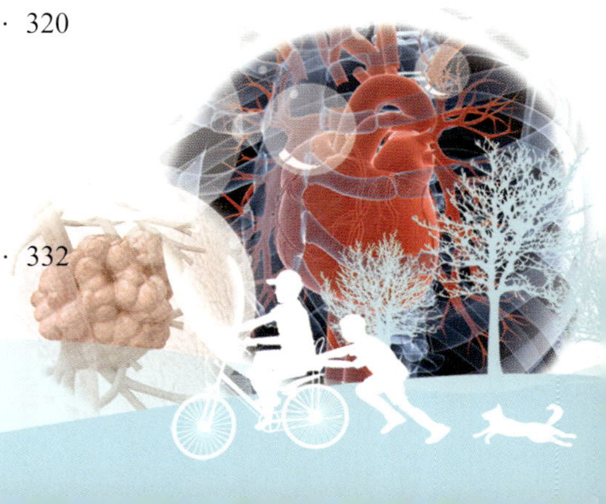

Small and Large Intestines, Peritoneum / 334
Liver, Biliary system and Pancreas / 336
• Terms for Test and Intervention 338
• Analysis and Meaning of Key Terms 339
• Abbreviations 343
• Exercises 345

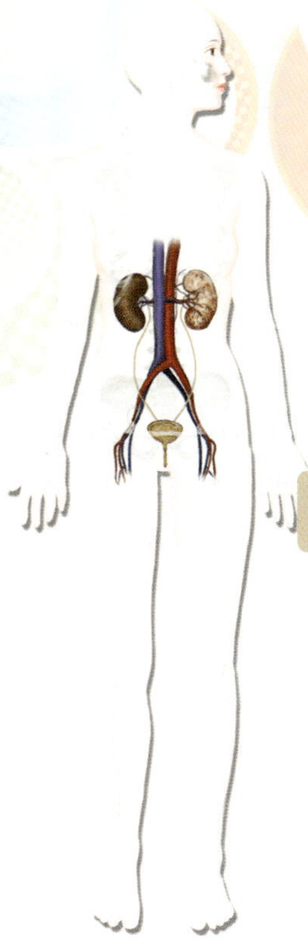

Chapter 16 Urinary System

• Prolog 348
• Anatomical Terms 348
• Terms for Symptoms and Diseases 354
Symptoms / 354 Diseases / 356
• Terms for Surgery and Treatment 359
• Terms for Test and Intervention 362
• Analysis and Meaning of Key Terms 365
• Abbreviations 366
• Exercises 368

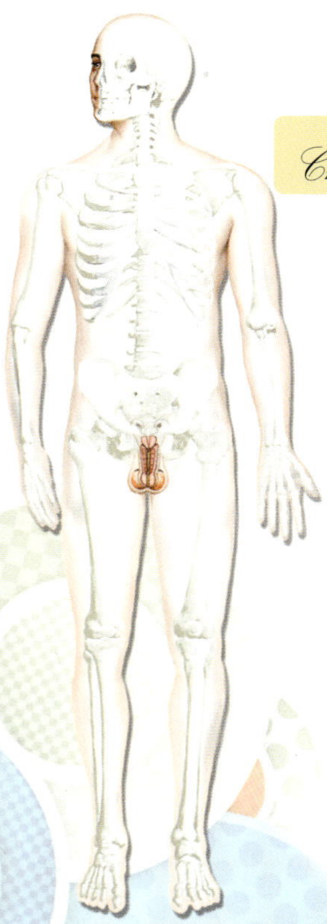

Chapter 17 Male Reproductive System

• Prolog 374
• Anatomical Terms 375
• Terms for Symptoms and Diseases 378
Sexually Transmitted Infections (STI) / 382
• Terms for Surgery and Treatment 383
• Terms for Test and Intervention 384
• Analysis and Meaning of Key Terms 385
• Abbreviations 387
• Exercises 387

Contents

Chapter 18 Female Reproductive System and Obstetrics

- Prolog 392
- Anatomical Terms 393
    - Vulva and Vagina / 393
    - Uterus and Pelvic Supporting Structure / 394
    - Ovaries and Fallopian Tubes / 396
    - Breast / 397
    - Menstrual Cycle / 397
- Terms for Symptoms and Diseases 397
    - Vulva and Vagina / 399
    - Uterus and Pelvic Supporting Structures / 399
    - Ovaries and Uterine Tubes / 400
    - Breasts / 401
- Terms for Surgery and Treatment 402
- Terms for Test and Intervention 403
- Analysis and Meaning of Key Terms 404
- Anatomical Terms in Obstetrics 406
- Terms for Symptoms and Diseases in Obstetrics 409
- Terms for Surgery and Treatment in Obstetrics 412
- Analysis and Meaning of Key Terms in Obstetrics 413
- Abbreviations 415
- Exercises 416

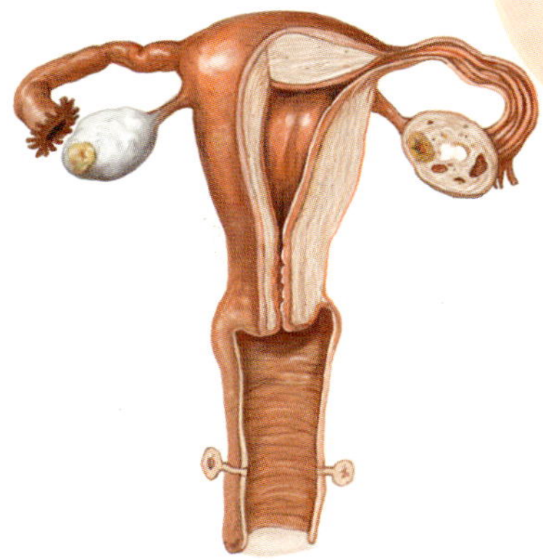

Index / 419

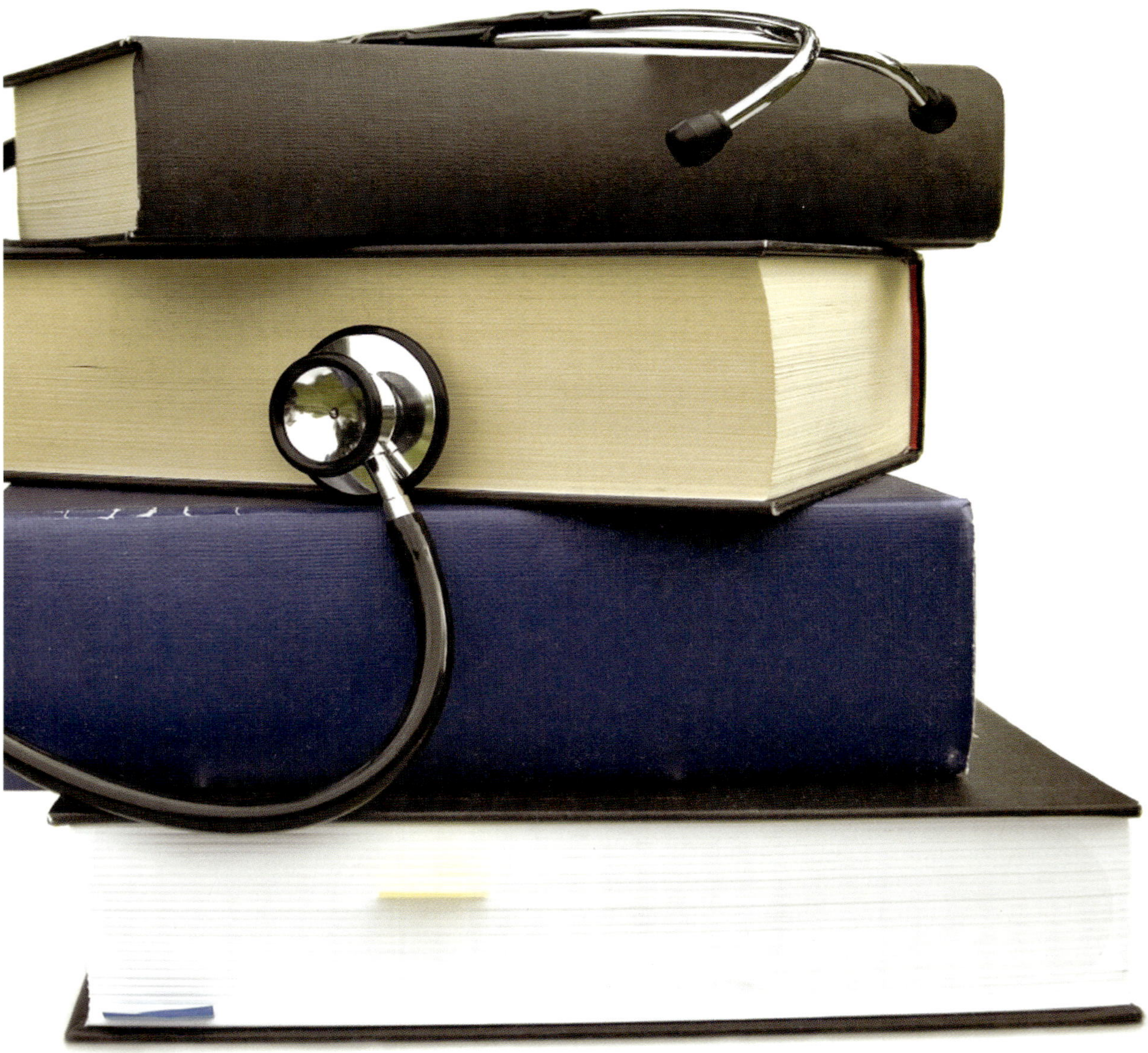

Chapter 1

Makeup of Medical Terminology

Chapter Contents

- Prolog
- Composition of Medical Terms
- The Combining Vowel
- Pronunciation Guide
- Singulars and Plurals
- Multiple Word Terms
- Exercises
- Medical Specialties
- Abbreviations for Diagnostic Procedures

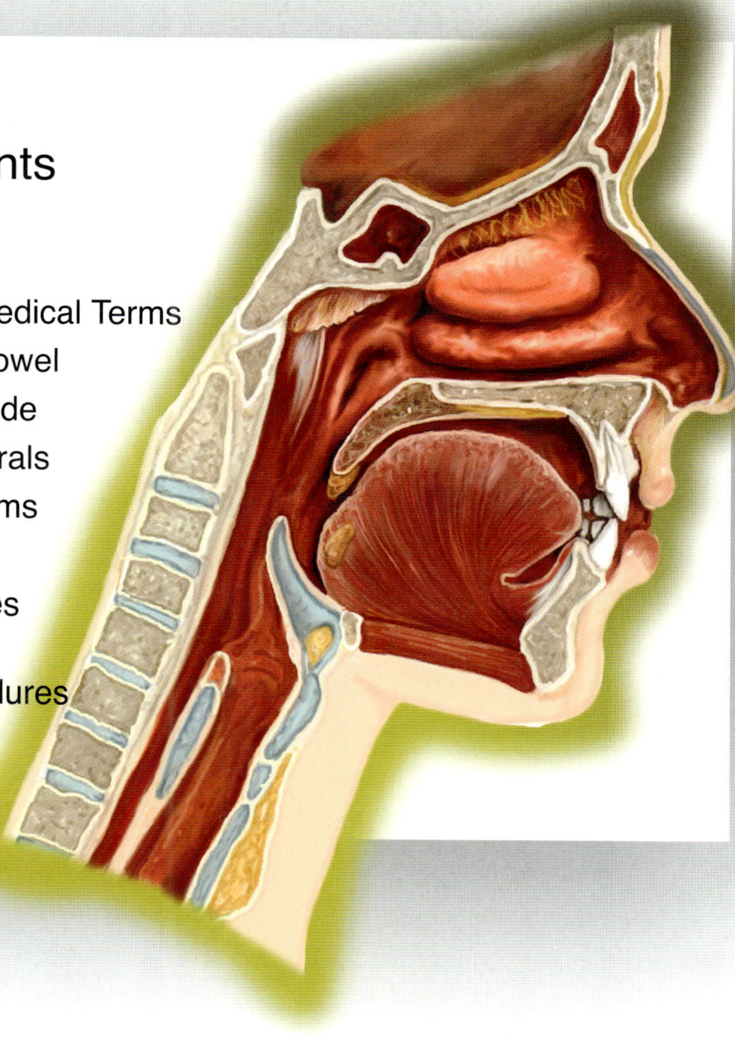

Learning Objectives

- Understand the need for medical terminology.
- Learn composition of medical terms.
- Analyze compos parts of medical terms.
- Understand how combining vowels are used.
- Learn singular and plural forms.

Prolog

A health record begins to build up using medical terminology when a patient calls on the health institution for service. Precise understanding and proper use of medical terminology is essential. Upon registration at the institution, the health professional records the patient' name, resident registration number, or ID number, contact infomation, insurance infomation and reason for visit. They also obtain the patient's health history and continue building up the record through test, diagnosis and treatment using medical terminology. When the patient is admitted and appropriate services are performed, the record is populated with details using standard medical terminology, and it becomes the basis for billing expenses incurred.

While standardization of the recording formats, codes and computerization would be desirable, individual health institutions are legally responsible for their own patients' health records. One such method is SOAP, which stands for Subjective, Objective, Assessment and Plan. The health service performer obtains the patient's subjective description of his/her symptoms. Then objective data is acquired through tests and measurements on the patient's body to use in diagnosis. In the assessment stage, all data is synthesized and the diagnosis is performed. Finally, treatment method, advice to the patient, additional tests, medication, etc. are determined. In all stages of SOAP appropriate and precise use of medical terminology is essential to build and maintain accurate health records.

Medical terminology is used to describe such things as parts of the body, locations, functions, diseases, surgical and clinical procedures, measurements and medical instruments. Each medical term is typically a combined word that can be expressed by multiple words. For example, '*gastroenteritis*' is a short form of saying '*inflammation of the stomach and intestines*'.

Each chapter deals with terminology belonging in each human body system. They are classified into terms for anatomic, pathology, diagnosis, surgery and treatment. Exercises are at the end of the chapter for the reader to review and test oneself.

Composition of Medical Terms

A medical term is typically made up of the following word elements: **prefix**, **root**, **suffix** and combining **vowel** that follows the root. However, not all terms have all four parts. Some terms don't have a prefix or a root, and others have multiple roots. And combining vowels don't always follow roots.

Analyzing each term by dividing it into composing elements vastly helps you understand, memorize and apply in actual use. As an example, when you learn 10 roots and 10 suffixes, theoretically you can compose 100 terms. Roots mostly refer to parts of the body (cells, tissues, organs, organ systems, organisms, etc.). Roots, suffixes and prefixes will be studied in detail in chapters 2, 3, 4 respectively.

Let's examine elements of some example terms by analysis.

[Ex. 1] When all four elements are used

endocrinology (study of the endocrine glands)

prefix	**endo-**	inside, within
root	**crin**	secretion
combining vowel	**-o-**	
suffix	**-logy**	study, science

[Ex. 2] When combining vowel is not necessary (typically the tail of the root or the head of the suffix is a vowel)

periarthritis (inflammation of the surrounding part of a joint)

prefix	**peri-**	vicinity, near, surrounding
root	**arthr**	joint
combining vowel		
suffix	**-itis**	inflammation

[Ex. 3] When there is no prefix

gastrology (study of the stomach)

prefix		
root	gastr	stomach
combining vowel	**-o-**	
suffix	**-logy**	study, science

some terms without prefix :

adenitis	inflammation of a gland
carditis	inflammation of the heart
hepatitis	inflammation of the liver
cardiology	study of the heart
hepatology	study of the liver

[Ex. 4] When the root and combining vowel are absent (a prefix and a suffix are combined)

neoplasm (new growth; typically abnormal growth meaning tumor)

prefix	**neo-**	new
root		
combining vowel		
suffix	**-plasm**	expansion, growth

metastasis (spread of the disease, usually tumor)

prefix	**meta-**	after, beyond, transcending
root		
combining vowel		
suffix	**-stasis**	being stationary or static

[Ex. 5] When multiple roots are combined (no prefix)

gastroenteritis (inflammation of stomach and intestines)

prefix		
root	**gastr**, **enter**	stomach, intestines
combining vowel	**-o-** (used only at the end of gastr)	
suffix	**-itis**	inflammation

The Combining Vowel

A combining vowel is used between a root and a suffix, or between two roots so as to facilitate pronuncing the resultant term. For example, the vowel -o- in '*gastrology*' helps in making smooth pronunciation between the root 'gastr' and the suffix '*-logy*'. A combining vowel is mostly used only when the suffix begins with a consonant. In most cases the combining vowel is -o-, however, -e- or -i- may be used instead.

In analysis of terms, a slash (/) is inserted between the root and the combining vowel. The resultant expression becomes a ***combining form***. For example, the combining form for the root 'gastr' is **gastr/o**. Combining form is used to indicate what combining vowel follows a specific root.

Generally, /o follows the root before the suffix :

hepatology (study of liver) = hepat/o (of liver) + -logy (study)

Occasionally /e follows the root before the suffix :

kinesthesia (perception of body movement) = kin/e (of movement) + esthesia (perceiving)

cholelith (gallstone) = chol/e (of gall) + -lith (stone)

Occasionally /i follows the root before the suffix :

dentiform (shape of a tooth) = dent/i (of tooth) + -form (shape)

bronchiectasis (enlargement of the lung airways) = bronch/i (of airways of the lung) + -ectasis (dilation, enlargement)

Sometimes no combining vowel is used because the suffix begins with a vowel :

gastritis (stomach inflammation) = gastr/o (of stomach) + -itis (inflammation)

When the root ends with a vowel and the suffix begins with the same vowel, one of them is discarded :

carditis (inflammation of the heart) = cardi/o (of heart) + -itis (inflammation)

kinesthesia (perception of body movement) = kin/e (of movement) + -esthesia (perceiving)

When the root ends with a vowel and the suffix begins with another vowel, a third vowel is inserted :

cardioesophageal (pertaining to junction of cardiac and esophagus) =
cardi/o (of heart) + esophag/o (esophagus, gullet) + -e- + -al (pertaining to)

When the prefix ends with a vowel and the root begins with another vowel, the vowel belonging to the prefix is discarded :

parenteral (not of intestine, intravenous) =
para (near, beside) + enter/o (of intestine) + -al (pertaining to)

Pronunciation Guide

For you to be able to use medical terms in real life, you must learn how to pronounce them. Each new term will be introduced with a phonetic notation as well as its meaning. Some terms can have more than one accepted pronunciation, so if a term is pronounced differently than the notation given in this book it's not necessarily incorrect.

Each term is divided into syllables and spelled phonetically to aid in pronunciation. Phonetic spelling is done with the spelling that is generally accepted to produce a particular sound. For example, pronunciation for 'nation' is spelled, with a hyphen (-) in the phonetic spelling between the two syllables, and the phonetically emphasized syllable (the first one in [**nay**-shun]) is noted in bold characters.

Syllable	Pronunciation	Example
short vowel a	ah	acute [ah-**kyout**]
long vowel a	ay	nation [**nay**-shun]
short vowel e	eh	hemoptisis [heh-**mop**-tih-sis]
long vowel e	ee	ileitis [**ill**-ee-**eye**-tis]
short vowel i	ih	adipose [**ad**-ih-pohs]
long vowel i	eye	ileitis [**ill**-ee-**eye**-tis]
long vowel o	oh	anorexia [**an**-oh-**reck**-see-ah]
long vowel u	you	acute [ah-**kyout**]
-tion	shun	nation [**nay**-shun]

In the following examples, consonants are shown to be pronounced in more than one way.

Consonant	Pronunciation	Example
c before a, o, u	k	cat, colon, cure, colposcopy
c before e, i, y	s	cervix, circle, cystocele
ch-	k	cholesterol, chronic, psychology
g before a, o, u	g	gallstone, gonad, gastrology
g before e, i	j	generic, geriatrics, giant
pn-	n	pneumatic, pneumonia
ps-	s	psychology
pt-	t	pterygium, ptosis
rh, rrh	r	rhythm, hemorrhoid
x- as first letter	z	xerosis

Singulars and Plurals

Plurals are formed in various ways, depending on the tail part of the term. Here are general rules and examples.

-is → -es

[Ex] diagnosis → diagnoses
pelvis → pelves
neurosis → neuroses
metastasis → metastases

-itis → -itides

[Ex] arthritis → arthritides
meningitis → meningitides

-us → -i

[Ex]	alveolus	→	alveoli
	bacillus	→	bacilli
	bronchus	→	bronchi
	embolus	→	emboli
	malleolus	→	malleoli

Exceptions to this rule, where -es is appended to

sinus	→	sinuses
virus	→	viruses

-a → -ae

[Ex]	bursa	→	bursae
	scapula	→	scapulae
	sclera	→	sclerae
	vena cava	→	venae cavae or vena cavae
	vertebra	→	vertebrae

-um → -a

[Ex]	atrium	→	atria
	capitulum	→	capitula
	diverticulum	→	diverticula
	ovum	→	ova
	septum	→	septa

-ix, -ex → -ices

[Ex]	apex	→	apices
	appendix	→	appendices
	calix	→	calices
	cervix	→	cervices
	cortex	→	cortices
	index	→	indices
	varix	→	varices

-ax → -aces

[Ex]	thorax	→	thoraces

-oma → -omas or -omata

[Ex]	adenoma	→	adenomas or adenomata
	carcinoma	→	carcinomas or carcinomata
	fibroma	→	fibromas or fibromata
	lipoma	→	lipomata

-nx → -nges

[Ex]	larynx	→	larynges
	meninx	→	meninges
	phalanx	→	phalanges

-on → -ons or -a

[Ex]	criterion	→	criteria
	ganglion	→	ganglions or ganglia

Multiple Word Terms

Sometimes a term consists of multiple words. In this case, the term typically doesn't have its components such as prefix, suffix and root combined into a term but spelled separately and may be given special meaning. When a term consists of more than two Greek or Latin words, you may simply memorize it as an idiom rather than find the meaning by analyzing.

vena cava (major vein that returns blood to the heart)

vena = vein   cava = heart

ductus deferens (sperm-carrying duct)

ductus = passage, duct   deferens = carrying-away (of sperm)

ductus deferens paravaginalis (sperm-carrying duct around vagina)

paravaginalis = of tissue around vagina

anorexia nervosa (nervous obsessive eating disorder)

anorexia = loss of appetite   nervosa = of nerve

Exercises

1. Divide the following terms into prefix, root/combining vowel and suffix.

Term	Prefix	Root/combining vowel	Suffix
① angiosarcoma		angi/o sarc/o	-oma
② autopsy		aut/o	-opsy
③ amniocentesis		amni/o	-centesis
④ bronchiole		bronch/i	-ole
⑤ bronchoscopy		bronch/o	-scopy
⑥ carcinogenic		carcin/o	-genic
⑦ cerebral		cerebr/o	-al
⑧ dermatitis		dermat/o	-itis
⑨ dermatology		dermat/o	-ology
⑩ diagnosis	dia-		-gnosis
⑪ enteritis		enter/o	-itis
⑫ gynecology		gynec/o	-logy
⑬ hyperplasia	hyper-		-plasia
⑭ metastasis	meta-		-stasis
⑮ ophthalmoscope		ophthalm/o	-scope
⑯ osteoid		oste/o	-oid
⑰ osteoporosis		oste/o por/o	-osis
⑱ panhysterectomy	pan-	hyster/o	-ectomy
⑲ pericardium	peri-	card/i	-ium
⑳ resection	re-	sect/o	-ion
㉑ renal		ren/o	-al
㉒ sarcoma		sarc/o	-oma
㉓ subhepatic	sub-	hepat/o	-ic
㉔ thrombocyte		thromb/o	-cyte
㉕ urology		ur/o	-logy

2. Change the following singulars into plurals.

① amniocentesis	amniocenteses
② bacterium	bacteria
③ bronchus	bronchi
④ diverticulum	diverticula, diverticulums
⑤ embolus	emboli
⑥ fibroma	fibromas, fibromata
⑦ meningitis	meningitides
⑧ metastasis	metastases
⑨ neurosis	neuroses
⑩ phalanx	phalanges, phalanxes
⑪ pubis	pubes
⑫ scapula	scapulae, scapulas
⑬ sarcoma	sarcomata, sarcomas
⑭ thorax	thoraces, thraxes
⑮ varix	varices
⑯ virus	viruses

3. Change the following plurals into singulars.

① acetabula	acetabulum
② bronchi	bronchus
③ calices	calix
④ carcinomas	carcinoma
⑤ diagnoses	diagnosis
⑥ ganglia	ganglion
⑦ indices	index
⑧ larynges	larynx
⑨ sclerae	sclera
⑩ septa	septum
⑪ sinuses	sinus
⑫ vertebrae	vertebra

Medical Specialties

Specialty	in the medical study of	Medical Doctor
Allergy and Immunology	hypersensitivity and resistance to disease	allergist, immunologist
Anesthetics	causing physical insensitivity for pain in surgery	anesthesiologist
Cardiology	heart and its functions	cardiologist
Cardiothoracic Surgery	operation of the chest or thoracic cavity	cardiotherapic surgeon
Dermatology	skin	dermatologist
Endocrinology	endocrine glands (blood and lymph)	endocrinologist
Gastroenterology	digestive organs (stomach and intestines)	gastroenterologist
General Surgery	surgery, usually of abdominal contents	general surgeon
Geriatrics	aging and aged persons, gerontology	geriatrician
Gynecology and Obstetrics	female reproductive system and childbirth	gynecologist / obstetrician
Hematology	blood and blood forming organs	hematologist
Hepatology	liver	hepatologist
Internal Medicine	diagnosis and nonsurgical treatment	physician
Interventional Radiology	surgery with the aid of radiological imaging	interventional radiologist
Microbiology	microscopic organisms	microbiologist
Neonatology	newborn babies	neonatologist
Nephrology	kidney	nephrologist
Neurology	nervous system	neurologist
Neurophysiology	functions of nervous system	neurophysiologist
Neuroradiology	radiology specializing in nervous system	neuroradiologist
Neurosurgery	surgery of the brain and other tissues	neurosurgeon
Nuclear Medicine	using radioisotopes in medicine	nuclear medicine physician
Occupational Medicine	prevention and treatment of occupational health	occupational physician
Ophthalmology	eyes	ophthalmologist
Orthopaedics	skeletal system (bones, muscles, ligaments)	orthopedic surgeon
Otorhinolaryngology	ear, nose and throat	otolaryngologists
Pathology	science of disease condition	pathologist
Pediatrics	babies and children	pediatrician
Pediatric Surgery	surgery involving babies and children	pediatric surgeon
Plastic Surgery	correction or restoration of form and function	plastic surgeon
Pneumology, Pulmonology	respiratory system	pulmonologist
Psychiatry	mental disorders	psychiatrist
Radiology	medical imaging including nuclear medicine	radiologist
Radiotherapy	radiation therapy, usually to treat cancer	radiation oncologist
Rheumatology	rheumatic diseases in joints, immune system	rheumatologist
Urology	male and female urinary tract	urologist
Venereology	sexually transmitted diseases	venereologist

Abbreviations for Diagnostic Procedures

Abbreviation	Full Term	Meaning
ADR	adverse drug reaction	harmful side effect due to medication
AP	anteroposterior	front to rear side of the body
Ba	barium	a metallic element used in medical imaging
bpm	beats per minute	heart beats per mimute
BP	blood pressure	
BUN	blood urea nitrogen	test result, an indication of kidney health
CBC	complete blood count	count of all cells and other parts in the blood
CT	computerized tomography	tomographic imaging using computerized x-rays
ECHO	echocardiography	sonogram of the heart using ultrasound
endo	endoscopy	looking inside the body
ESR	erythrocyte sedimentation rate	rate of red blood cell sedimentation rate
Fluor	fluoroscopy	x-ray imaging technique using fluroroscope
HEM	hematuria	presence of blood cells in urine
Hct, hemat, hmt	hematocrit	volume % of red blood cells in blood
ID	intradermal	inside or between the layers of the skin
IM	intramuscular	within a muscle
IMF	immunofluorescence	detecting antigen or antibody using fluorescence
IV	intravenous	into a vein (usually for injection)
LAP	laparoscopy	examination of abdominal cavity using laparoscopy
lat	lateral	side
MRA	magnetic resonance angiography	MRI using substance injected in blood vessels
MRI	magnetic resonance imaging	imaging technique using magnetism and radiowaves
NI	nuclear imaging	imaging technique using radioactive substance
NM	nuclear medicine	study of nuclear imaging
obl	oblique	slant, at an angle other than normal or parallel
PLC	platelet count	count of platelets in the blood
PA	posteroanterior	rear to front side of the body
PET	positron emission tomography	a tomographic technique to assess body functions
PT	prothrombin time	blood clotting time measurement
RIA	radioimmunoassay	measurement of antigens using radioactive substances
RP	radiopharmaceuticals	radioactive drugs used in diagnosis or therapy
RBC	red blood cell count	count of red blood cells in blood
RR	respiratory rate	breathing rate per minute
SC	subcutaneous	under the skin
SPECT	single photon emission computerized tomography	tomographic imaging technique using gamma rays
TPR	temperature, pulse, respiration	vital signs usually included in medical chart
TEE	transesophageal echocardiography	echocardiography using probe in esophagus
UA, U/A	urinalysis	examination of the urine
WBC	white blood cell count	count of white blood cells in blood

Chapter 2

Roots of Body Systems

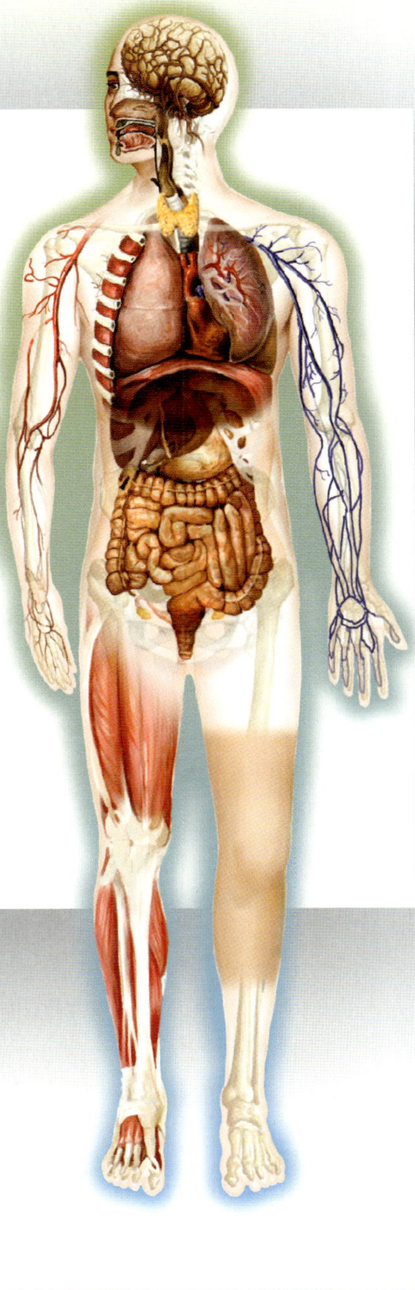

Chapter Contents

- Prolog
- Anatomy and Physiology
- Organization of Human Body
- Anatomical Roots
- Exercises

Learning Objectives

- Define anatomy and physiology.
- Understand levels of human body organization.
- Name the basic body systems.
- Learn and use anatomical roots.

Prolog

We will define anatomy and physiology, and understand the various levels of body organization starting from cell, the smallest unit at the lowest level of the body, ending in the human body. Human body is classified into a dozen physiological body systems, and roots are listed for each system.

Roots are introduced in combining forms. They will be the basis for understanding terms in subsequent chapters.

Anatomy and Physiology

Anatomy is the study of the structure of the human body. We will learn the construction of the skeleton, and the structure and characteristics of each system of the body. Histology is a subset of anatomy in that it is the study of cells and tissues. Physiology is the study of functions of anatomical system or part of the body. As an example, how food ingested is digested, absorbed and converted into energy, will be understood in physiology. Pathology examines the causes, conditions, symptoms and prognoses of abnormal structures and functions of the body systems.

Memory key

- Anatomy is the study of the structure, and physiology is the study of functions. Pathology is the study of diseased or abnormal structure and functions.

Organization of Human Body

Human body is constructed with many parts composed of cells that perform various functions. A cell is the unit at the lowest level that can perform various functions.

Tissues such as muscles are consist of cells and at the next level up. Next, organs such as stomach and intestines are constructed with tissues. An organ system comprists of organs like stomach and intestines which are a part of the digestive system. At the highest level, the human body is constructed with organ systems.

Human body is commonly classified into skeletal, muscular, integumentary, respiratory, digestive, endocrine, nervous, eyes and ears, cardiovascular, lymphatic and immune, urinary, and reproductive systems.

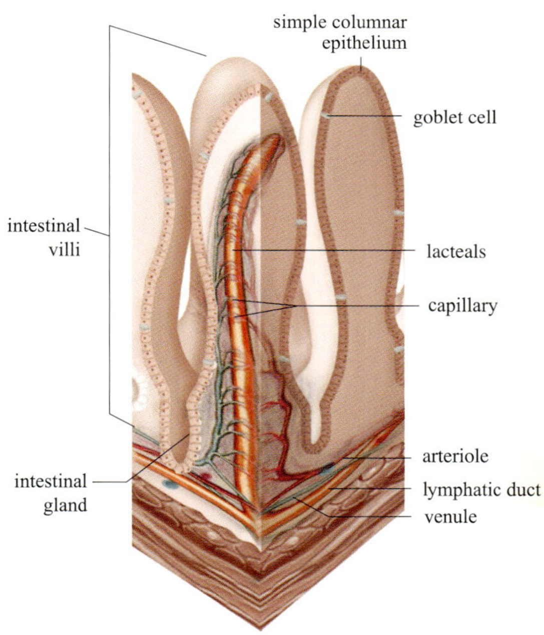

Figure 2-1 Intestinal villous cells

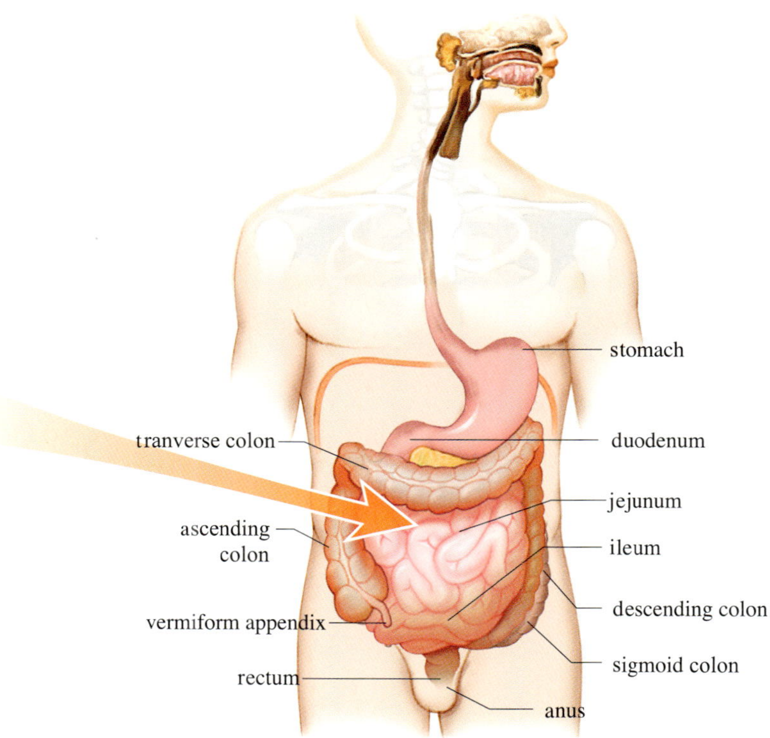

Figure 2-2 Organs in digestive system

Anatomical Roots

Skeletal System

Root	Meaning
arthr/o, articul/o	joint
chondr/o	cartilage
crani/o	skull
cost/o	rib
myel/o	bone marrow
oste/o	bone
pelv/o	pelvis
spin/o	backbone, spine
vertebr/o, spondyl/o	vertebra

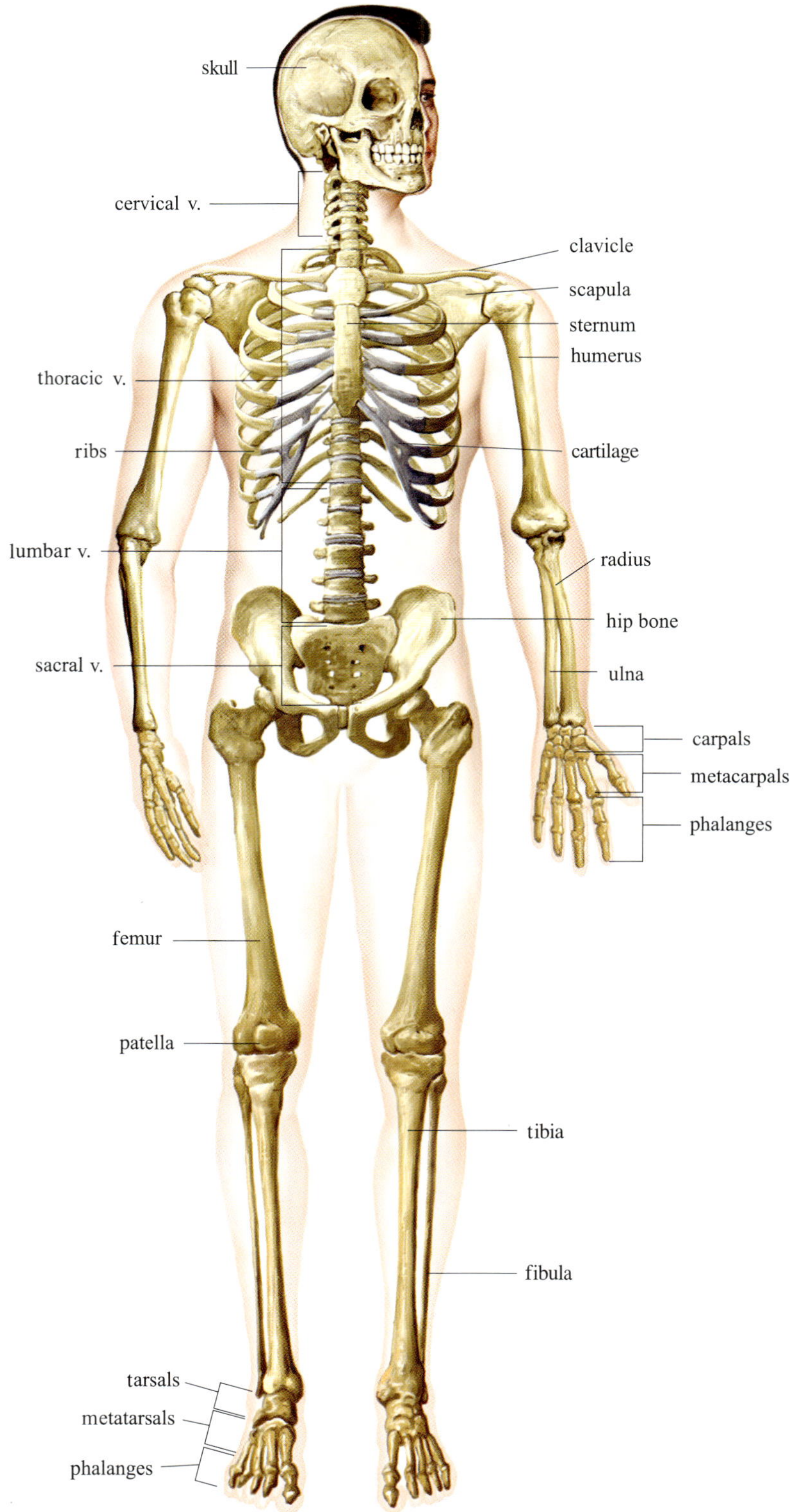

Figure 2-3 Terms of skeletal system

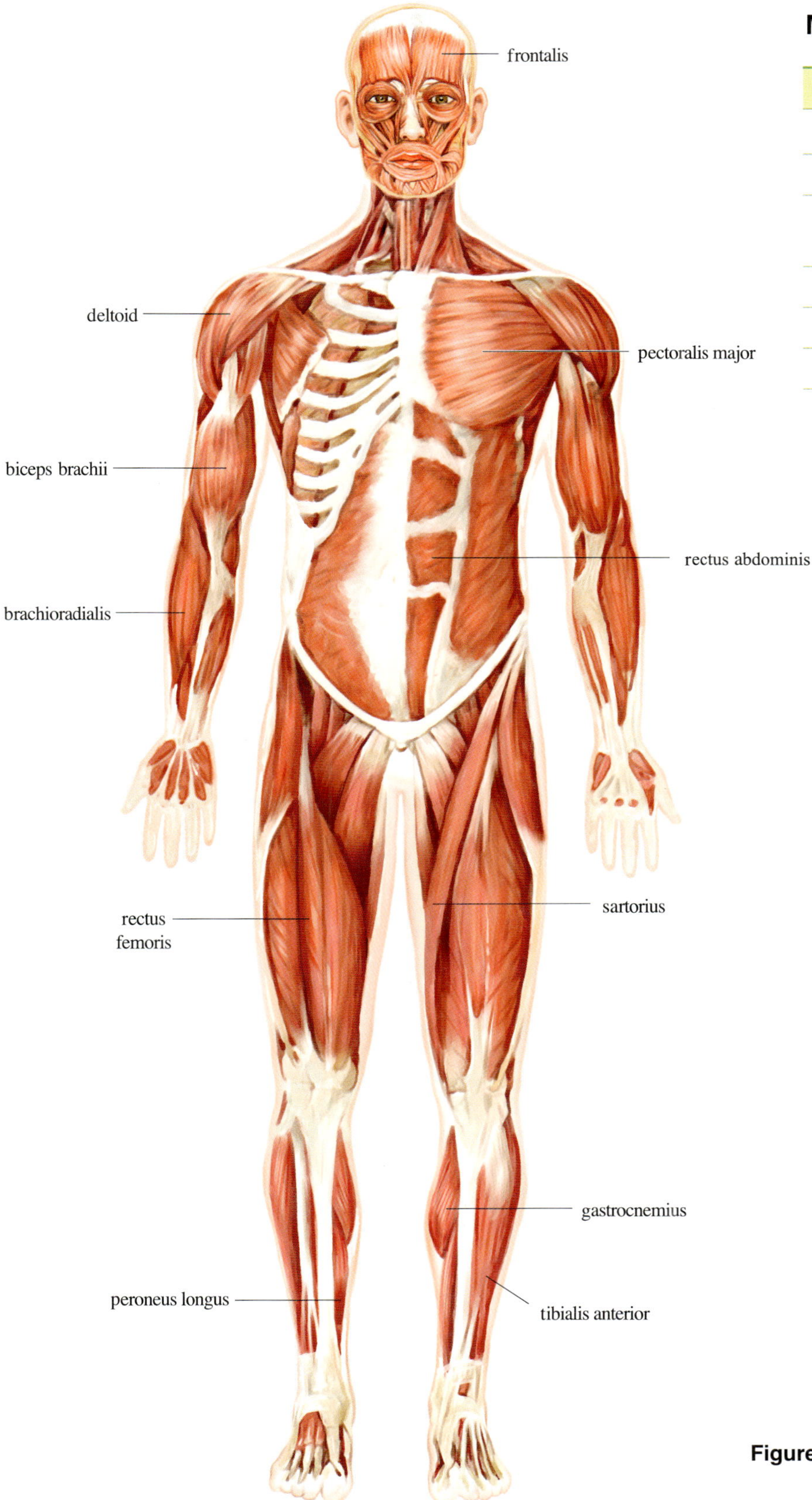

Muscular System

Root	Meaning
fasci/o	fascia
lei/o	smooth
my/o, muscul/o, myos/o	muscle
sarc/o	flesh
tend/o, tendin/o	tendon
ton/o	tone or tension

Figure 2-4 Terms of muscular system

Integumentary System

Root	Meaning
adip/o, lip/o, steat/o	fat
axill/o	armpit
cili/o, pil/o	hair
derm/o, dermat/o, cutane/o	skin
diaphor/o	profuse sweating
hidr/o	sweat
kerat/o	hard, cornea
onych/o, ungu/o	nail
plas/o	formation
squam/o	scale
xer/o	dryness

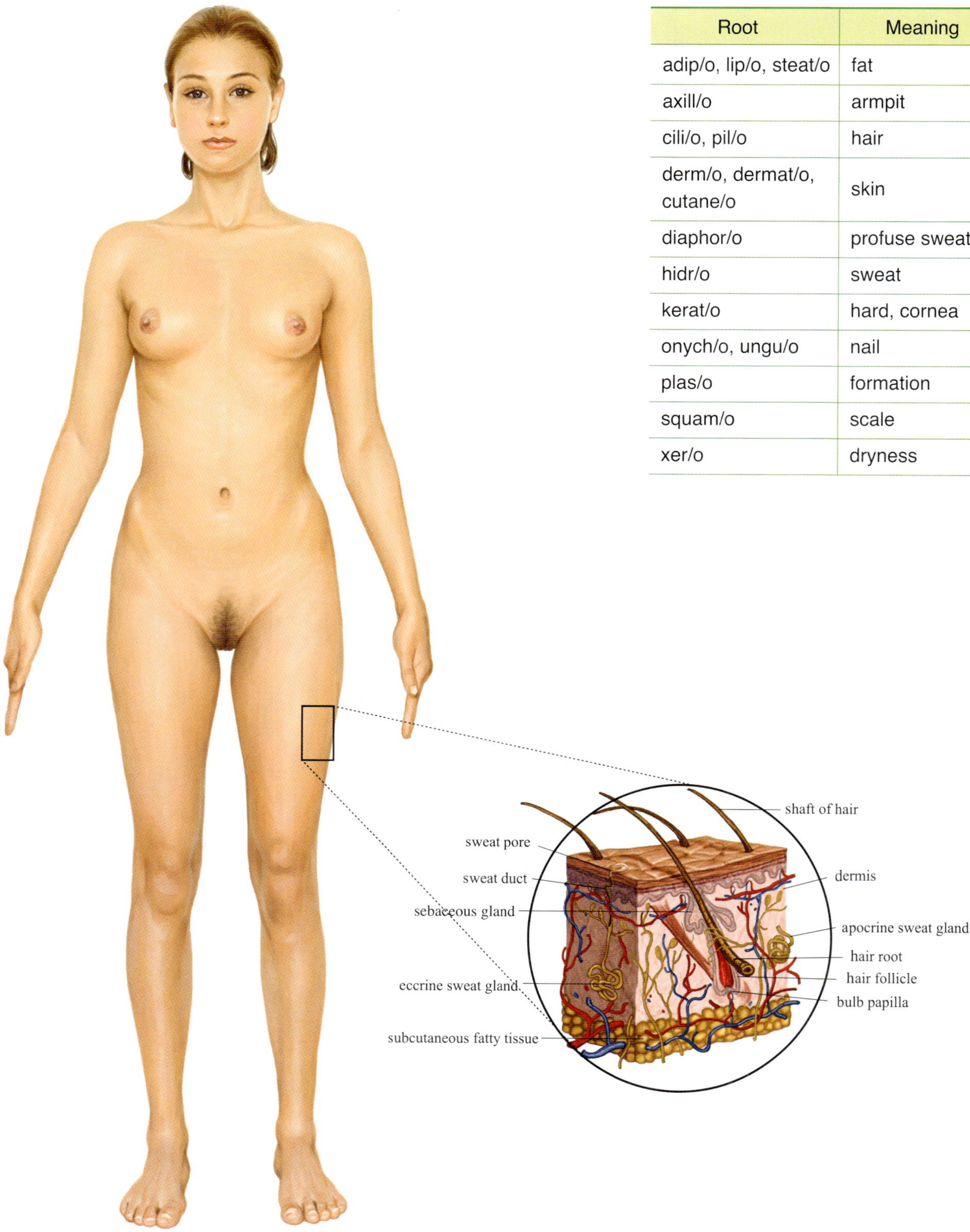

Figure 2-5 Terms of integumentary system

Respiratory System

Root	Meaning
alveol/o	air sac, alveolus
bronch/o, bronchi/o	bronchus
bronchiol/o	small bronchial tubes
capn/o, carb/o	carbon dioxide
laryng/o	voice box, larynx
lob/o	lobe
nas/o, rhin/o	nose
or/o	mouth
ox/o	oxygen
pharyng/o, /i	throat, pharynx
phren/o, /i	diaphragm
pleur/o	pleura
pneum/o, pneumon/o	air
pulmon/o	lungs
sinus/o	sinus
spir/o	breathing
thorac/o, /i	chest
trache/o	windpipe, trachea

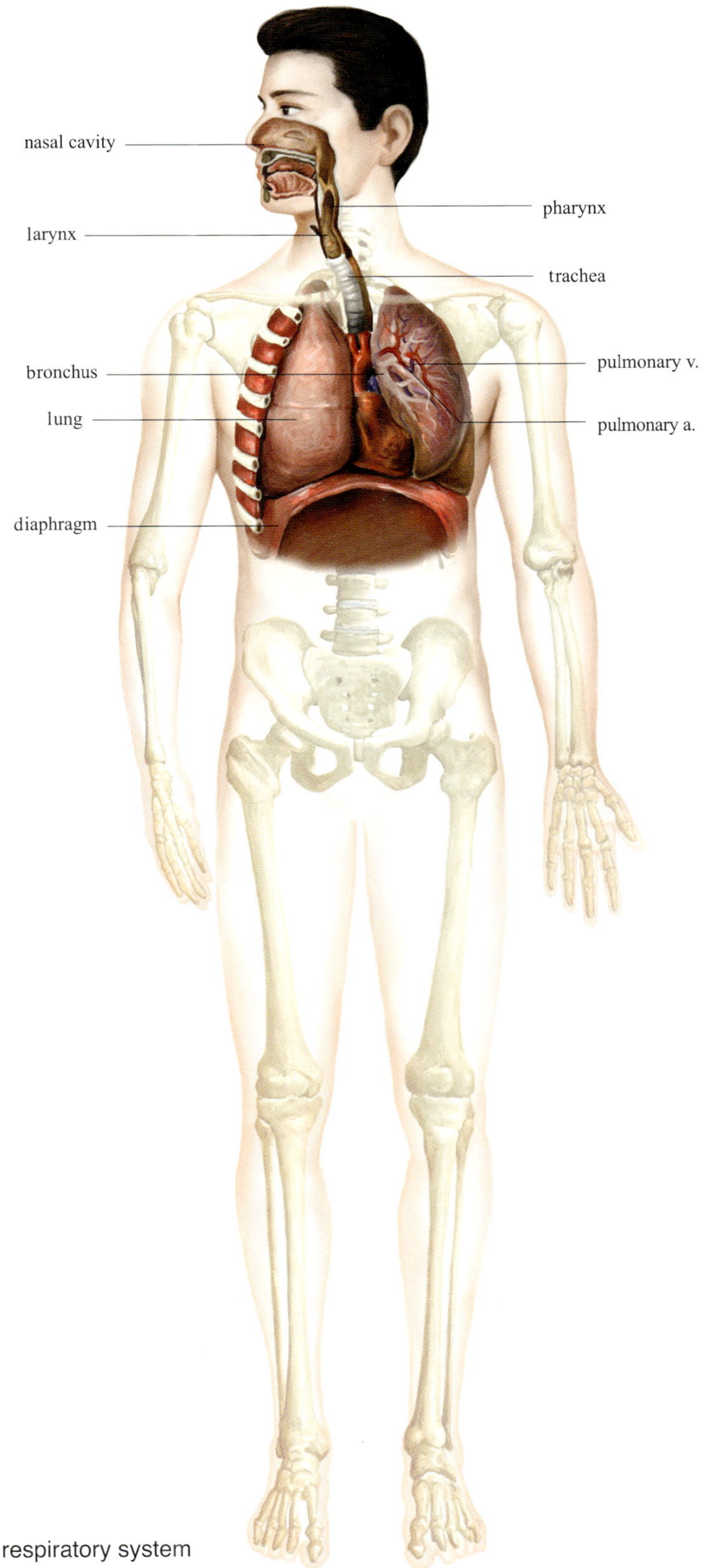

Figure 2-6 Terms of respiratory system

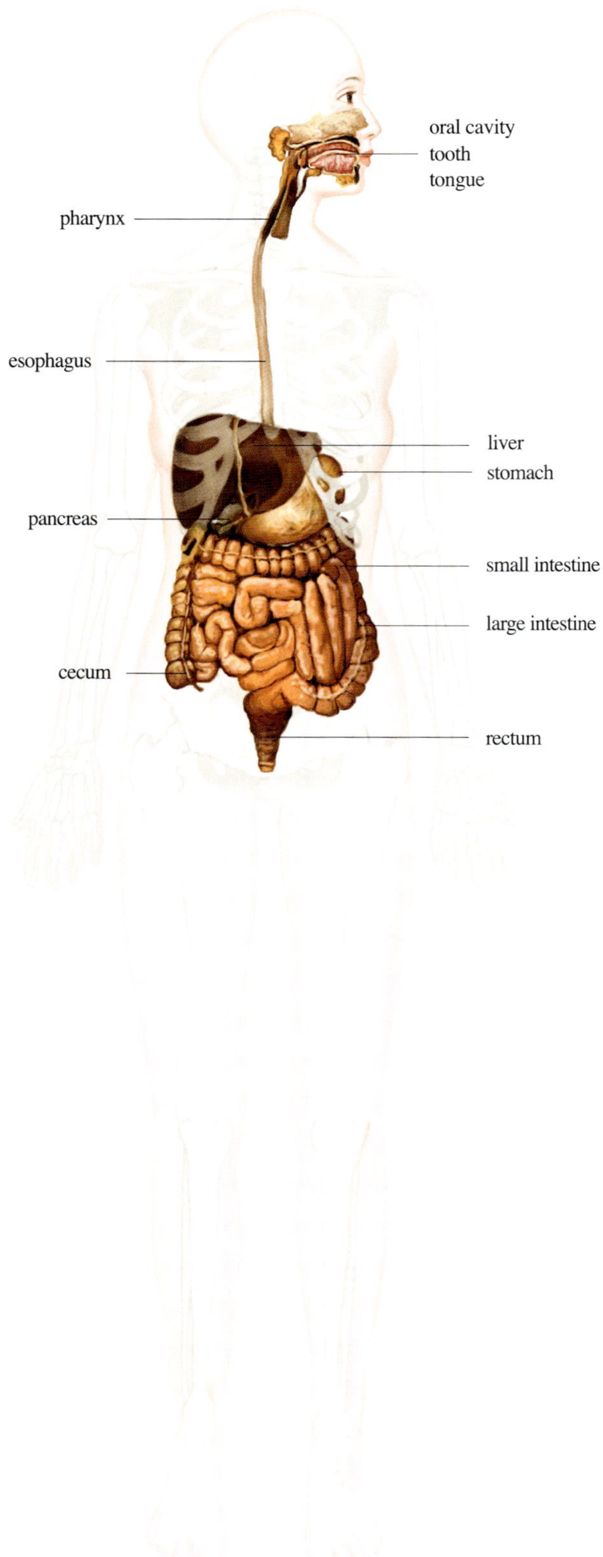

Digestive System

Root	Meaning
abdomin/o, lapar/o, celi/o	abdomen
an/o	anus
appendic/o	appendix
bil/i, chol/o	bile, gall
bucc/o	cheek
cheil/o	lips
choled/o	common bile duct
col/o	large intestine; colon
dent/i	teeth
duoden/o	duodenum
enter/o	small intestine
esophag/o	esophagus
gastr/o	stomach
gingiv/o	gum
gloss/o, lingu/o	tongue
hepat/o, hepatic/o	liver
herni/o	hernia
ile/o	ileum
lith/o	stone
or/o, stomat/o	mouth
pharyng/o	throat, pharynx (also part of the respiratory system)
rect/o	rectum
sial/o	saliva

Figure 2-7 Terms of digestive system

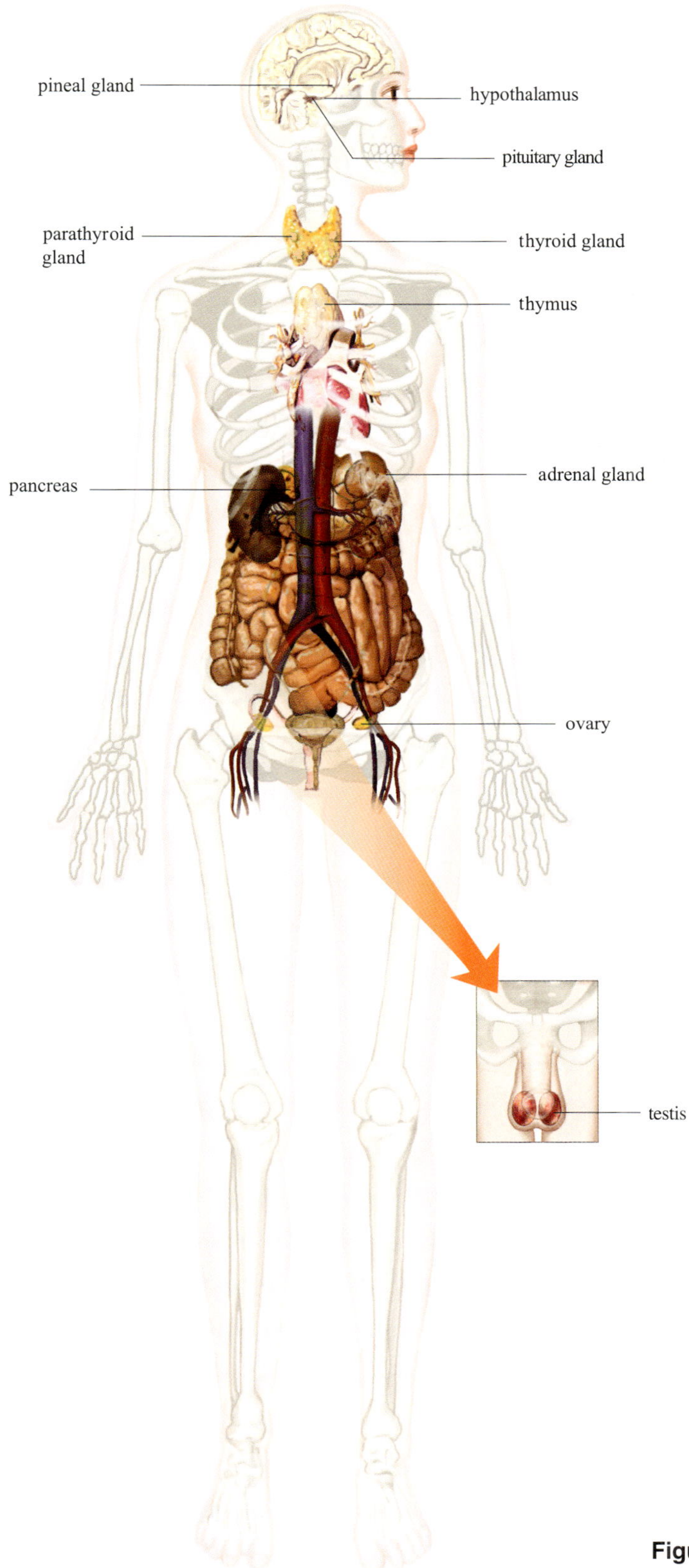

Endocrine System

Root	Meaning
aden/o	gland
adren/o	adrenal gland
andr/o	male
crin/o	to secrete
dips/o	thirst
gluc/o, glyc/o, glycos/o	sugar, sweet
hormon/o	hormone
pancreat/o	pancreas
parathyroid/o	parathyroid gland
pituitar/o	pituitary gland
thym/o	thymus
thyr/o, thyroid/o	thyroid gland

Figure 2-8 Terms of endocrine system

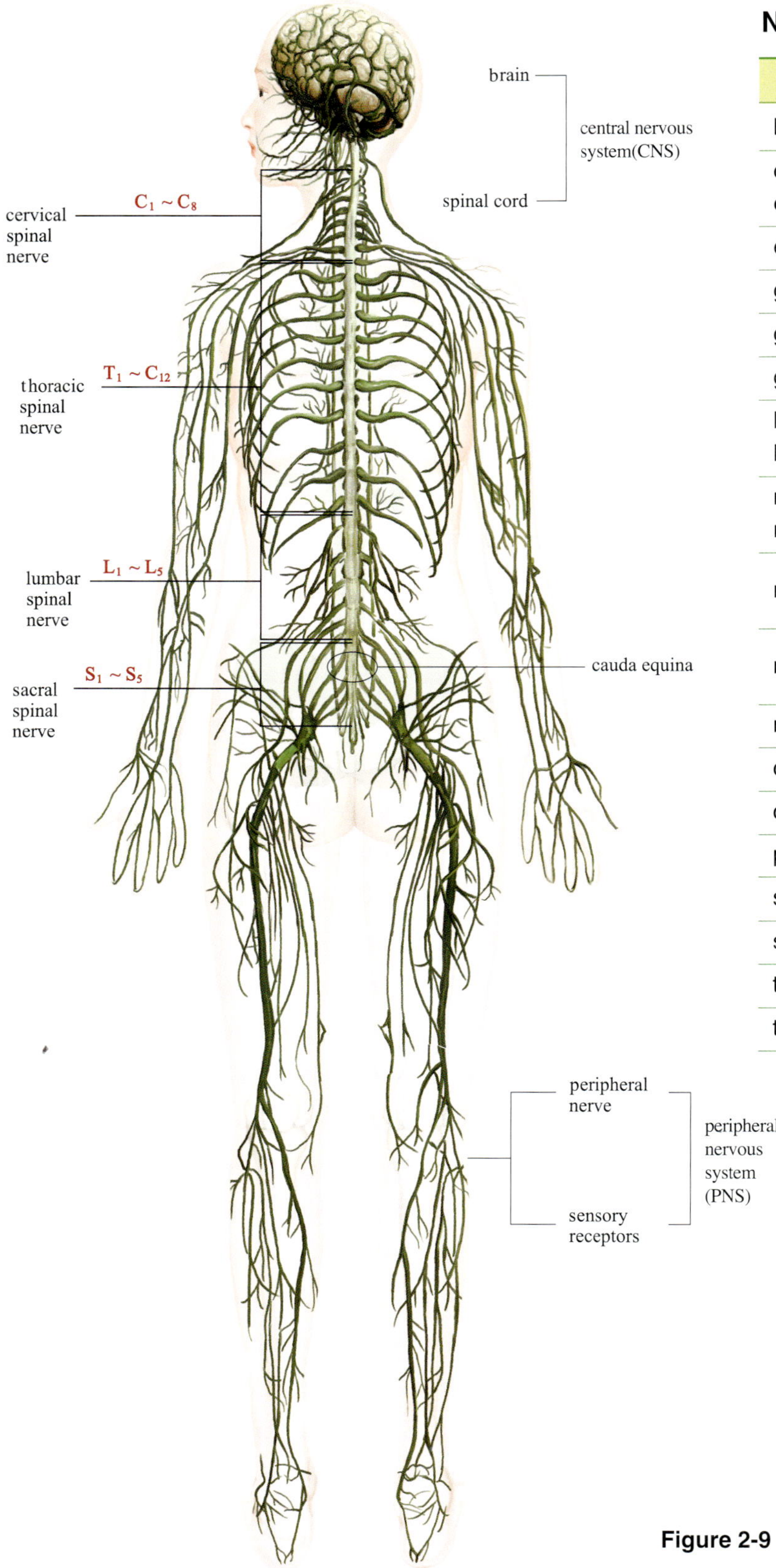

Nervous System

Root	Meaning
blephar/o	eyelid
cerebr/o, encephal/o	brain
esthesi/o	sensation
gangli/o	ganglion
gli/o	glue
gnos/o	gnosia
kinesi/o, kin/o, kin/e	movement
mening/o, meningi/o	meninges, membrane
myel/o	spinal cord/ bone marrow
narc/o	stupor, numb, sleep
neur/o	nerve
ophthalm/o, ocul/o	eye
ot/o	ear
phas/o	speech
somn/o	sleep
stere/o	three dimension
tax/o	order, coordination
thalam/o	thalamus

Figure 2-9 Terms of nervous system

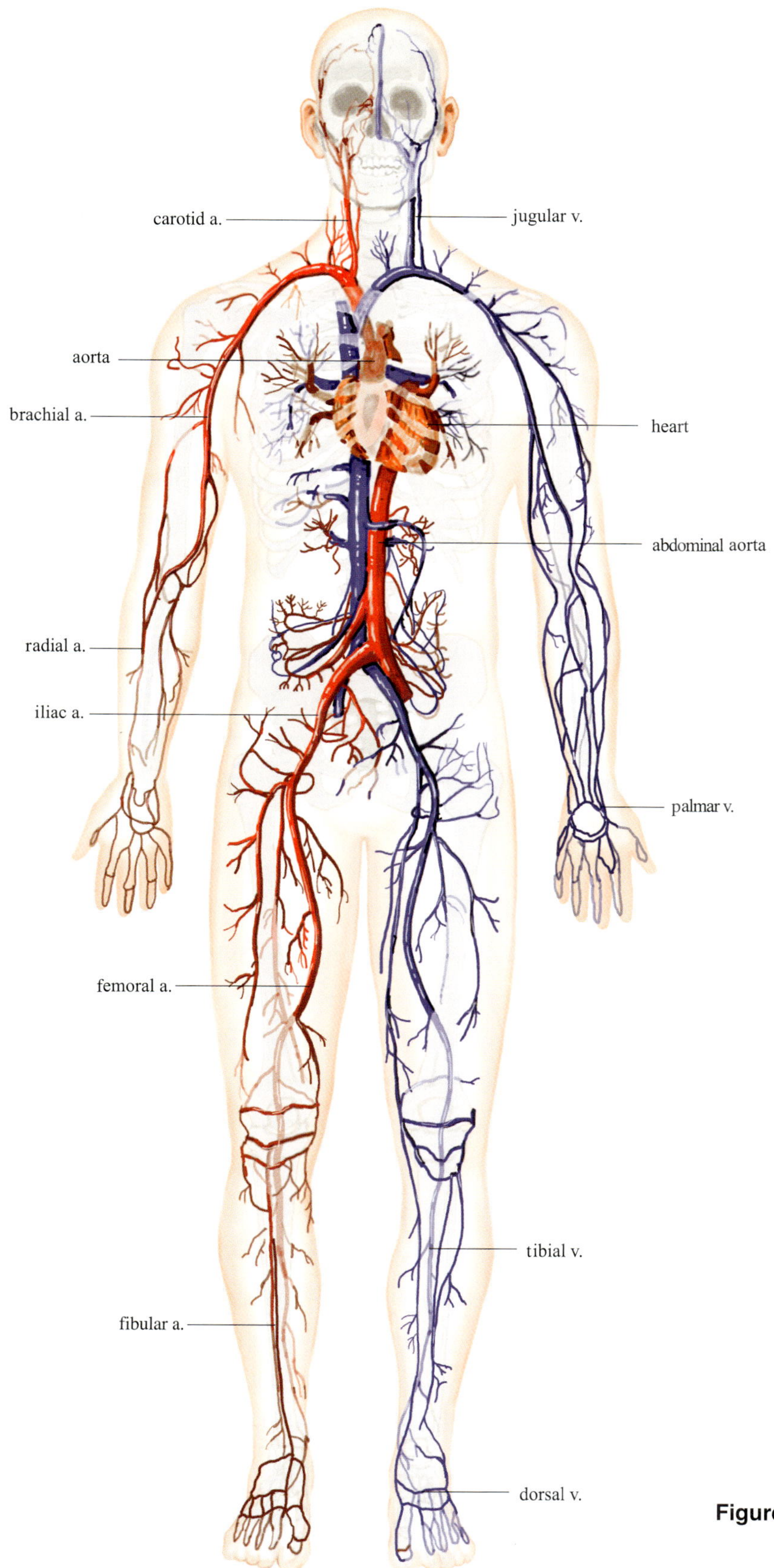

Circulatory System

Root	Meaning
angi/o, vascul/o, vas/o	blood vessel
aort/o	aorta
arteri/o	artery
ather/o	fatty deposit
atri/o	atrium
cardi/o	heart
coron/o	crown
hem/o, hemat/o	blood
pector/o	chest
sphygm/o	pulse
thromb/o	blood clot
varic/o	swollen vein
ven/o, phleb/o	vein
ventricul/o	ventricle

Figure 2-10 Terms of circulatory system

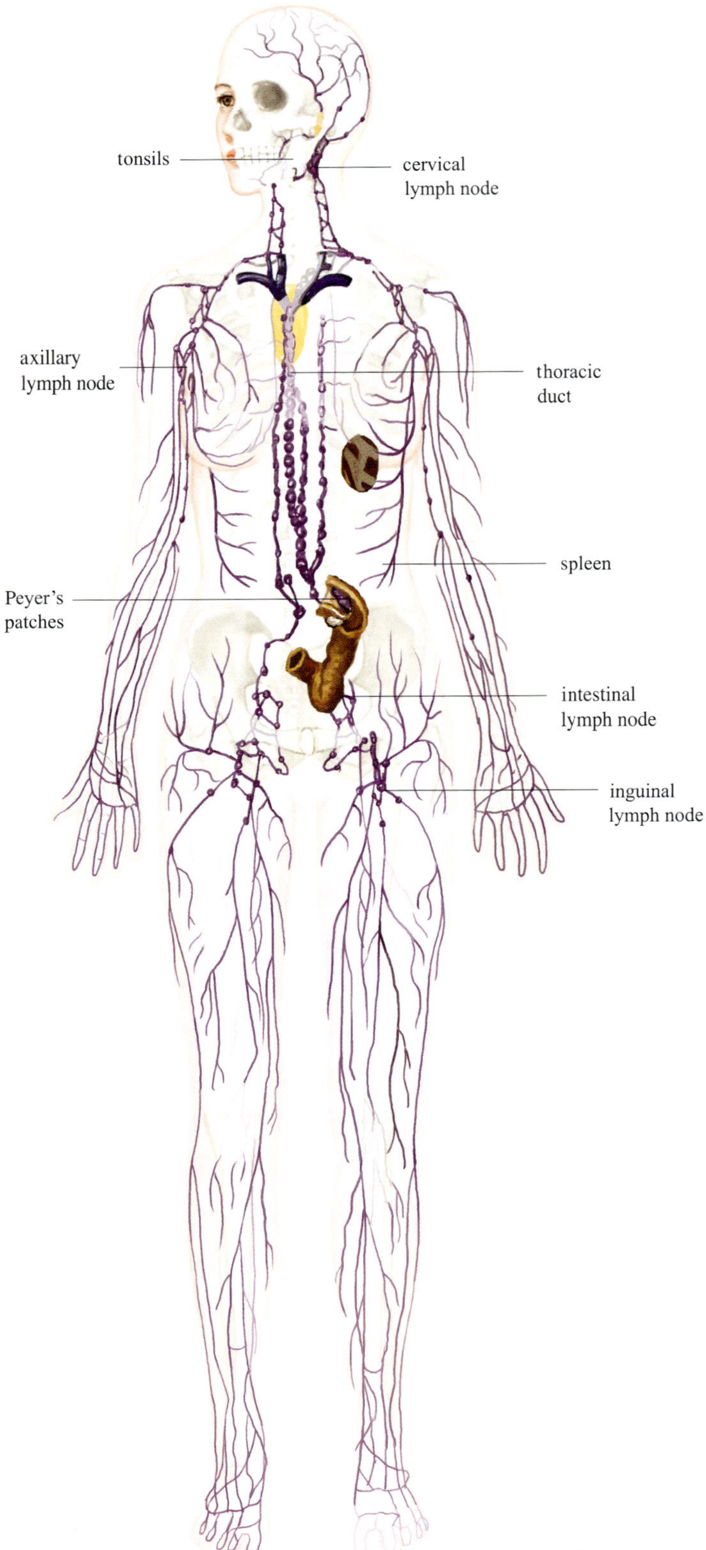

Lymphatic and Immune Systems

Root	Meaning
adenoid/o	adenoids
blast/o, -blasto	germ or bud
immun/o	safe, protection
lymph/o	lymph
lymphaden/o	lymph glands, lymph nodes
lymphangi/o	lymph vessels
phag/o	to eat, swallow
reticul/o	net
splen/o	spleen
thym/o	thymus gland
tonsill/o	tonsils

Figure 2-11 Terms of lymphatic and immune systems

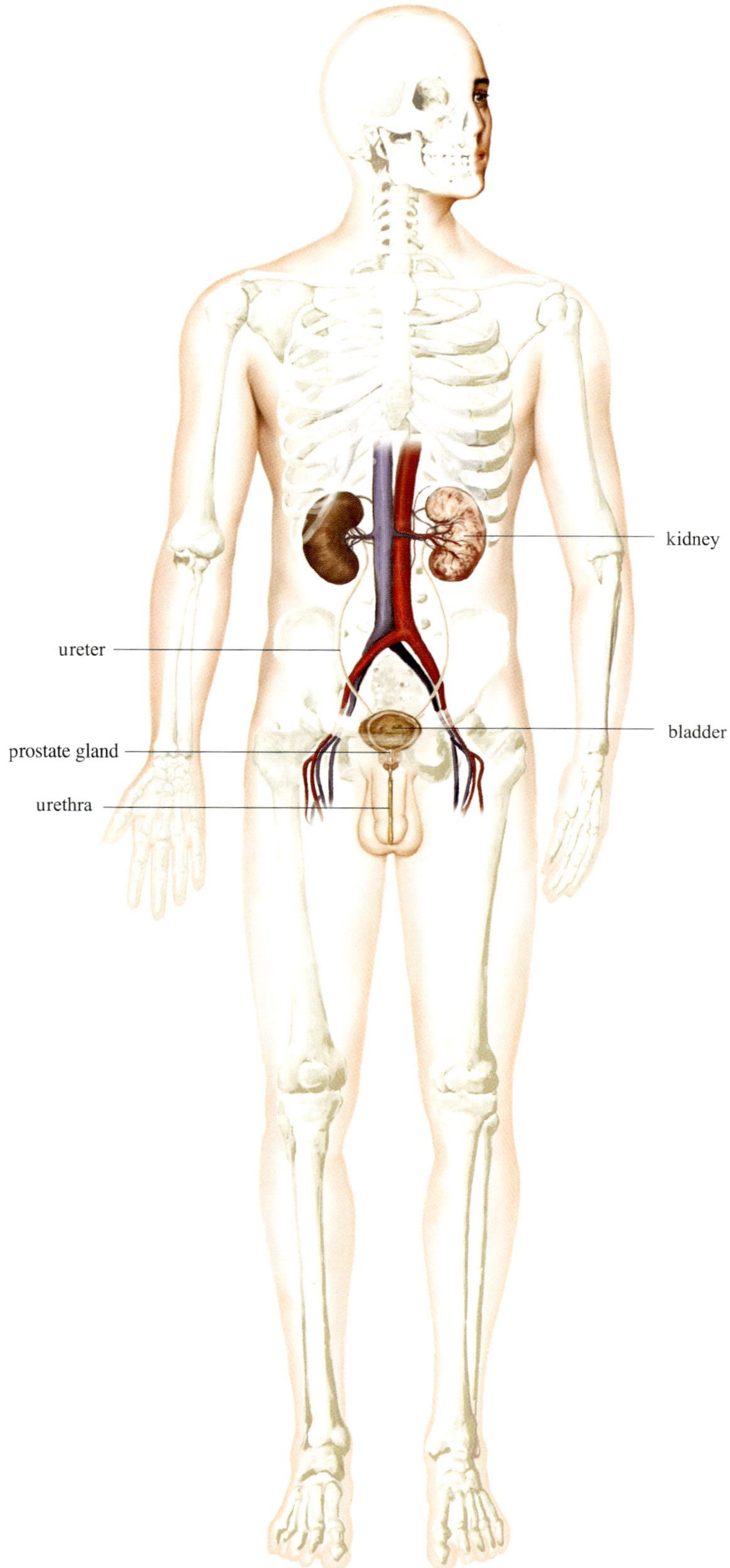

Urinary System

Root	Meaning
albumin/o	protein
bacteri/o	bacteria
cyst/o	bladder, sac
dips/o	thirst
glomerul/o	glomerulus
gluc/o, glyc/o, glycos/o	sugar, sweet
ket/o, keton/o	ketone bodies, aceton
meat/o	opening
pyel/o	basin, pelvis
py/o	pus
ren/o, nephr/o	kidneys
ureter/o	ureters
urethr/o	urethra
ur/o, urin/o	urine

Figure 2-12 Terms of urinary system

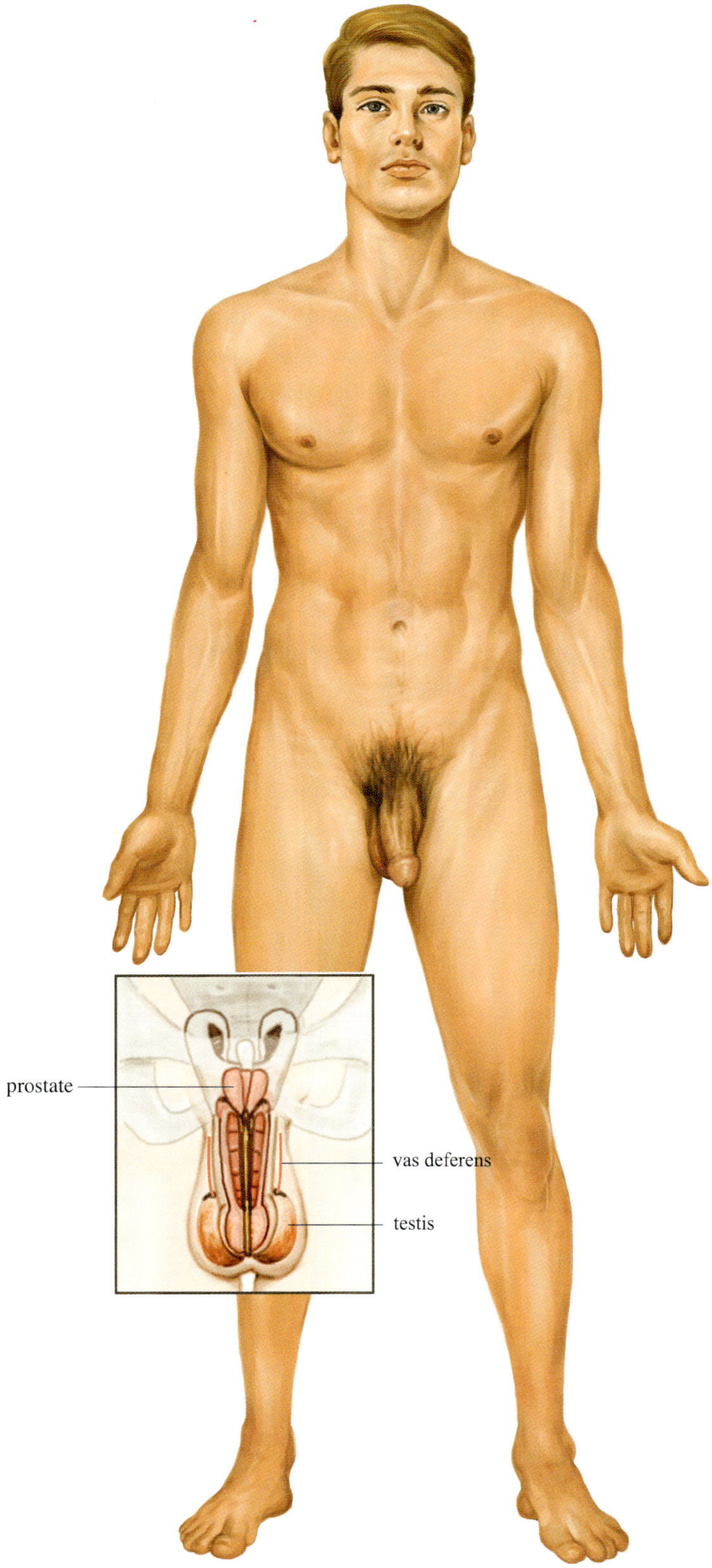

Male Reproductive System

Root	Meaning
balan/o	glans penis
epididym/o	epididymis
orchid/o, orch/o, test/o, testicul/o	testicle; testis
perine/o	perineum
phall/o	penis
prostat/o	prostate gland
sperm/o	sperm
vas/o	ductus (vas) deferens

Figure 2-13 Terms of male reproductive system

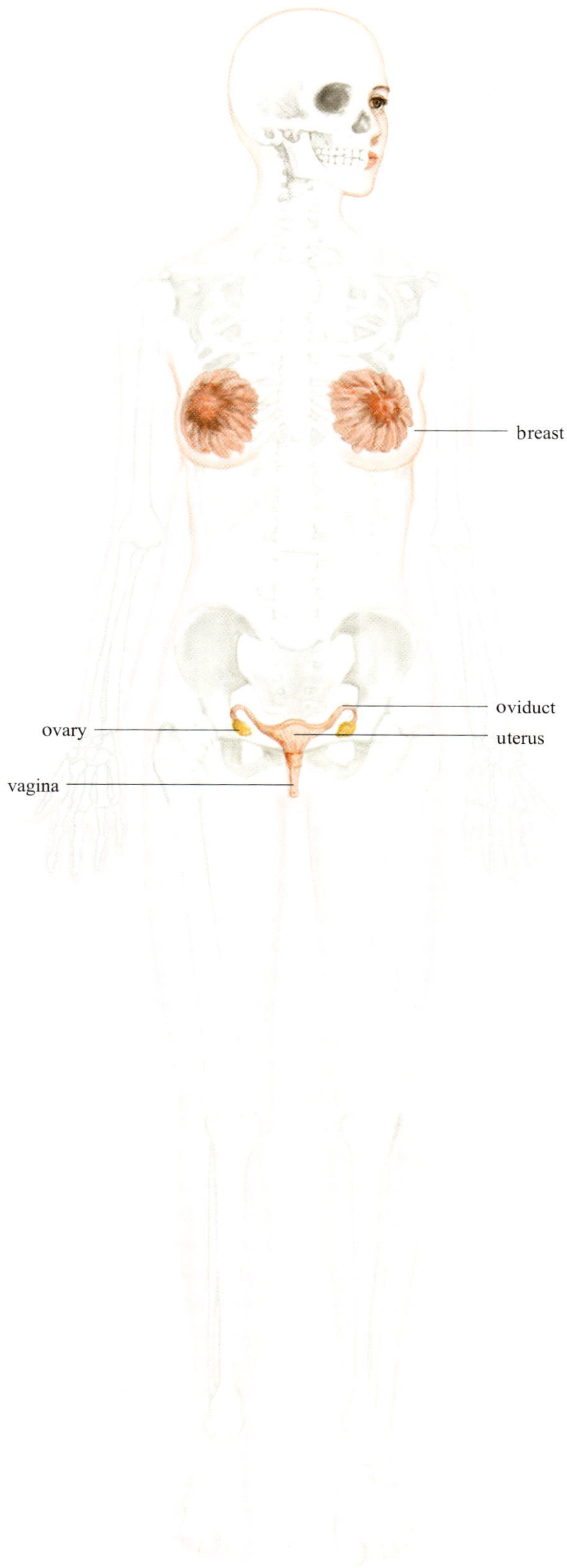

Female Reproductive System

Root	Meaning
cervic/o	neck or cervix
colp/o, vagin/o	vagina
episi/o, vulv/o	vulva
gynec/o	female
lact/o	milk
mast/o, mamm/o	breast
men/o	menstruation
oophor/o, ovari/o	ovary
ov/i, ov/o	egg
salping/o	fallopian tubes; uterine tubes
toc/o	labor or birth
uter/o, hyster/o, metr/o	uterus

Figure 2-14 Terms of female reproductive system

Exercises

1. Write the meaning of the following combining forms :

① arthr/o joint

② cyst/o sac of fluid, bladder

③ encephal/o brain

④ bronchi/o bronch/o broncus, air passage

⑤ hemat/o blood

⑥ oste/o bone

⑦ nephr/o kidney

⑧ blephar/o eyelid

⑨ rhin/o nose

⑩ arteri/o artery (as opposed to vein)

⑪ neur/o nerve

⑫ tonsil/o tonsil

⑬ bi/o life

⑭ ophthalm/o eye

⑮ viscer/o internal organs

2. Write combining forms that mean the following words :

① ears ot/o

② rectum rect/o

③ stomach gastr/o

④ vessel angi/o

⑤ fat adip/o, lip/o

⑥ heart cardi/o

⑦ cell cyt/o

⑧ hair cili/o

⑨ spleen splen/o

⑩ pathology path/o

⑪ abdomen abdomin/o

⑫ spinal cord myel/o

⑬ windpipe; trachea trachi/o

⑭ liver hepat/o

⑮ brain cephal/o

3. Write combining forms of the following roots :

① armpit axill/o

② nail onych/o

③ skull crani/o

④ eye ophthalm/o

⑤ colon col/o

⑥ ductus deferens vas/o

⑦ vein ven/o, phleb/o

⑧ chest thorac/o

⑨ epididymis epididym/o

⑩ head crani/o

⑪ cartilage chondr/o

⑫ tendon tend/o, tendin/o

⑬ small intestine enter/o

⑭ tongue gloss/o, lingu/o

⑮ thyroid gland thyroid/o

⑯ lung pneum/o, pulmon/o

⑰ lymph vessels lymphangi/o

⑱ testicle orchid/o, test/o, testicul/o

⑲ ovary oophor/o, ovari/o

4. Explain the difference between anatomy and physiology.

① antomy

A study of the parts of the body

② physiology

A study of how the body parts work

5. List all human body systems, and list 3 organs for each system.

① Integumentary system — nail, hair, skin

② Skeletal system — skull, joint, cartilage

③ Muscular system — muscle, tendon, fascia

④ Nervous system — brain, spinal cord, eye

⑤ Endocrine system — pituitary gland, thyroid gland, adrenal gland

⑥ Circulatory system — artery, vein, blood

⑦ Lymphatic and immune systems — adenoids, spleen, tonsils

⑧ Respiratory system — lungs, trachea, bronchus

⑨ Digestive system — esophagus, stomach, liver

⑩ Urinary system — bladder, kidney, urethra

⑪ Male reproductive system — epididymis, testis, prostate

⑫ Female reproductive system — ovary, fallopian tube, uterus

Chapter 3

Suffixes

Chapter Contents

- Prolog
- General Suffixes
- Adjectival Suffixes
- Suffixes used to Indicate Pathological Conditions
- Suffixes used to Indicate Diagnostic Procedures
- Suffixes used to Indicate Surgical Procedures
- Exercises

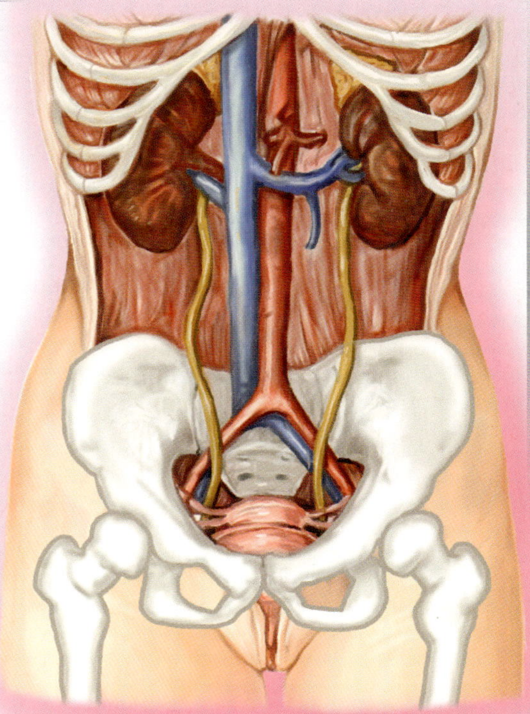

Learning Objectives

- Learn spelling and meaning of suffixes.
- Distinguish suffixes that signify pathological conditions from other types.
- Understand suffixes pertaining to diagnostic and surgical procedures.
- Identify suffixes used to convert medical nouns to adjectives.
- Analyze, define, spell and pronounce medical terms in the chapter.

Prolog

Suffixes are classified into following types :

① **General Suffixes** : These are common suffixes widely used in medical terms.

② **Adjectival Suffixes** : Adjectival suffixes describe special qualities or relationships. These may precede terms in noun form.

③ **Suffixes used to Indicate Pathologic Conditions** : Suffixes that describe diseases, signs, abnormalities, etc.

④ **Suffixes used to Indicate Diagnostic Procedures** : Suffixes that describe procedures to diagnose symptoms displayed by patients.

⑤ **Suffixes used to Indicate Surgical Procedures** : Suffixes that describe standardized surgical procedures performed based on diagnosed pathological conditions.

General Suffixes

Term	Pronunciation	Term Analysis	Meaning
-cyte :		cell	
adipocyte	[**ad**-ih-poh-sight]	adip/o = fat	fat cell
histiocyte	[**hiss**-tee-oh-sight]	histi/o = tissue	tissue cell
leukocyte	[**lyou**-ko-sight]	leuk/o = white	white blood cell

Term	Pronunciation	Term Analysis	Meaning
-er, -or, -ician, -ist :		performer	
donor	[**doh**-nor]	don/o = donation	organ donor
practitioner	[prack-**ti**-shun-er]	practition/o = practice	practicing physician
physician	[fih-**zih**-shun]	physi/o = nature, function	doctor of internal medicine
neurologist	[new-**rol**-oh-jist]	neur/o = nerve	medical specialist in neurology
pharmacist	[**farm**-ah-sist]	pharmac/o = drug	one who specializes in drugs
-iatrics, -iatry :		(study of) treatment	
geriatrics	[je-ri-**at**-ricks]	ger/o = old age	study of health in old persons
pediatrics	[pe-di-**at**-ricks]	ped/o = child	study of medicine in children
-ion :		state, process	
section	[**seck**-shun]	sect/o = to cut	process of cutting
-ium :		structure, tissue	
pericardium	[peh-rih-**kar**-dee-uhm]	peri- = around; card/i = heart	membrane surrounding the heart
-logy :		study of	
hepatology	[hep-ah-**tol**-oh-jee]	hepat/o = liver	study of liver, gallbladder, pancreas
physiology	[fiz-ee-**ol**-oh-jee]	physi/o = nature, function	study of functions of living things
-logist :		one that specializes in	
ophthalmologist	[off-thal-moh-**loh**-jist]	ophthalm/o = eye	medical specialist in the eyes
radiologist	[ray-dee-oh-**loh**-jist]	radi/o = radiation	medical specialist in radiology
-plasia :		formation, development	
chondroplasia	[kon-droh-**play**-zee-ah]	chondr/o = cartilage	formation of cartilage

Term	Pronunciation	Term Analysis	Meaning
-poiesis :		production, manufacture, formation	
hematopoiesis	[he-ma-to-**po**-ee-sis]	hemat/o = blood	production process of blood cells
-rrhea :		discharge, flow	
diarrhea	[dye-a-**ree**-a]	dia- = through, across	watery fecal discharge
-trophic, -trophy :		development, growth, nutrition	
thyrotrophic hormone	[thigh-roh-**troh**-fick]	thyr/o = thyroid gland	thyroid gland hormone

Adjectival Suffixes

Term	Pronunciation	Term Analysis	Meaning
-genic :		produced by, producing	
carcinogenic	[kar-sih-noh-**jen**-ick]	carcin/o = cancer	causing cancer
-oid :		resembling	
osteoid	[**os**-tee-oyd]	oste/o = bone	resembling bone
-icle, -ole, -ula, -ule :		small	
bronchiole	[**brong**-kee-ohl]	bronchi/o = bronchus	small branch of bronchus
venule	[**ven**-youl]	ven/o = vein	small vein
-ac, -al, -ar, -ary, -eal, -ic, -ous, -tic :		pertaining to	
cardiac	[**kar**-dee-ack]	cardi/o = heart	pertaining to the heart
renal	[**ree**-nal]	ren/o = kidney	pertaining to the kidney
neutral	[**nyou**-tral]	neutr/o = mid	positioning in the middle
mammary	[**mam**-ah-ree]	mamm/o = breast	pertaining to the breast
pharyngeal	[far-**in**-jee-al]	pharyng/o = throat, pharynx	pertaining to the throat
laryngeal	[lar-**in**-jee-al]	laryng/o = larynx, voice box	pertaining to larynx
gastric	[**gas**-trick]	gastr/o = stomach	pertaining to the stomach
venous	[**vee**-nus]	ven/o = vein	pertaining to the vein

Suffixes used to Indicate Pathological Conditions

Term	Pronunciation	Term Analysis	Meaning
-algia, -dynia :		pain	
arthralgia	[arth-**ral**-jee-ah]	arthr/o = join	joint pain
cephalgia	[sef-**al**-jee-ah]	cephal/o = head	headache
myalgia	[mye-**al**-gee-ah]	my/o = muscle	pain in muscle
neuralgia	[nyou-**ral**-jee-ah]	neur/o = nerve	pain of nerve
otalgia	[oh-**tal**-gee-ah]	ot/o = ear	earache
gastrodynia	[gas-troh-**din**-ee-ah]	gastr/o = stomach	stomach pain
mastodynia	[mas-toh-**din**-ee-ah]	mast/o = breast	breast pain
-cele :		hernia	
cystocele	[**sis**-toh-seel]	cyst/o = bladder	hernia of the bladder into the vagina
rectocele	[**reck**-toh-seel]	rect/o = rectum	hernia of the rectum into the vagina
encephalocele	[en-**sef**-ah-loh-seel]	encephal/o = brain	hernia of the brain
-ectasis, -ectasia :		expansion or dilation	
bronchiectasis	[brong-kee-**eck**-tay-sis]	bronch/o = breathing branch	dilation of bronchial tubes
-emesis :		vomiting	
hematemesis	[hee-mah-**tem**-eh-sis]	hemat/o = blood	vomiting of blood
-emia :		blood condition	
anemia	[ah-**nee**-me-ah]	an- = not, lacking	shortage of red blood cells or hemoglobin
glycemia	[glye-**see**-mee-ah]	glyc/o = sugar, glucose	glucose level in the blood
leukemia	[**lyou**-ke-me-ah]	leuk/o = white	malignancy in blood or blood-forming tissues
-genesis :		origin or production	
ovogenesis	[oh-voh-**jen**-eh-sys]	ov/o = ovum	formation of ovum
spermatogenesis	[sper-mah-toh-**jen**-eh-sis]	spermat/o = sperm cells	production of sperms

Term	Pronunciation	Term Analysis	Meaning
-ia, -ism :		state of, condition	
pneumonia	[new-**moh**-nee-ah]	pneumon/o = lung	condition or inflammation of the lung
-iasis :		formation or process of	
mydriasis	[mid-**rye**-ah-sys]	mydr/o = wide (eye)	dilated pupil of the eye
-itis :		inflammation	
enteritis	[en-ter-**eye**-tis]	enter/o = small intestine	inflammation of small intestine
stomatitis	[sto-mah-**tye**-tis]	stomat/o = mouth	inflammation of the mouth
spondylitis	[spon-dih-**lye**-tis]	spondyl/o = vertebra	inflammation of vertebra
-lysis :		destruction, separation, breakdown	
hemolysis	[hee-**mo**-lih-sis]	hem/o = blood	breakdown of blood
-malacia :		softening	
cerebromalacia	[ser-eh-broh-mah-**lay**-shee-ah]	cerebr/o = brain	softening of the brain
chondromalacia-cia	[kon-droh-mah-**lay**-shee-ah]	chondr/o = cartilage	softening of cartilage
-megaly :		enlargement	
visceromegaly	[**vis**-er-oh-meg-ah-lee]	viscer/o = internal organs	enlargement of internal organs
-oma :		tumor, mass	
lipoma	[lih-**poh**-mah]	lip/o = fat	tumor containing fat
myoma	[my-**oh**-mah]	my/o = muscle	tumor of muscle
-osis :		abnormal condition or increase	
nephrosis	[neh-**froh**-sis]	nephr/o = kidney	abnormal condition of the kidney
-pathy :		disease in process	
ureteropathy	[you-ree-ter-**op**-pah-thee]	ureter/o = ureter	disease of the ureter
-penia :		decrease, deficiency	
cytopenia	[sigh-toh-**pee**-nee-ah]	cyt/o = cell	deficiency of cells

Term	Pronunciation	Term Analysis	Meaning
-phil, -philia :		attraction for	
hemophilia	[heh-moh-**fih**-lee-ah]	hem/o = blood	condition of impaired blood-clotting ability
-phobia :		irrational fear	
acrophobia	[ack-roh-**foh**-bee-ah]	acr/o = sharp, top, extremities	fear of heights
-ptosis :		drooping, prolapsed, sagging	
blepharoptosis	[blef-ah-rop-**toh**-sis]	blephar/o = eyelid	drooping eyelid
nephroptosis	[nef-rop-**toh**-sis]	nephr/o = kidney	drooping kidney
-ptysis :		spitting, vomitting	
hemoptysis	[he-**mop**-tih-sis]	hem/o = blood	spitting up of blood
-rrhage; -rrhagia :		bursting forth	
hemorrhage	[**hem**-or-ridge]	hem/o = blood	bleeding
gastrorrhagia	[gas-troh-**ray**-jee-ah]	gastr/o = stomach	bleeding from the stomach
-rrhea :		flow, discharge	
otorrhea	[oh-toh-**ree**-ah]	ot/o = ear	discharge from the ear
-rrhexis :		rupture	
splenorrhexis	[splee-nor-**eck**-sis]	splen/o = spleen	ruptured spleen
-sclerosis :		hardening	
arteriosclerosis	[ar-tee-ree-oh-skleh-**roh**-sis]	arteri/o = artery	hardening of the arteries
-spasm :		sudden, involuntary contraction	
blepharospasm	[**blef**-ah-roh-spazm]	blephar/o = eyelid	sudden, involuntary contraction of the eyelid
-stenosis :		narrowing, stricture	
phlebostenosis	[fleb-oh-steh-**noh**-sis]	phleb/o = vein	narrowing of a vein
-y :		condition or process	
neuropathy	[new-**roh**-pah-thee]	neur/o = nerve; path/o = disease	disease process of the nerve

Suffixes used to Indicate Diagnostic Procedures

Term	Pronunciation	Term Analysis	Meaning
-gram :		record writing	
lymphangiogram	[lim-**fan**-jee-oh-gram]	lymphangi/o = lymph vessel	record of the lymph vessel
-graph :		instrument used to record	
cardiograph	[**kar**-dee-oh-graf]	cardi/o = heart	instrument used to record heart activity
-graphy :		process of recording, producing images	
mammography	[mam-**og**-rah-fee]	mamm/o = breast	producing images of the breast
myelography	[my-eh-**log**-rah-ree]	myel/o = spinal cord	producing images of the spinal cord
tomography	[toh-**mog**-rah-fee]	tom/o = to cut, sectioning	computerized imaging by sectioning
-meter :		instrument used to measure	
craniometer	[kray-nee-**om**-eh-ter]	crani/o = skull	instrument used to measure the skull
-metry :		to measure, measurement	
pelvimetry	[pel-**vim**-eh-tree]	pelv/i = pelvis	measurement of the pelvis
-opsy :		to view	
biopsy	[**bye**-op-see]	bi/o = life	removing and visually examining a living tissue
-scope :		instrument used to visually examine inside	
bronchoscope	[**brong**-koh-skope]	bronch/o = bronchus	endoscope for bronchial tubes
-scopy :		process of visually examining (a body cavity or organ)	
bronchoscopy	[brong-**kos**-koh-pee]	bronch/o = bronchus	process of visually examining the bronchus

Suffixes used to Indicate Surgical Procedures

Term	Pronunciation	Term Analysis	Meaning
-centesis :		surgical puncture to remove fluid	
abdominocentesis	[ab-dom-ih-noh-sen-**tee**-sis]	abdomin/o = abdomen	surgical puncture to remove fluid from the abdomen
thoracocentesis	[thoh-rah-koh-sen-**tee**-sis]	thorac/o = chest	surgical puncture of the chest wall to remove excess fluid from around the lungs
-desis :		surgical binding, fusion	
arthrodesis	[ar-throh-**dee**-sis]	arthr/o = joint	surgical fusion of a joint
-ectomy :		excision, surgical removal	
oophorectomy	[oh-of-oh-**reck**-toh-mee]	oophor/o = ovary	excision of the ovary
nephrectomy	[nef-**reck**-toh-mee]	nephr/o = kidney	excision of the kidney
tonsillectomy	[ton-sih-**leck**-toh-mee]	tonsill/o = tonsils	excision of the tonsils
-pexy :		surgical fixation	
nephropexy	[**nef**-roh-peck-see]	nephr/o = kidney	surgical fixation of the kidney
-plasty :		surgical reconstruction, surgical repair	
orchidoplasty	[**or**-kid-oh-plas-tee]	orchid/o = testicle	surgical reconstruction of the testicle
-rrhaphy :		suture, sewing	
colporrhaphy	[kol-**por**-ah-fee]	colp/o = vagina	suturing of the vagina
-stasis :		stoppage, stopping, controlling	
hemostasis	[he-moh-**stay**-sis]	hem/o = blood	stoppage of bleeding
-stomy :		creation of new opening	
colostomy	[koh-**loh**-stoh-mee]	col/o = colon	incision into colon to create an opening for drainage of feces

Term	Pronunciation	Term Analysis	Meaning
-stomy :		creation of new opening	
tracheostomy	[tray-kee-**os**-toh-mee]	trache/o = trachea	making a new opening into the trachea
-tome :		instrument used to cut	
myotome	[**my**-oh-tohm]	my/o = muscle	instrument used to cut muscle
-tomy :		surgical process of cutting, incision	
tenotomy	[teh-**not**-oh-mee]	ten/o = tendon	process of cutting a tendon

Exercises

1. Write the meaning of the following suffixes :

① -ac	pertaining to
② -algia	pain
③ -cele	hernia
④ -centesis	surgical puncture to remove fluid
⑤ -ectomy	removal, excision, resection
⑥ -gram	record
⑦ -ism	process, condition
⑧ -itis	inflammation
⑨ -logist	specialist
⑩ -malacia	softening
⑪ -megaly	enlargement
⑫ -opsy	view of, visual examination
⑬ -penia	deficiency
⑭ -phobia	excessive fear
⑮ -ptosis	drooping, prolapse
⑯ -rrhaphy	suturing
⑰ -pexy	surgical fixation
⑱ -spasm	sudden, involuntary contraction
⑲ -stomy	creation of an opening

2. Write examples of words using the following suffixes :

① -ary	mammary	binary	
② -atrics	geriatrics	pediatrics	
③ -cele	cystocele	rectocele	
④ -dynia	gastrodynia	mastodynia	
⑤ -genesis	ovogenesis	spermatogenesis	
⑥ -graphy	mammography	tomography	
⑦ -ium	pericardium	endometrium	
⑧ -logy	biology	physiology	
⑨ -lysis	hemolysis	analysis	paralysis
⑩ -meter	craniometer	sphygmometer	manometer
⑪ -oma	sarcoma	lipoma	
⑫ -osis	nephrosis	psychosis	osteoporosis
⑬ -phil, philia	hemophilia	neutrophil	
⑭ -plasty	orchidoplasty	rhinoplasty	
⑮ -rrhagia	gastrorrhagia	metrorrhagia	
⑯ -rrhea	otorrhea	diarrhea	
⑰ -scopy	endoscopy	bronchoscopy	
⑱ -stasis	hemostasis	metastasis	
⑲ -tomy	tenotomy	gastrotomy	anatomy
⑳ -ule	venule	nodule	

Chapter 4

Prefixes

Chapter Contents

- Prolog
- Negative Prefixes
- Prefixes Referring to Direction, Position, Posture, etc.
- Prefixes Related to Time
- Prefixes Referring to Numbers and Measurements
- Miscellaneous Prefixes
- Prefixes with Similar or Opposite Meaning
- Exercises

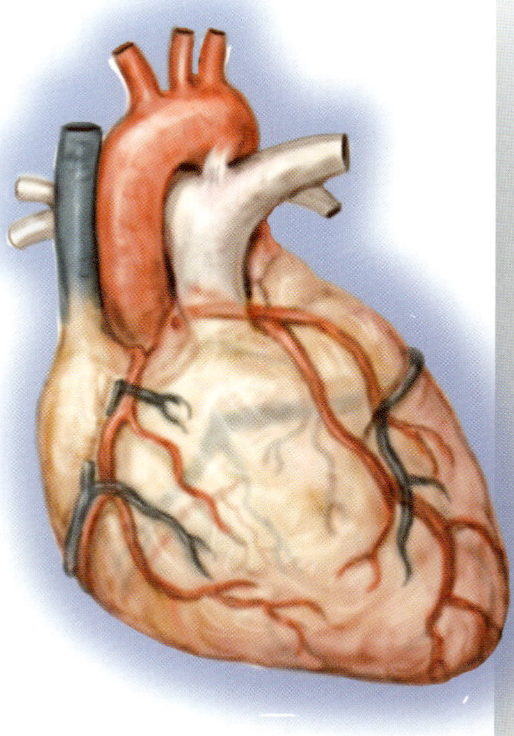

Learning Objectives

- Learn meaning of prefixes.
- Distinguish prefixes that signify direction, position and posture from those of negation and number.
- Identify prefixes with same or similar meaning.
- Identify prefixes that are opposite in meaning.
- Analyze, define, spell and pronounce medical terms in the chapter.

Prolog

A prefix tells us "how" with respect to the combined root and/or suffix of the term. Prefixes are classified into the following types :

① **Negative Prefixes** : These mean not, against or lacking, etc.

② **Prefixes Referring to Direction, Position, Posture, etc.** : These signify spatial concepts including fore, aft, side, near, far, in, out, etc.

③ **Prefixes Related to Time** : These indicate time related concepts including early/late, fast/slow, before/after, etc.

④ **Prefixes Referring to Numbers and Measurements** : These signify quantitative concepts such as few/many, singular/plural, how much, etc.

⑤ **Miscellaneous Prefixes** : Other prefixes that are frequently used in medical terms.

Negative Prefixes

Term	Pronunciation	Term Analysis	Meaning
a-, an- :		no, not, lack of	
aseptic	[ay-**sehp**-tick]	-ic = pertaining to; sept/o = infection	free from infectious material
anemia	[ah-**nee**-me-ah]	-emia = blood condition	lack of red blood cells (RBCs) or hemoglobin (Hgb)

Term	Pronunciation	Term Analysis	Meaning
anti- :		against	
antibiotic	[an-tih-bye-**oh**-tick]	bi/o = life; -tic = pertaining to	drug used to kill harmful bacteria
contra- :		against, opposite	
contralateral	[kon-trah-**lat**-ter-al]	-al = pertaining to; later/o = side	pertaining to opposite side of the body
de- :		from, down, not	
dehydration	[dee-hyed-**ray**-shun]	hydr/o = water; -ation = action, process	loss of water
in- :		not	
indigestible	[in-dih-**jes**-tih-bl]	-ible = able to be; digest/o = digestion	not capable of being digested

Prefixes Referring to Direction, Position, Posture, etc.

Term	Pronunciation	Term Analysis	Meaning
ab- :		away from	
abduction	[ab-**duck**-shun]	-ion = process; duct/o = to draw, carry	process of drawing away from
ad- :		toward	
adduction	[ah-**duck**-shun]	-ion = process; duct/o = to draw	process of drawing toward
circum- :		around	
circumduction	[ser-kum-**duck**-shun]	-ion = process; duct/o = to draw	process of moving a body part in a circular motion
dia- :		through, complete	
diameter	[dye-**am**-eh-ter]	-meter = measurement	measurement from edge to edge of a circle
diagnosis	[dye-ag-**noh**-sis]	-gnosis = knowledge	finding the nature and cause of anomaly

Term	Pronunciation	Term Analysis	Meaning
ecto- :		outside	
ectogenous	[eck-**toh**-jeh-nus]	-genous = produced by	generated outside the host
en-, endo- :		within	
endoscope	[en-**doh**-skohp]	-scope = visual instrument	instrument used to visually examine inside the body
epi- :		upon, on, above	
epigastric	[ep-ih-**gas**-trick]	-ic = pertaining to; gastr/o = stomach	pertaining to upon the stomach
e-, ec-, ecto-, ex-, exo-, extra- :		out, outward, outside	
eversion	[ee-**ver**-zhun]	-version = process of turning	process of turning inside out; turning outward
excision	[eck-**sih**-zhun]	-ion = process; cis/o = cut	process of cutting out
extraocular	[ecks-trah-**ock**-you-lar]	-ar = pertaining to; ocul/o = eye	pertaining to outside the eye
hyper- :		excessive, above	
hyperplasia	[high-per-**play**-zee-ah]	-plasia = formation, development	excessive formation, enlargement
hypo- :		below, under, deficient	
hypogastric	[high-poh-**gas**-trick]	-ic = pertaining to; gastr/o = stomach	pertaining to below the stomach
in- :		in, into	
incision	[in-**sih**-zhun]	-ion = process; cis/o = cut	process of cutting into
inversion	[in-**ver**-zhun]	-version = process of turning	process of turning inward
infra- :		below, beneath	
infracostal	[in-frah-**kos**-tal]	-al = pertaining to; cost/o = rib	pertaining to below the ribs

Term	Pronunciation	Term Analysis	Meaning
inter- :		between	
intercellular	[in-ter-**sel**-you-lar]	-ar = pertaining to; cellul/o = cell	pertaining to between the cells
intra- :		within	
intracranial	[in-trah-**kray**-nee-al]	-al= pertaining to; crani/o = skull	pertaining to within the skull
meta- :		beyond	
metamorphosis	[meh-tah-mor-**foh**-sis]	morph/o = shape, form	transformation in shape or function
metaplasia	[met-ah-**play**-zee-ah]	plasia = formation, development	change in formation
metastasis	[meh-**tas**-tah-sis]	-stasis = stopping, controlling	beyond control; spread of cancer from one organ to another
para- :		beside, near	
paranasal	[par-ah-**nay**-sal]	-al = pertaining to; nas/o = nose	pertaining to near the nose
per- :		through	
percutaneous	[per-kyou-**tay**-nee-us]	-ous = pertaining to; cutane/o = skin	pertaining to through the skin
peri- :		around	
perineuritis	[per-ih-nyou-**rye**-tis]	-itis = inflammation; neur/o = nerve	inflammation around a nerve
post- :		after	
postmortem	[pohst-**mor**-tehm]	-mortem = death	after death
pre- :		before, in front of	
prenatal	[pre-**nay**-tal]	-al = pertaining to; nat/o = birth	pertaining to before birth
pro- :		before	
prodrome	[**proh**-drohm]	-drome = to run	early symptom before the onset of disease.
prognosis	[prohg-**noh**-sis]	-gnosis = knowledge	forecast for the future of the disease

Term	Pronunciation	Term Analysis	Meaning
retro- :		back, behind	
retroversion	[ret-roh-**ver**-zhun]	-version = turning	backward turning or tipping of an organ
sub- :		under, below	
subcutaneous	[sub-kyou-**tay**-nee-us]	-ous= pertaining to; cutane/o = skin	pertaining to under the skin
sublingual	[sub-**ling**-gwahl]	-al = pertaining to; lingu/o = tongue	pertaining to under the tongue
super-, supra- :		above	
suprarenal	[soo-prah-**ree**-nal]	-al= pertaining to; ren/o = kidney	pertaining to above the kidney
trans- :		across	
transection	[tran-**seck**-shun]	-ion = process; sect/o = cut	a transverse cut (view)
ultra- :		beyond	
ultrasonography	[ul-trah-son-**og**-rah-fee]	-graphy = process of recording; son/o = sound	process of recording using ultrasound

Prefixes Related to Time

Term	Pronunciation	Term Analysis	Meaning
ante-, pre-, pro- :		before	
antenatal	[an-tee-**nay**-tal]	-al = pertaining to; nat/o = birth	pertaining to before birth
brady- :		slow	
bradycardia	[brad-ee-**kar**-dee-ah]	-ia = condition or state of; cardi/o = heart	state of slow heartbeat
chron-, chrono- :		time	
chronobiology	[kroh-no-bye-**ol**-oh-jee]	biology = study of living things	study of the effect of time on biological system

Term	Pronunciation	Term Analysis	Meaning
tachy- :		fast, rapid	
tachycardia	[tack-ee-**kar**-dee-ah]	-ia = condition; cardi/o = heart	fast heartbeat
tachypnea	[tack-**eep**-nee-ah]	-ia = condition; pne/o = lung	fast breathblood-clotting ability
re- :		again, back	
reconstruction	[ree-const-**ruck**-shun]	-ion = process; construct/o = build	process of restoring or rebuilding
relapse	[ree-**laps**]	lapse = slip, failure, decline, fall	recurrence of disease

Prefixes Referring to Numbers and Measurements

Term	Pronunciation	Term Analysis	Meaning
bi-, di- :		two	
bilateral	[bye-**lat**-er-al]	-al = pertaining to; later/o = side	pertaining to two sides
dissection	[dye-**seck**-shun]	-ion = process; sect/o = to cut	to cut into two pieces
hemi-, semi- :		half	
hemigastrectomy	[hem-ee-gas-**treck**-toh-mee]	-ectomy = excision; gastr/o = stomach	excision of half the stomach
semicomatose	[sem-ee-**koh**-mah-tohs]	semi- = half; comat/o = deep sleep	in mildly unconscious state
hect-, hecto- :		hundred, 100	
hectogram	[**heck**-to-gram]	gram = a unit of weight	100 grams
hept (a)-, sept- :		seven	
heptadactylism	[hep-tah-**dack**-tih-lism]	-dactyl = digit	having seven fingers on a hand
hex (a)- :		six	
hexadactylism	[heck-sah-**dack**-tih-lism]	-dectyl = digit	having six fingers on a hand

Term	Pronunciation	Term Analysis	Meaning
kil-, kilo- :		thousand, 1,000	
kilometer	[**kih**-lo-mee-ter]	meter = a unit of length	1,000 meters
mega- :		million, large	
megadont	[**meg**-a-dont]	dont = tooth	having large teeth
giga- :		billion	
gigantism	[jeye-**gan**-tism]	-ism = condition	being abnormally large
mono-, monus-, uni- :		one	
monocyte	[**mon**-oh-sight]	-cyte = cell	white blood cell with a single nucleus
unilateral	[you-nih-**lat**-er-al]	-al = pertaining to; later/o = side	pertaining to one side
multi-, poly- :		many	
multiform	[**mul**-tih-form]	-form = shape	having many shapes
polyadenoma	[pol-ih-ad-eh-**noh**-mah]	-oma = tumor; -aden/o = gland	tumor of many glands
nona-, novem- :		nine	
nonan	[**non**-nan]	-an = belonging to	occurring every ninth (day)
nulli-, nullus- :		null, none	
nullipara	[nul-**lih**-pah-rah]	-para = giving birth	woman who has not given birth
oct (a)-, octi- :		eight	
octipara	[**ock**-ti-pah-rah]	-para = giving birth	woman who has given birth to 8 children
olig (o)- :		few, deficient	
oliguria	[oh-li-**goo**-ree-ah]	-uria = unine condition	decreased urine production
pan-, pant (o)- :		all, whole	
panangiitis	[pan-an-jee-**eye**-tis]	angi/o = vessel; -itis = inflammation	inflammation of all blood vessels
pent (a)-, quinqu (e)- :		five	
pentagon	[**pen**-tah-gon]	-gon = angled shape	polygon with 5 sides

Term	Pronunciation	Term Analysis	Meaning
quadri-, tetra- :		four	
quadrilateral	[kwad-rih-**lat**-er-al]	-al = pertaining to; later/o = side	pertaining to four sides
tri-, ter- :		three	
tricuspid	[try-**kus**-pid]	-cuspid = sharp point, projection	having three cusps or projections

Miscellaneous Prefixes

Term	Pronunciation	Term Analysis	Meaning
ana- :		apart, up	
anatomy	[ah-**nat**-oh-mee]	-tomy = process of cutting	study of the structure of the body
auto- :		self	
autopsy	[**aw**-top-see]	-opsy = to view	dissection (of human) to find the cause of death necropsy = dissection (of animal) to find the cause of death
con- :		together	
concrescence	[kon-**kreh**-sans]	crescence = rise, growth	merging and growing together (of 2 teeth)
dys- :		bad, abonormal, difficult, painful	
dysplasia	[dis-**play**-see-ah]	-plasia = formation, development	abnormal development
eu- :		normal, good	
euphoria	[you-**foh**-ree-ah]	-phoria = feeling, mental state	feeling of happiness or satisfaction
macr (o)- :		large	
macrocephalia	[mack-roh-seh-**fay**-lee-ah]	-ia = state of, condition	having excessively large head

Term	Pronunciation	Term Analysis	Meaning
micr (o)- :		small	
microscope	[**mye**-kroh-skohp]	-scope = instrument	instrument used to view very small objects
mal- :		bad	
malaise	[mah-**layz**]	-aise = ease, comfort	feeling of uneasiness or discomfort
malnutrition	[mahl-nyou-**tri**-shun]		lack of nutrition
neo- :		new	
neoplasm	[**nee**-oh-plazm]	-plasm = formation, development	abnormal new growth, tumor
pan- :		all	
panhysterectomy	[pan-hiss-ter-**eck**-toh-mee]	-ectomy = excision; hyster/o = uterus	excision of all of the uterus
syn-, sym- :		together, with, joined	
synarthrotic	[sin-ar-**throh**-tick]	-tic = pertaining to; arthr/o = joint	as a type of joint in which the bones are joined
symmetry	[**sim**-eh-tree]	-metry = process of measuring	being similar in measurement on opposite side

Prefixes with Similar or Opposite Meaning

Prefixes with same or similar meaning

prefix	meaning
• ante-, pre-, pro-	before
• anti-, contra-	against
• circum-, peri-	around
• dys-, mal-	bad
• e-, ex-, extra-	outside
• endo-, intra	within
• epi-, hyper-, supra-	above
• hypo-, infra-, sub-	below

Prefixes with opposite meaning

prefix	meaning
{ ab-	away from
ad-	toward
{ ante-, pre-, pro-	before
post-	after
{ ecto-, ex-, extra-	outside
endo-, in-, intra-	within, inward
{ hyper-, supra-, epi-, ultra	above
hypo-, infra-, sub-	below
{ tachy-	fast
brady-	slow
{ hyper-	excessive
hypo-	deficient
{ macro-	large
micro-	small
{ ana-	apart
syn-	together, with, joined

Exercises

1. Write the meaning of the following prefixes, and give examples by combining with roots and/or suffixes :

Prefix	Meaning	Examples
① a-	no, not	apathy, aseptic
② an-	not, lacking	analgesic, anemia
③ ab-	away from	abduction, abnormal
④ anti-	against	antibody, antibiotic
⑤ ante-	before, in front of	antenatal, antepartum, anterior
⑥ bi-	two, double	binary, bilateral
⑦ brady-	slow	bradycardia
⑧ dys-	bad, difficult, abnormal	dysplasia, dysfuction
⑨ endo-	inside, within	endoscope, endocrinology
⑩ epi-	above, upon, outside of	epigastric, epidermis
⑪ exo-	out, away from	exoskeleton, exocytosis
⑫ extra-	outside, beyond	extraocular, extracellular
⑬ hyper-	above, excessive	hyperplasia, hypertension
⑭ intra-	within	intracranial, intravenous
⑮ mal-	bad	malaise, malnutrition
⑯ meta-	beyond, changed	metastasis, metamorphosis
⑰ micro-	small	microscope, microbiology
⑱ neo-	new	neoplasm, neonatal
⑲ para-	near, alongside, abnormal	paranasal, paraphilia, paraplegia
⑳ poly-	many	polyadenoma, polymyositis
㉑ post-	after, behind	postmortem, posterior
㉒ pre-	before, in front of	prenatal, prematurity
㉓ quadri-	four, square	quadrilateral, quadriceps
㉔ re-	again, backward	relapse, reconstruction
㉕ supra-	above, over	suprarenal, supraorbital
㉖ syn-	together, with	synarthrosis, synesthesia

㉗ tachy-	fast	tachycardia, tachypnea
㉘ ultra	beyond, excessive	ultrasonography

2. Write prefixes that have opposite meaning to the following :

① ad-	ab-
② post-	ante-, pre-
③ endo-	ex-, ecto-
④ hypo-	hyper-, supra-
⑤ brady-	tachy-
⑥ micro-	macro-
⑦ syn-	ana-

3. Write prefixes that have same or similar meaning to the following :

① anti-	contra-
② circum-	peri-
③ dys-	mal-
④ endo-	intra-
⑤ epi-	supra-
⑥ infra-	sub-

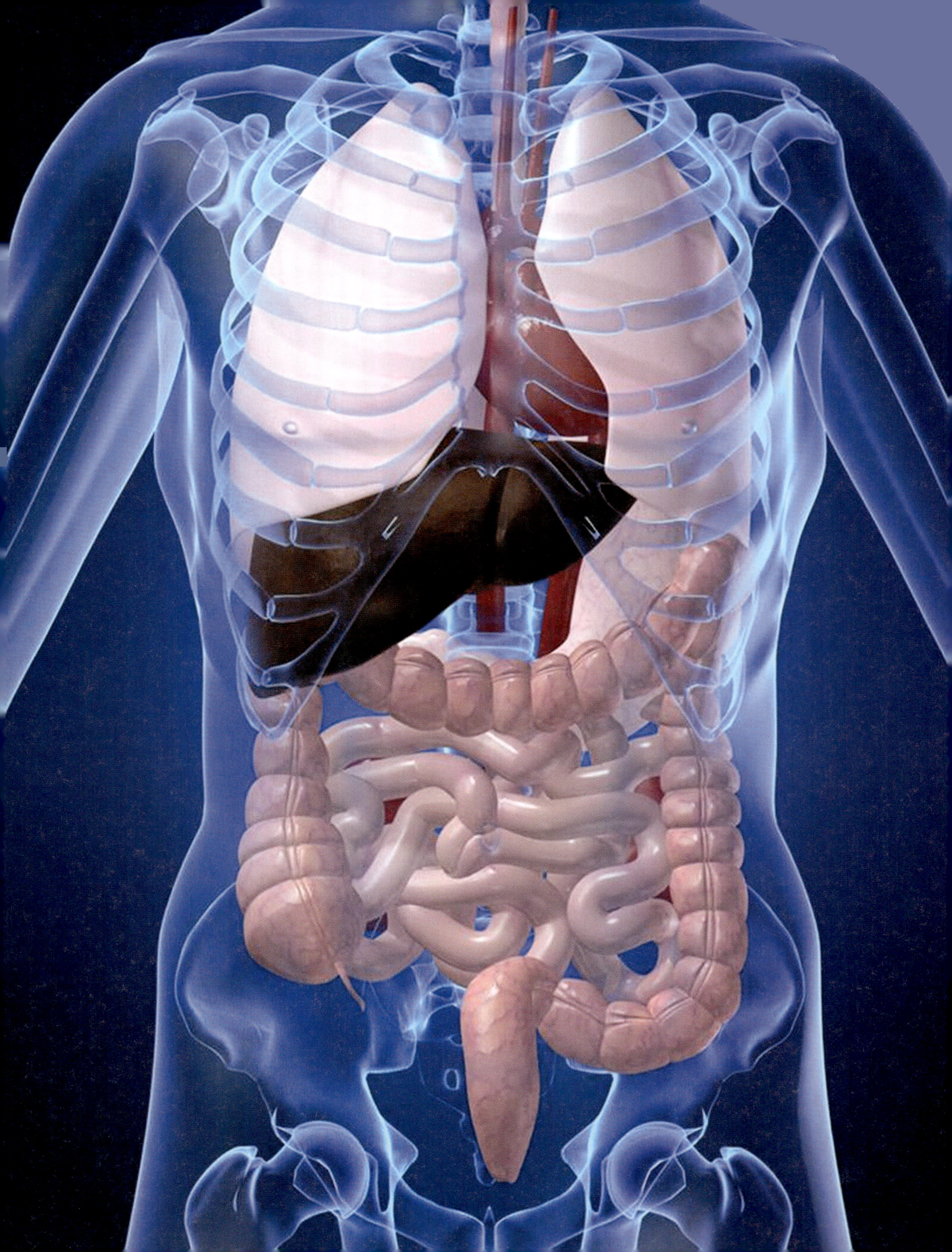

Chapter 5

Body Organization

Chapter Contents

- Prolog
- Terms for Cavities in the Body
- Terms for Direction and Motion of the Body
- Analysis and Meaning of Key Terms
- Abbreviations
- Exercises

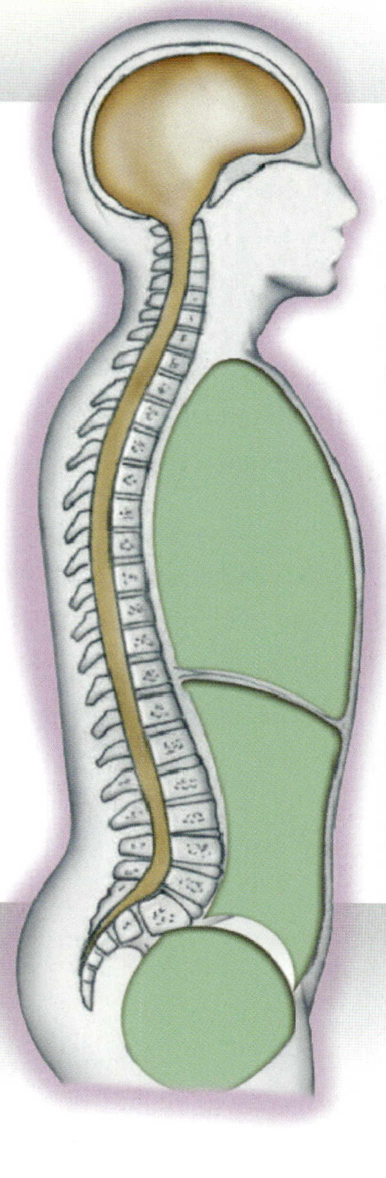

Learning Objectives

- Define anatomical position.
- Learn terms for cavities and organs in the body.
- Correctly define terms for directions, abdominopelvic regions and quadrants.
- Correctly locate body cavities, abdominopelvic regions and quadrants.
- Analyze, define, spell and pronounce medical terms.
- Define abbreviations for body organizations.

Prolog

On the earth we live in, we need directional terms such as east and west. So do we need directional terms to describe locations in the body. However, it is not a simple matter to describe directions because a person can have a variety of positions such as standing up, lying down, sitting down, etc. This led to the development of the standard concept, the **anatomical position** (see Figure 5-1).

In the anatomical position, the body is standing up straight, arms straight by the side with head, palms and feet facing forward. We define directional terms as well as locations based on the anatomical position.

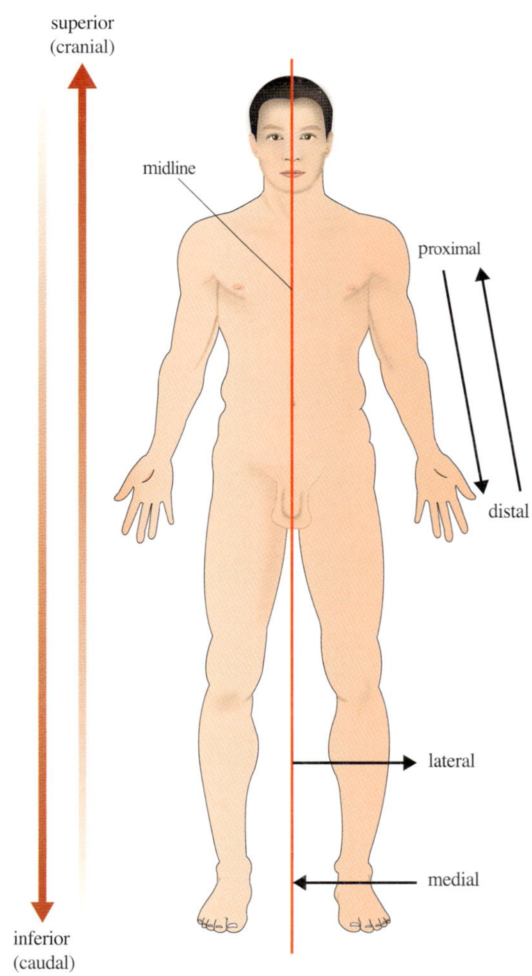

Figure 5-1 Anatomical position

Memory key

- In the anatomical position, the body stands up straight, arms straight by the side with head, palms and feet facing forward.

Terms for Cavities in the Body

The body includes two main cavities — the back (dorsal) cavity and the front (ventral) cavity. These can be subdivided into smaller cavities. The dorsal cavity consists of the cranial cavity and the spinal cavity. The cranial cavity contains the brain, and the spinal cavity contains the spinal cord. The ventral cavity consists of the thoracic, abdominal and pelvic cavities.

The diaphragm is the main respiratory muscle and separates the thoracic and the abdominal cavities. The thoracic cavity contains the lungs, trachea, heart, aorta and esophagus. The abdominal cavity contains digestive organs such as stomach, small and large intestines, liver, gallbladder and pancreas, as well as spleen, kidneys and ureters. In the pelvic cavity are reproductive and urinary organs (excluding kidneys and ureters which belong in the abdominal cavity). Sometimes we call the abdominal and pelvic cavities combined as the abdominopelvic cavity (see Figure 5-2).

Memory key

- The two main cavities are dorsal and ventral.
- The dorsal cavity consists of the cranial cavity and the spinal cavity.
- The ventral cavity consists of the thoracic, abdominal and pelvic cavities.

Body Cavities

The body cavity is the space in the body that contains internal viscera.

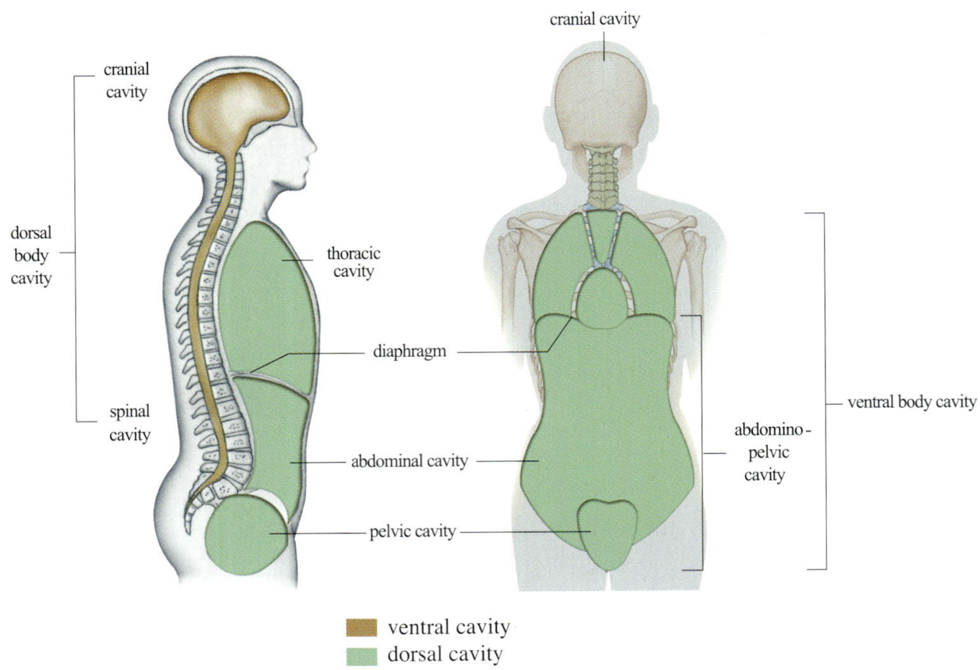

Figure 5-2 Divisions of body cavities

Dorsal cavity

- **Cranial cavity**

  The cranial cavity is the space in the skull that contains the brain.

- **Spinal cavity**

  The spinal cavity is the space in the spine that contains spinal nerve.

Ventral cavity

- **Thoracic cavity**

  The thoracic cavity is the space in the body that contains internal viscera.

- **Abdominal cavity**

  The abdominal cavity is the space surrounded by the abdominal wall.

- **Pelvic cavity**

  The pelvic cavity is the space surrounded by the pelvic walls.

Table 5-1 Major organs in body cavities

Body Cavity	Organs Contained
cranial cavity	brain, pituitary gland
thoracic cavity	lungs, heart, esophagus, trachea, bronchus, thymus gland, aorta
abdominal cavity	stomach, small intestine, large intestine, spleen, liver, gallbladder, pancreas, kidneys, ureters
pelvic cavity	urinary bladder, urethra, uterus, vagina
spinal cavity	spinal cord

Abdominopelvic Regions and Quadrants

The abdominopelvic area of the body can be divided into 9 regions or 4 quadrants for the purpose of describing locations of organs within the cavity.

Figure 5-3 illustrates the four quadrants as follows :

Right upper quadrant (RUQ)

Includes liver (right lobe), gallbladder, a part of pancreas, parts of small and large intestines.

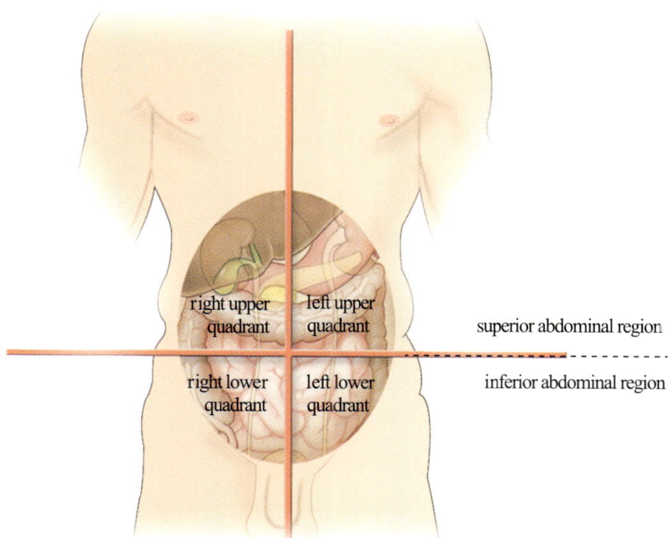

Figure 5-3 Abdominopelvic quadrants

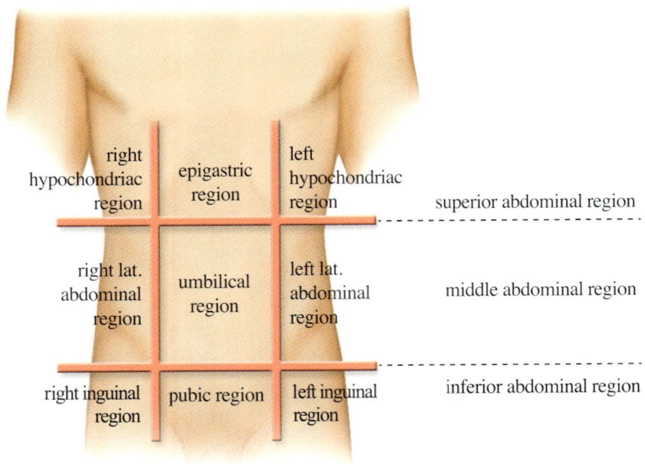

Figure 5-4 Nine abdominopelvic regions

Left upper quadrant (LUQ)

Includes liver (left lobe), stomach, spleen, a part of pancreas, parts of small and large intestines.

Right lower quadrant (RLQ)

Includes parts of small and large intestines, right uterine tube, right ovary, appendix, right ureter.

Left lower quadrant (LLQ)

Includes parts of small and large intestines, left uterine tube, left ovary, right ureter.

Figure 5-4 illustrates the nine regions.

Anatomical Planes

The anatomical position is a standardized position that has been developed in order to clearly describe the human anatomical regions and body structure (see Figure 5-1). In the anatomical position, the body can be divided by the imaginary body planes — frontal, sagittal, transverse planes (see Figure 5-5).

Frontal plane

This plane divides the body into anterior (front) and posterior (back) portions.

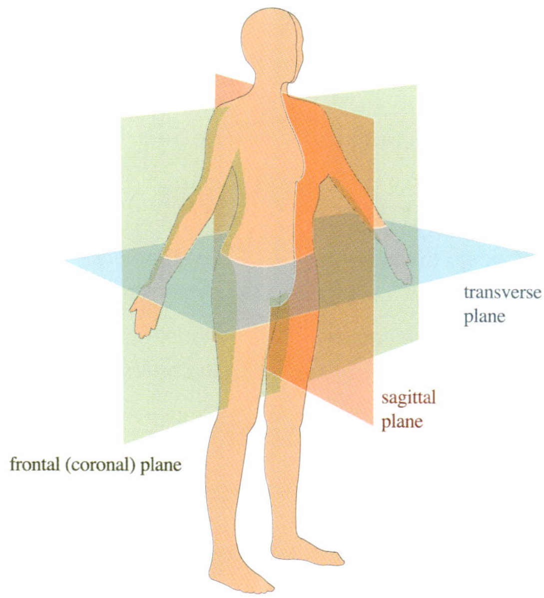

Figure 5-5 Anatomical planes

It is also called coronal plane since it is the plane of the coronal suture.

Sagittal plane

This plane is parallel to the median plane, which divides the body into left and right symmetrically. If the sagittal plane divides the body into equal portions, it becomes the median plane and is called a midsagittal plane.

Transverse plane

This plane is parallel to the ground plane and also called horizontal plane. It is also called cross-sectional (or transverse) plane since the body or the structure is divided into superior and inferior portions.

Terms for Direction and Motion of the Body

The following table lists directional terms of the body (see Figure 5-6).

Directional Term	Definition	Example
central	pertaining to the center	Brain belongs in the central nevous system
peripheral	away from the center	Peripheral nerves are away from the brain and spinal cord.
superior or cranial	above, toward the head	Cranial nerves originate in the head.
inferior or caudal	below, toward the feet or tail	Caudal anesthesia is injected in the lower spine.
proximal	1. nearer to the attachment to the trunk 2. nearer to the point of origin	The elbow is proximal to the wrist. The stomach is proximal to the intestines.
distal	1. farther from the attachment to the trunk 2. farther from the origin	The ankle is distal to the knee. The stomach is distal to the throat.
anterior or ventral	front surface, belly side	The thoracic cavity is anterior to the spinal cavity.
posterior or dorsal	back surface	The spinal cavity is posterior to the thoracic cavity.
medial	toward the midline (centerline)	The big toe is medial to the small toe.
lateral	away from the midline	The small toe is lateral to the big toe.
supine	1. lying on the back with the face up 2. palm facing the front	The patient may be placed in the supine position.
prone	lying on the abdomen with face down	The patient may be placed in the prone position.
superficial	near the surface of the body	The skin is superficial to the internal organs.
deep	farther from the surface of the body	Muscles are deep to the skin.
plantar	sole of the foot	Plantar is to the foot what palm is to the hand.
dorsum	upper portion of the hand or the foot	The dorsum of the foot is the top portion.

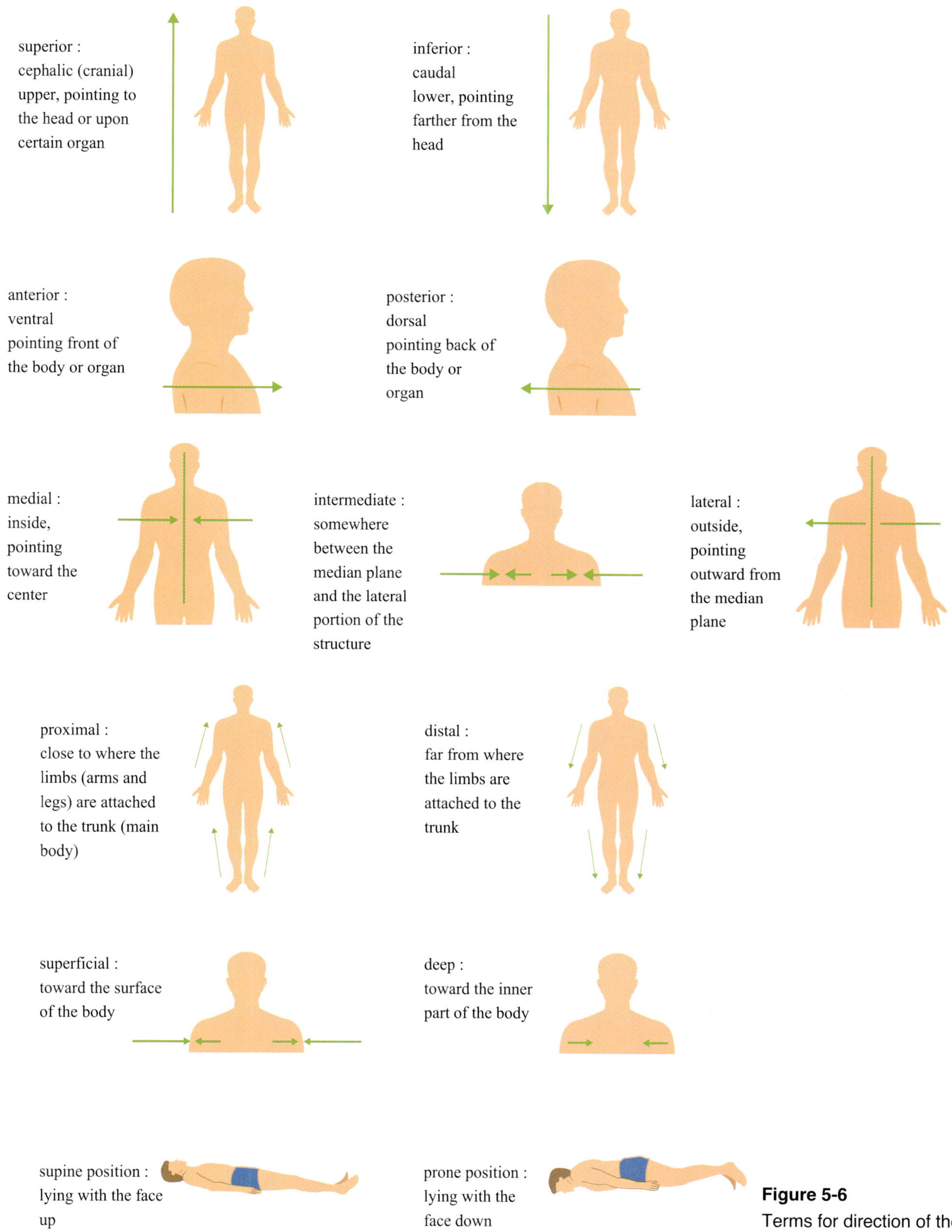

Figure 5-6
Terms for direction of the body

Figure 5-7 illustrates terms for body motion.

flexion
Bending a limb, resulting in decreasing the angle about the transverse axis of the joint.

extension
Bending a limb, resulting in increasing the angle about the transverse axis of the joint.

adduction
Moving a limb toward the median plane.

abduction
Moving a limb away from the median plane.

rotation
Moving a limb about the longitudinal axis centered at the joint.

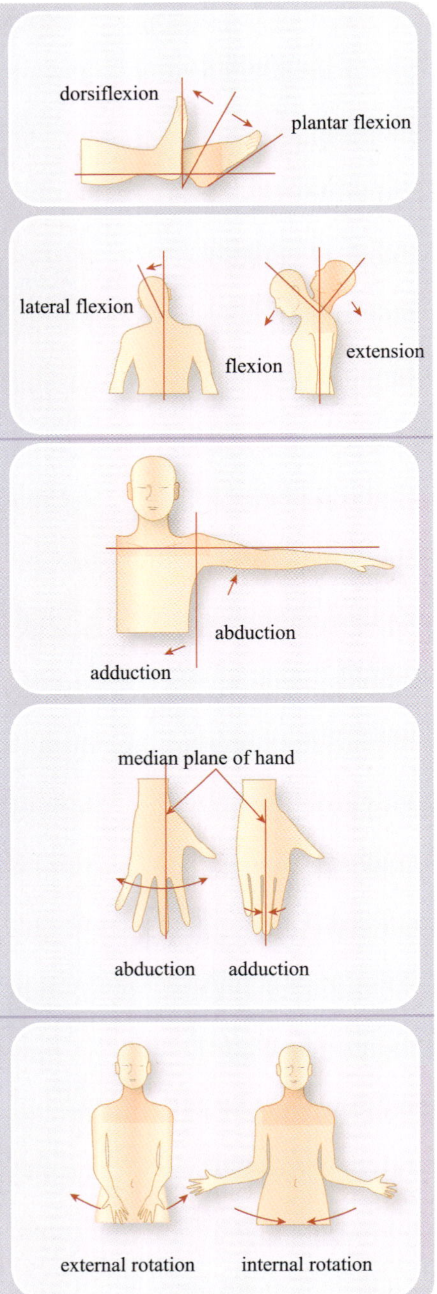

Figure 5-7 Terms for motion of the body

circumduction
Moving a limb in a conical shape with the apex being at the joint attached to the trunk.

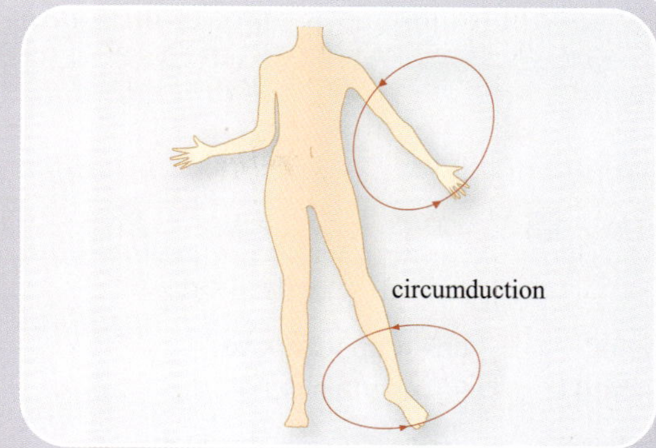

pronation
Twisting an arm resulting in the palm facing backward.

supination
Twisting an arm resulting in the palm facing forward.

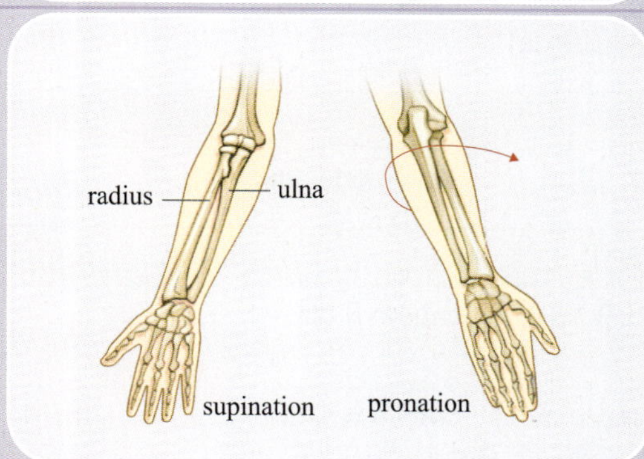

inversion
Moving the leg and the foot so the sole faces inward.

eversion
Moving the leg and the foot so the sole faces outward.

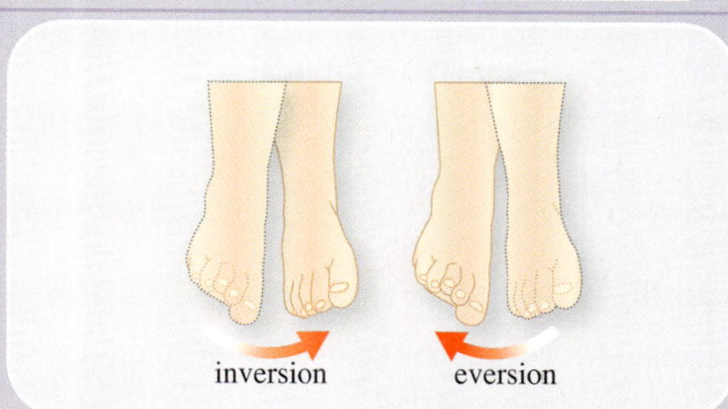

protraction
Moving the jaw or shoulder forward.

retraction
Moving the jaw or shoulder backward.

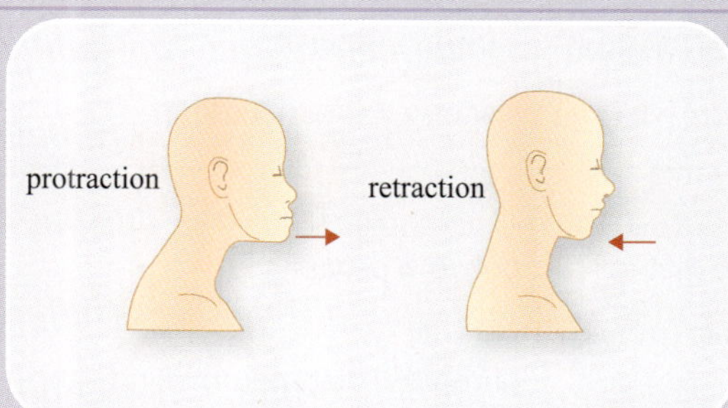

elevation
Moving the shoulder up.

depression
Moving the shoulder down.

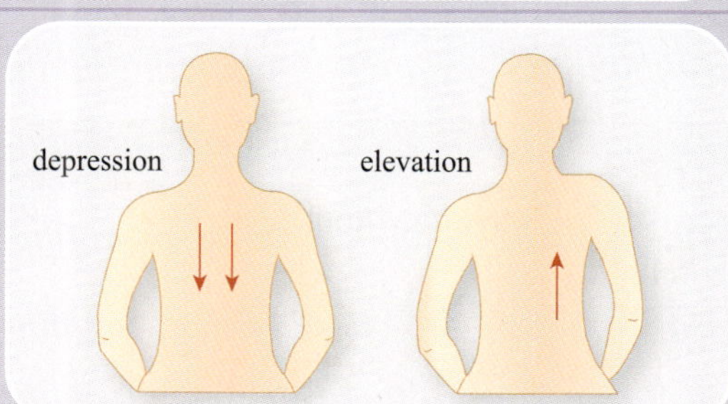

Analysis and Meaning of Key Terms

Term	Term Analysis	Meaning
	gastr/o	stomach
epigastric [èpəgǽstrik]	epi- = upon, above; -ic = pertaining to	pertaining to upon the stomach
hypogastric [hàipougǽstrik]	hypo- = below, deficient	pertaining to below the stomach
	ili/o	hip
iliac	-ac = pertaining to	pertaining to the hip
	-al	pertaining to
caudal [kɔ́:dəl]	caud/o = tail	pertaining to the tail; toward the tail
cranial [kréiniəl]	crani/o = skull	pertaining to blow the stomach
dorsal [dɔ́:rsəl]	dors/o = back	pertaining to the back
inguinal [íŋgwənəl]	inguin/o = groin	pertaining to the groin
medial [mí:diəl]	medi/o = middle	pertaining to the middle
proximal [prάksəməl]	proxim/o = near, close	pertaining to that which is near the point of reference
spinal [spáinl]	spin/o = spine, spinal column, backbone	pertaining to the spine
ventral [véntrəl]	ventr/o = front	pertaining to the front
visceral [vísərəl]	viscer/o = internal organ	pertaining to internal organs
	-ic	pertaining to
pelvic [pélvik]	pelv/o = pelvis	pertaining to the pelvis
phrenic [frénik]	phren/i, phren/o = diaphragm, mind	pertaining to the diaphragm
thoracic [θɔ:rǽsik]	thorac/o = chest, thorax	pertaining to the chest
	-ior	pertaining to
anterior [æntíəriər]	anter/o = front	toward the front side

Term	Term Analysis	Meaning
	-ior	pertaining to
inferior [infíəriər]	infer/o = below downward	toward the lower side
posterior [pɑstíəriər]	poster/o = back	toward the rear side
superior [səpíəriər]	super/o = above, toward the head	toward the upper (head) side

Abbreviations

Abbreviation	Full Term	Meaning
AE	above elbow	above the elbow toward the attachment of the arm
AP	anterior-posterior	from front to back
BE	below elbow	below the elbow
BK	below knee	below the knee toward the feet
LE	lower extremity	leg
LLQ	left lower quadrant	lef lower quadrant of the abdominopelvic cavity
Lt.	left	
LUQ	left upper quadrant	left upper quadrant of the abdominopelvic cavity
PA	posterior-anterior	from back to front
Post-op	post-operation	after surgery
Pre-op	pre-operation	before surgery
RLQ	right lower quadrant	right lower quadrant of the abdominopelvic cavity
RUQ	right upper quadrant	right upper quadrant of the abdominopelvic cavity
Rt.	right	
UE	upper extremity	arm

Exercises

1. Write terms that have opposite meaning to the following :

① Anterior ⟺ Posterior

② Cranial ⟺ Caudal

③ Distal ⟺ Proximal

④ Dorsal ⟺ Ventral

⑤ Inferior ⟺ Superior

⑥ Lateral ⟺ Medial

⑦ Superficial ⟺ Deep

⑧ Supine ⟺ Prone

2. Write full term for the following abbreviations :

① LLQ (left lower quadrant)

② LUQ (left upper quadrant)

③ RLQ (right lower quadrant)

④ RUQ (right upper quadrant)

3. Fill in the blanks for the following figure :

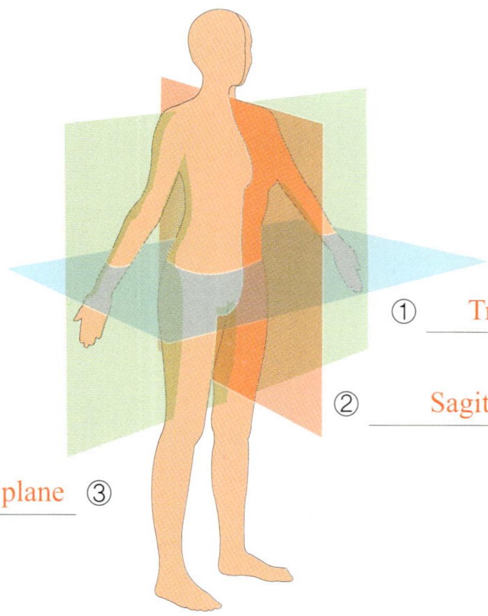

① Transverse plane

② Sagittal plane

Frontal(coronal) plane ③

Chapter 6

Integumentary System

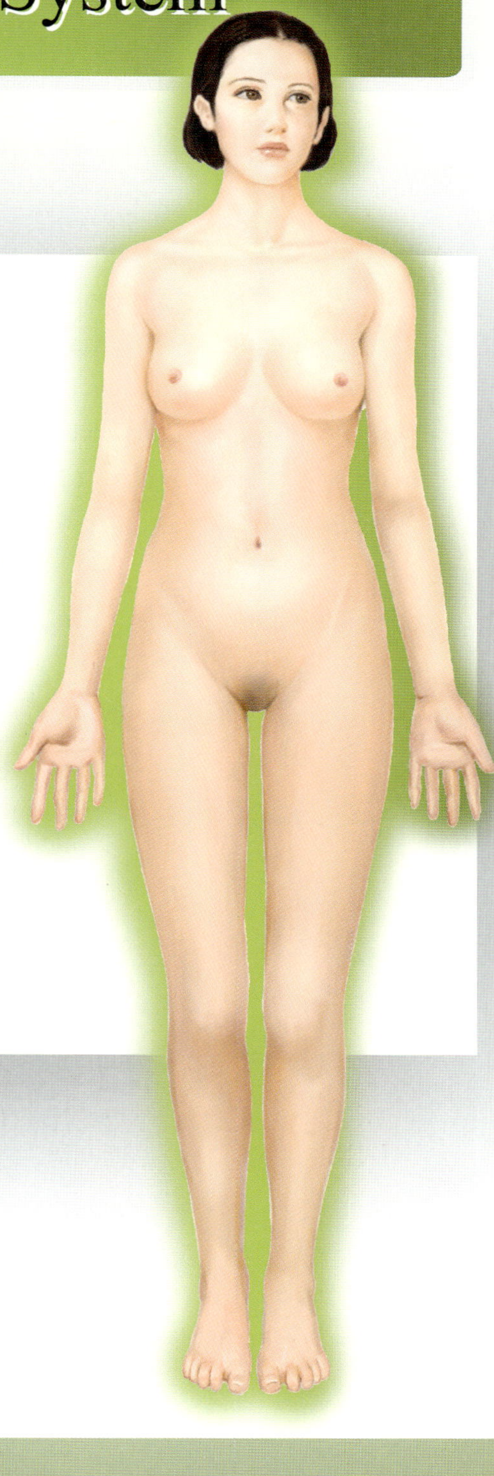

Chapter Contents

- Prolog
- Anatomical Terms
- Terms for Symptoms and Diseases
- Terms for Surgery and Treatment
- Terms for Test and Intervention
- Analysis and Meaning of Key Terms
- Abbreviations
- Exercises

Learning Objectives

- Learn integumentary tissue structures and their functions.
- Be familiar with symptoms arising in integumentary tissues.
- Learn terms for diagnostic methods appropriate for skin diseases.
- Analyze, define, spell and pronounce medical terms used for the skin.
- Define abbreviations for the integumentary system.

Prolog

The skin is the largest organ in the body and it is composed of epidermis and dermis as well as hair, nails and skin glands as appendage.

The layers of the skin cover the body as a membrane to protect the body from external environment. As an organ by itself, the skin performs various, physiologically important functions to protect and regulate inner organs. The area of the skin coverage is almost 2 m^2 and its thickness averages about 1.5 mm.

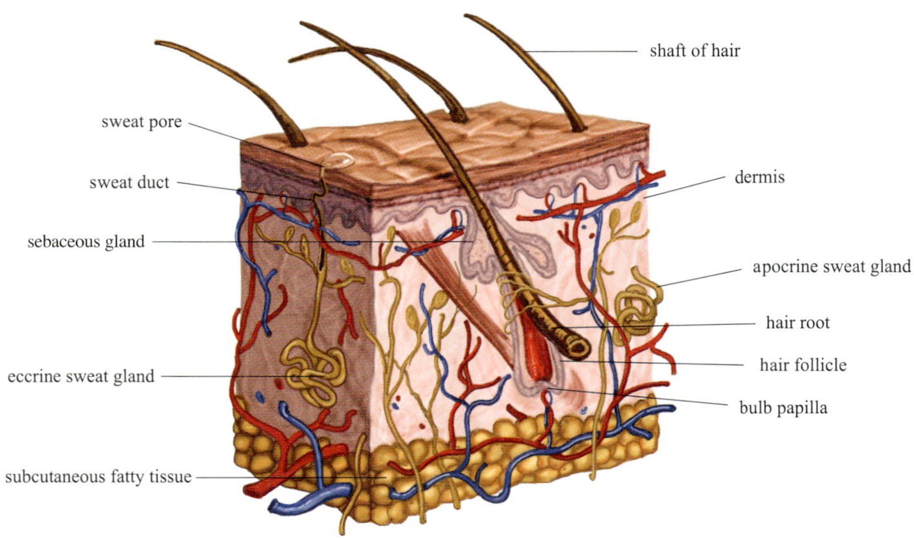

Figure 6-1 Structure of the skin

Anatomical Terms

Being the largest organ in our body, the skin typically weighs about 4 kg. As the protective layer, it regulates body temperature, senses and transmits outer signals, minimizes loss of water. It can sense pain, external temperature, pressure and touch.

Memory key

- The skin is composed of epidermis, dermis and subcutaneous fatty tissue.

Epidermis

Epidermis is the superficial layer and consists of stratified squamous epithelial tissue that contains no blood vessel. Epidermic layers are classified and ordered from the most superficial layer as follows : stratum corneum, stratum lucidum, stratum granulosum, stratum spinosum and stratum basale. Epidermic layer consists of keratinocyte, melanocyte, Langerhans cells and Merkel cells. The stratum basale (the base layer) cells divide and migrate to the upper layers and harden. This physiological cycle of keratinization (or cornification) continues indefinitely to protect the underlying tissues.

Stratum corneum

This is the most superficial layer filled by cells without nucleus. This layer consists of keratinocytes that become corneous and lifeless after cell divisions, which continuously shred and fall off the main body.

Stratum lucidum

Just under the stratum corneum, this layer consists of tiny transparent, lifeless cells without nucleus. This lucidous layer is not easily identified except on the palms of the hands and soles of the feet.

Stratum granulosum

This layer has cells containing small visible granules which are in the process of becoming the keratin.

Stratum spinosum

Also called papillary layer, several layers of cells are built up with keratinocytes migrated from stratum basale.

Stratum basale

The deepest layer of the epidermis, this layer consists of densely and orderly arranged young cells that have nucleus. As a membrane that cover epithelial cells it is located at the border with the interstitial tissue.

Melanocyte

As a skin layer that lie in stratum basale, it generates melanine which determines the skin color.

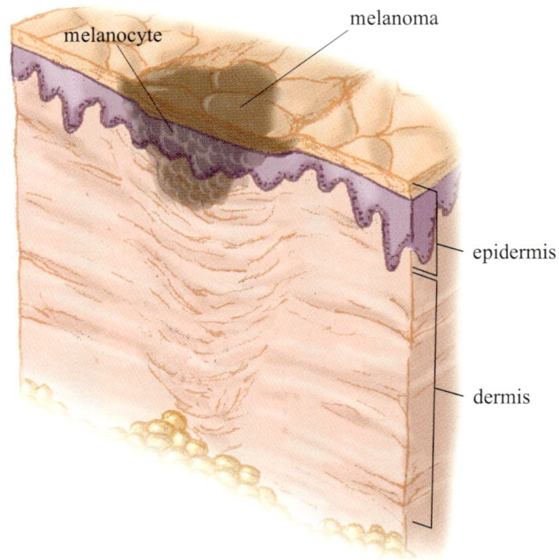

Figure 6-2 Melanin

Dermis

Dermis consists of collageneous and elastic fibers, macrophages, fat cells, fibroblasts, mast cells, etc. It contains blood vessels, nerves, sweat glands, sebaceous glands, hair follicles, hair roots, lymphatic vessels, etc.

Stratum papillarosum

As the superficial layer of dermis, this meets with epidermis and occupies about 1/5 of the whole dermis. The papillary cells are arranged in a particular pattern on the surface of the skin, especially on the palms and soles — which we commonly call fingerprints.

Stratum reticularosum

As the deep layer of dermis, the constructing fibers form relatively thick reticles which are more densely and orderly arranged. The fiber lines run parallel with the surface of the skin which tend to make various patterns of wrinkles depending on location, called Langer's lines.

Memory key

- Dermis is a tissue that include hair follicles, blood vessels, nerves, glands, etc. It consists of fibroblasts, macrophages, mast cells, plasma cells, etc. that reinforce and protect the skin.

Subcutaneous Tissue

Subcutaneous tissue lies between dermis and muscles and as a retiform tissue is tightly connected to dermis. It contains fatty tissue which varies depending on the region of the body. Fatty tissue is better developed in women than men, and is well developed in the abdomen and hip areas of both sexes.

Skin Appendage

Hair, finger nails, toe nails, sebaceous and sweat glands are appendage organs to the skin.

Hair

Hair, comprised of epithelial cells, grows off the hair follicle which is formed in the indented place of the skin and penetrate outward through dermis and epidermis. It is a part of first-line defense for the body, and connected to sebaceous gland and arrector pili muscle. The hair cells start from the follicle and get old to become keratinized epithelial cells which comprise the hair shaft. Hair is made up of hair shaft, hair root inside the skin and hair bulb. The hair bulb is the basal part of the root in the hair follicle which gets nutrition through the blood vessels in the dermis.

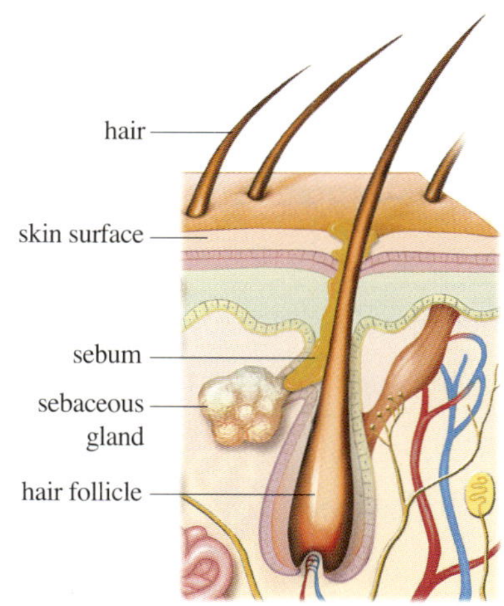

Figure 6-3 Hair

Nails

Finger nails and toe nails consist mainly of keratin and are formed through keratinization of the epidermis. New nail cells are generated through cell divisions at the lunula and grow toward the tip of finger or toe along the nailbed. Finger nails grow at the rate of roughly 1 mm per week.

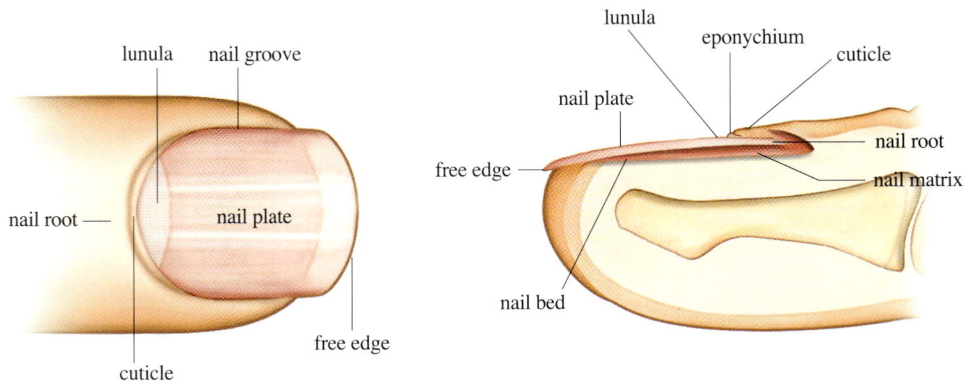

Figure 6-4 Structure of a nail

Glands

The skin glands are important to the maintenance of skin's health and function. The glands secrete through ducts onto the surface and keep the skin soft and waterproof. There are sebaceous glands and sweat glands.

Sebaceous glands

A sebaceous gland is a holocrine gland that secretes sebum onto the hair shaft. Sebum is mostly made up of oil and migrate from the hair shaft onto the skin surface to enhance lubricating and waterproofing functions of the keratinous layer.

Memory key

- Sebaceous glands secrete sebum to lubricate and enrich the skin and hair.

Sebum

Semifluid oil secreted by the sebaceous gland which spread onto the skin surface and hair to form oil film. This maintains the skin and hair soft and pliable.

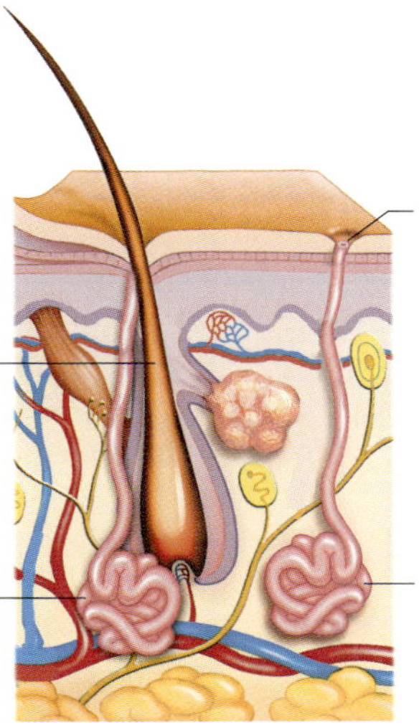

Figure 6-5 Sweat glands

Sweat glands

Sweat glands are distributed in dermis or subcutaneous fatty tissue. They excrete sweat in order to control body temperature through evaporation, and remove harmful materials from the body. They are classified into eccrine sweat glands and apocrine glands.

Sweat

Sweat is salty and, being at pH levels of 4.5 ~ 7.5, contains albumin, water, sodium chloride, urea and other chemicals. Sweat secreted by the glands helps lower the temperature by evaporation and excrete harmful impurities from the body. Governed by sympathetic nerves, sweat is secreted whenever the body temperature is elevated from normal level.

Memory key

- Sweat glands are distributed in dermis or subcutaneous tissue.

Eccrine sweat glands

These are the typical sweat glands distributed throughout the surface of the body. They are more populated especially on the forehead, the back, palms, soles, armpits, the groin and nose.

Apocrine glands

These glands are much larger than eccrine glands and located at open hair follicles at armpits, the pubic region, nipples, ear canals, etc. Sweat from these glands contains substances that diffuse characteristic odors that indicate gender, race and individual differences, so these are also called body odor glands. The sweat is at pH levels of 5.5 ~ 6.5 and rich in protein, which harbors bacteria that generate the bad odor.

Ceruminous glands

Ceruminous glands are special glands only found in external auditory canals. They secrete cerumen (earwax) to protect the inside of the ear from infections.

Terms for Symptoms and Diseases

Papule

A papule is a circumscribed elevation of skin under 1cm in diameter, slightly brighter than the surrounding area. It can occur as rash, allergic cluster or initial symptom of pimples. (see Figure 6-6(a) ①)

Erythema

Erythema is indicated by red macules (spots) on the skin or mucous membranes, caused by hyperemia of superficial capillaries. This can occur in patients with measles, scarlet fever, etc. ②

Eruption

Characteristic flares or bumps occur rapidly in affected lesions due to viral infections or side effects of drugs. ③

Nodule

Similar to papules but larger and deeper, a nodule is of medium scale between papules and tumors. A small circular mass is felt as a hard bump. Unlike papules, nodules encroach on dermis and subcutaneous layers as well as epidermis. ④

Cyst

Cyst is a cluster of cells that group together to form a sac with a normal or abnormal membrane containing fluid or semi-solid matter. A cyst causes the surface to protuberate and encroaches on epidermis, dermis and subcutaneous layers. ⑤

Pustule

A pustule is a small round protuberance of the epidermis containing white, yellow or greenish yellow hemorrhagic pyogenic fluid. If the pustule is left untreated for long and allowed to encroach on the dermis, a scar will remain after cure. ⑥

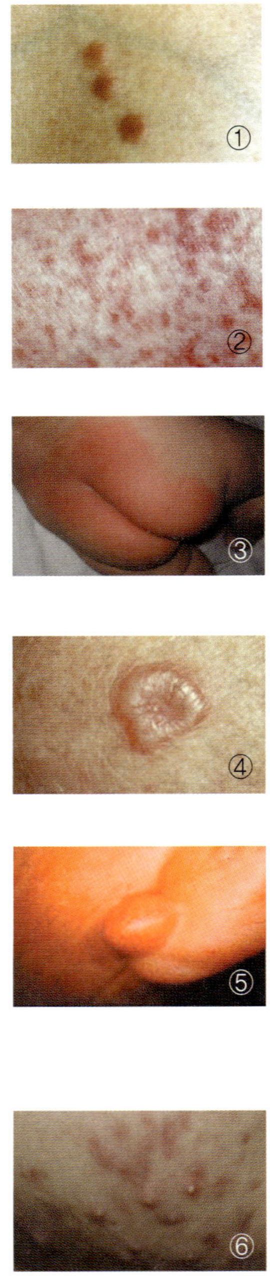

Figure 6-6(a)
Skin diseases

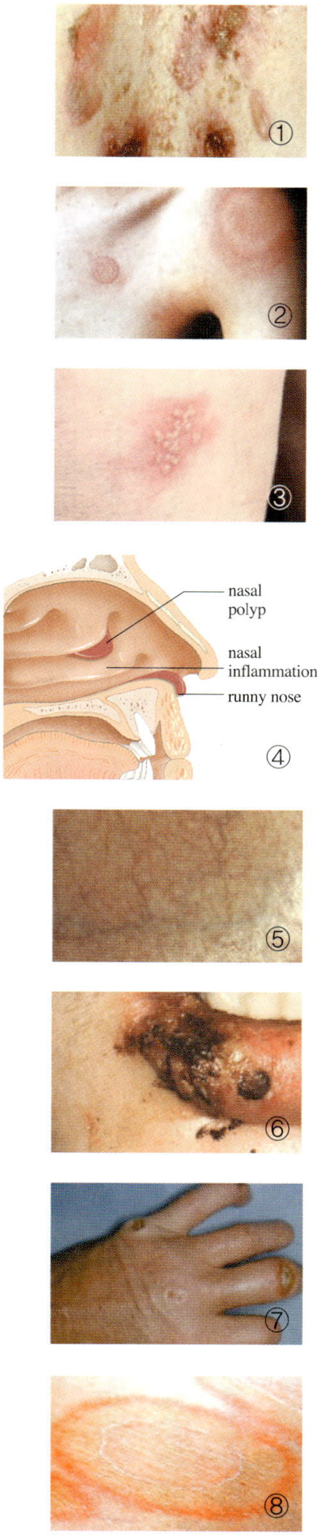

Figure 6-6(b)
Skin diseases

Erosion

A discontinuity of the skin exhibiting gradual destruction and loss of the epidermis, erosion is a moist and scarlet lesion of the skin. (see Figure 6-6(b) ①)

Wheal

Flat-topped elevation of the skin of various size, it is an edematous rash accompanying itching. ②

Vesicle

A vesicle is an epidermal elevation with thin walls containing clear fluid. A small vesicle is a bleb under 1 cm in diameter, and a large one exceeding that size is a bulla existing between dermis and epidermis. ③

Polyp

A polyp is an abnormal growth of tissue forming a nodule or ganglion projecting typically from a mucous membrane. ④

Atrophy

With atrophy, the skin loses tissue and thins due to degenerative changes in the dermis. The aging skin loses resilience and wrinkles. ⑤

Crust

Serum, pus, or blood usually mixed with epithelial debris hardened by drying. ⑥

Scleroderma

This is a sclerosis (hardening) of the skin due to some chronic dermatologic or other disorder. ⑦

Scale

Scale is keratinocytes in the superficial layer that visibly separate from the epidermis in powder form or in coagulated, squamous form. ⑧

Hyperkeratosis

This is thickening of the stratum corneum due to excessive keratinization, often caused by lack of vitamin A or excessive physical stimulation on the skin.

Abrasion

Excoriation of the skin by mechanical wound, continuous rubbing, scratches, etc. (see Figure 6-6(c) ①)

Fissure

A fissure is a crack in the skin that is usually narrow but deep, in a dry or moist condition, due to loss of resilience caused by a disease or a wound. It frequently appears with inflammation of the lips or athlete's foot. ②

Purpura

Characterized by bleeding in the tissues, purpura is red or purple discolored macules visible on the epidermis. It is caused by bleeding underneath the skin or mucous membrane and effluence of red blood cells. ③

Petechia

Petechia is a flare caused by bleeding underneath the skin or mucous membrane varying in size. The bleeding is spotty and in purple-red color. ④

Ulcer

An ulcer is a discontinuity of the skin or mucous membrane exhibiting death of the epidermis and often portions of the dermis caused by inflammation, inducing pain. The affected area is of round or irregular shape. ⑤

Keloid

Keloid is a type of visible scar, displayed as an elevated and hardened lump on normal skin due to excessive production of collagen, the connective tissue in the dermis layer while an incision or wound is slowly being healed. Individual disposition of the patient is considered to be the important factor in causing the condition. ⑥

Lichenification

With lichenification, the skin thickens and hardens like leather due to drying of epidermis and part of dermis and losing softness, and wrinkles become conspicuous. This often occurs on the skin affected by chronic pruritic dermatitis. ⑦

Itch

Itch is a sensation that causes the desire or urge to scratch or rub. It is due to various external stimulations sensed by cutaneous nerves. ⑧

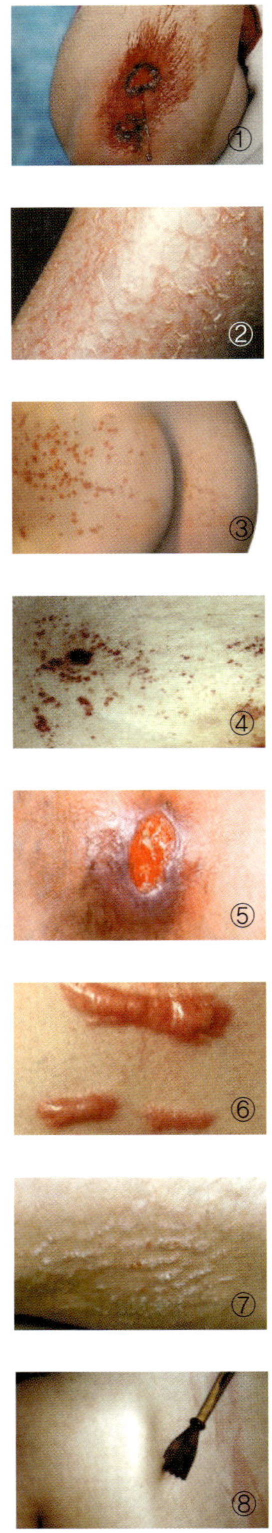

Figure 6-6(c)
Skin diseases

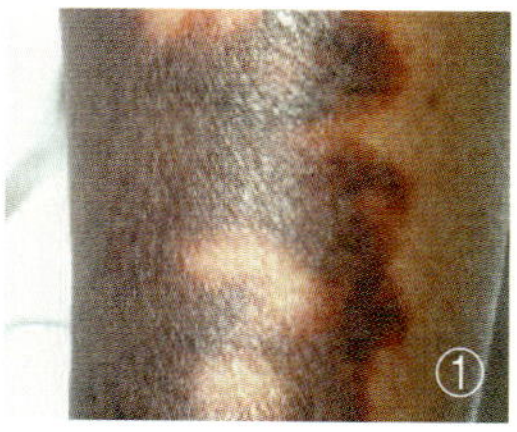

Ecchymosis

Caused by seepage of blood due to damage to vessels in subcutaneous tissue or mucous membrane, ecchymosis appears in round or random macules of blue or purple color. The spots exceed 3 mm in diameter and larger than petechia. (see Figure 6-6(d) ①)

Pruritus

Pruritus is the sensation of desire or urge to scratch or rub. It accompanies various types of dermatitis.

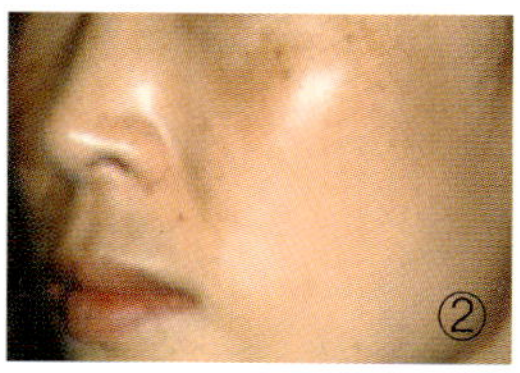

Chloasma

This is a tan or dark skin discoloration on the forehead, cheek or nose that occur more often in women, especially pregnant or taking oral contraceptives. ②

Melanoderma

Darkening of the skin due to excessive production of melanin pigment when there is increase in melanocytes' activity.

Leukoderma

This is a cutaneous condition with localized loss of pigmentation of the skin due to several types of envionmental or pathological factors.

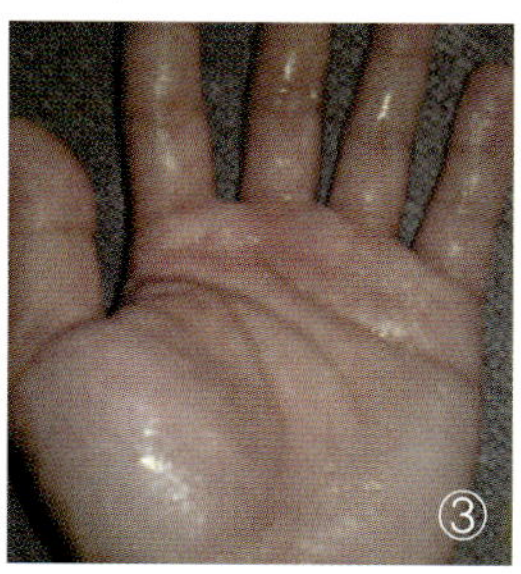

Hyperhidrosis

Hyperhidrosis is the condition characterized by abnormally increased sweating, in excess of that required for regulation of body temperature. Systemic hyperhidrosis may be caused by endocrine disturbance. Local hyperhidrosis may be caused by sympathetic nerve disorder. ③

Anhidrosis

This is a condition of decreased or inhibited sweating.

Bromhidrosis

This is an abnormal condition of apocrine sweat glands that emit displeasing odor. The odor is generated by bacteria that decompose substances contained in the sweat.

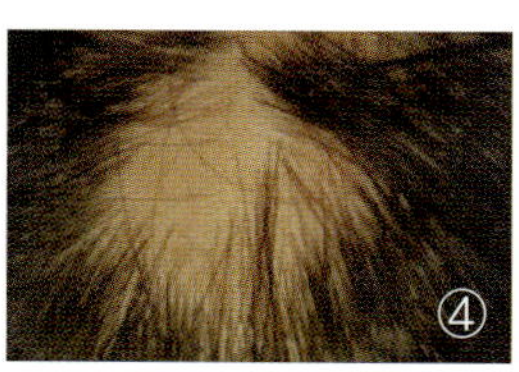

Figure 6-6(d)
Skin diseases

Alopecia

Alopecia is a condition of general or local hair loss due to normal aging, endocrine disturbance, side effects of medication, anticancer drugs or skin diseases. ④

Rosacea

In patients with rosacea, the nose, forehead and cheek turn red due to hyperemia of superficial capillaries. (see Figure 6-6(e) ①)

Frostbite

Frostbite is the medical condition in which localized damage is caused to skin and other tissues due to freezing, where the affected portion may die and ulcerate. ②

Burn

This is skin damage due to heat, electricity, chemicals, radiation, gas, etc. The degree of burn is determined by the condition, exposure of the tissue to the source, and the nature and cause of the damage. ③

- First-degree burn : The affected area has flares and swelling but no blisters.
- Second-degree burn : The depth of burn involves upper portion of dermis, and the affected area may have blisters as well as flares and swelling, causing severe pain.
- Third-degree burn : The damage extends deep into the dermis.
- Fourth-degree burn : The depth of burn extends down to the muscle.

Acne

Acne occurs through complex activities of hormone and bacteria in the sebaceous glands. It is most common on the face, upper part of the back and the chest where sebaceous glands are densely populated. Open and closed comedos, papules, pustules and nodules are characteristic of acne. In severe cases cystic acne affects deeper skin tissues by forming inflammatory tunnels and pyogenic cysts. ④

Comedo

A comedo is the blockage of the opening of the hair follicle, usually meaning acne. There are open and closed types of comedones. In an open type comedo it is open to air that oxidize the sebum that turns black. In a closed type, the sebum is closed by skin and kept light in color. ⑤

Eczema

Eczema is a chronic cutaneous inflammation of unknown cause. It usually starts with flares, red macules, blisters, swelling or oozing accompanied by

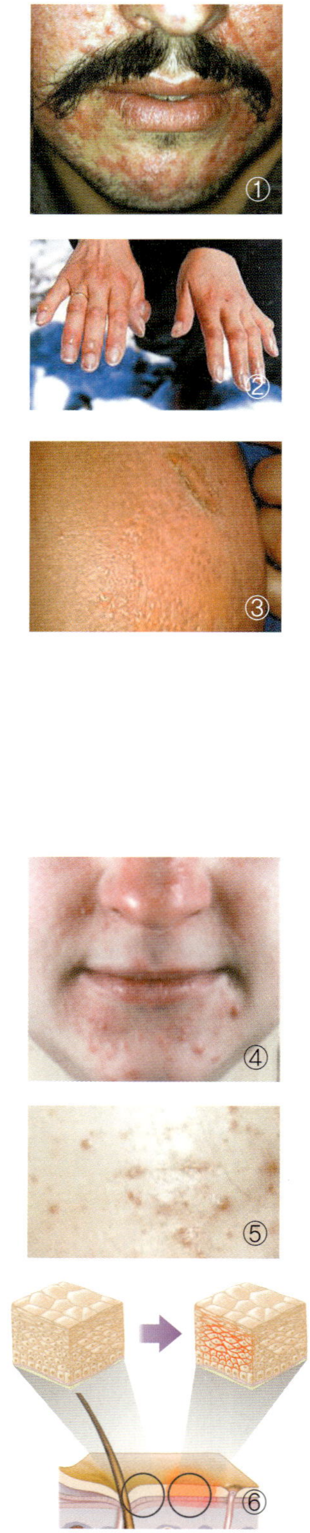

Figure 6-6(e)
Skin diseases

itching sensation. In chronic stage, crust, hypertrophy and lichenification can occur. Sudden temperature changes, humidity, mental stress, fabric detergents and fragrances can aggravate the condition. ⑥

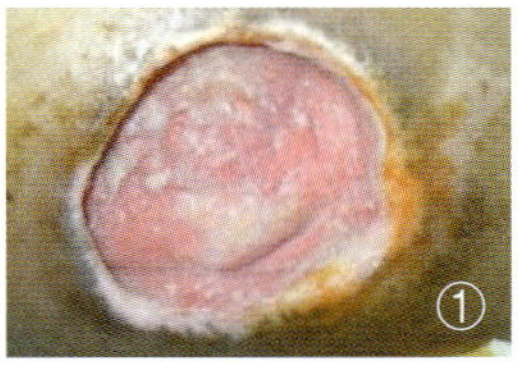

Decubitus, Bedsore

When a patient lies in bed for a long time motionless, blood circulation in the skin compressed under the body is inhibited, which can cause necrosis of the cutaneous tissue of the affected area. The affected area tends to be where bones protrude and press the surrounding flesh — knees, heels, sacrum, shoulder blade, etc. (see Figure 6-6(f) ①)

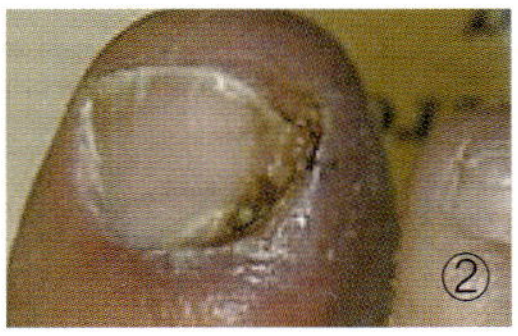

Onychia

Onychia is inflammation of the skin surrounding fingernails and toenails due to infection. Acute and chronic conditions exist. ②

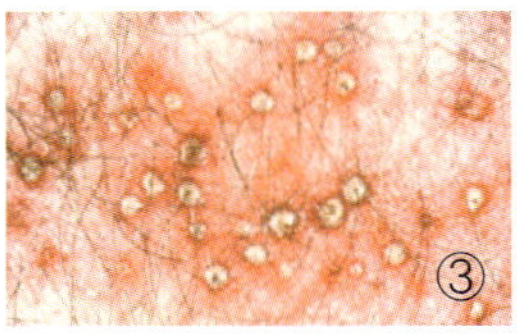

Folliculitis

Pyogenic inflammation due to staphylococcus infection of hair follicles. ③

Dermatitis

Dermatitis is typically eczematous inflammation of the skin with eruptions in multiple cutaneous layers. Its outbreak may occur due to allergens, other diseases or simply by itself. Acute and chronic conditions exist, and proper treatment depends on the cause.

- actinic dermatitis : dermatitis due to photosensitivity
- allergic dermatitis : dermatitis due to allergic reaction
- atopic dermatitis : dermatitis due to unknown cause, similar to eczema
- contact dermatitis : dermatitis due to contact with allergens

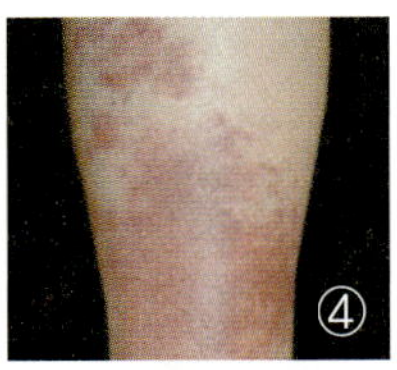

Erysipelas

Contagious disease transmitted through contact, affecting cutaneous and subcutaneous tissues due to streptococcus infection. The affected area flares and swells. ④

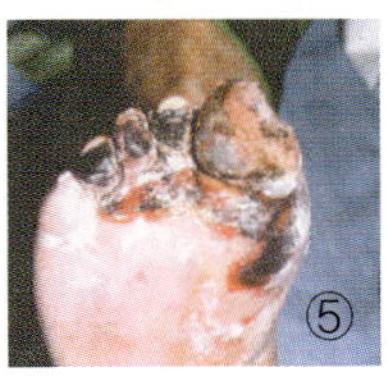

Figure 6-6(f)
Skin diseases

Gangrene

Gangrene is a condition with necrosis of a considerable mass of body tissue due to lack of blood supply or bacterial infection. ⑤

Albinism

Due to congenital lack of skin pigmentation, the patient's hair, skin or pupils appear white or colorless. The condition may affect the whole body as well as locally.

Impetigo

Impetigo is a highly contagious bacterial skin infection. It is primarily caused by *Staphylococcus aureus* or group A *Streptococcus* infection. It is most common among pre-school children, however, adults with itch sensation that accompany skin disease such as eczematous condition are also susceptible.

Pemphigus

Pemphigus is a rare group of blistering autoimmune diseases that affect the skin and mucous membranes. In pemphigus, autoantibodies form against desmosomes which are the glue that attaches adjacent epidermal cells. (see Figure 6-6(g) ①)

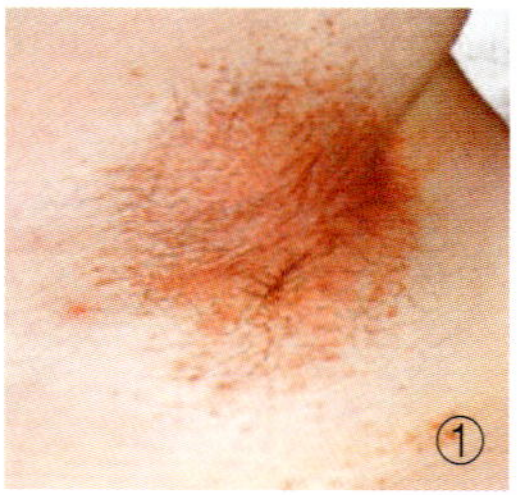

Herpes simplex

This is infection by herpes simplex virus, mostly through direct contact. It has affinity to skin and nerves and causes blisters on the skin or mucous membrane and accompanying pain. Genital herpes is contracted through sexual contact or during childbirth at birth canal. ②

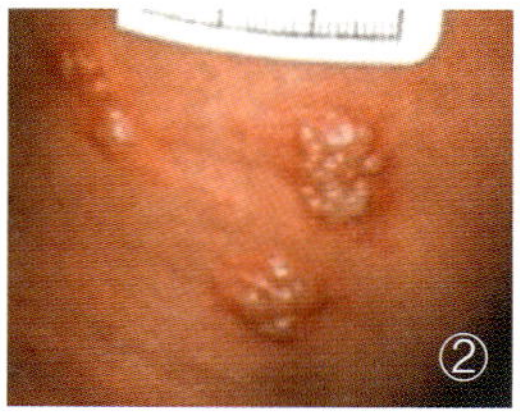

Herpes zoster

This is an acute viral disease caused by revitalized varicella zoster virus usually dormant in adults. In the vicinity of the viral inflammation of the cranial or spinal nerves, a cluster of small blisters form in the affected area accompanied by severe pain. ③

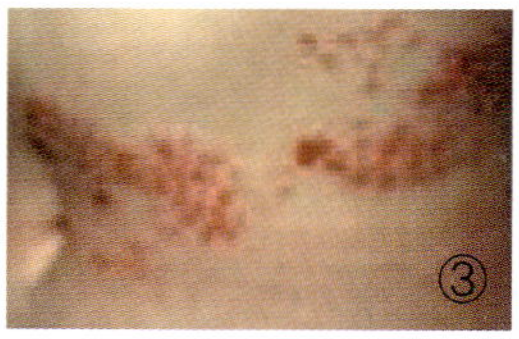

Memory key

- Herpes simplex is a highly contagious viral infection, and herpes zoster exhibit a cluster of blisters accompanied by severe pain.

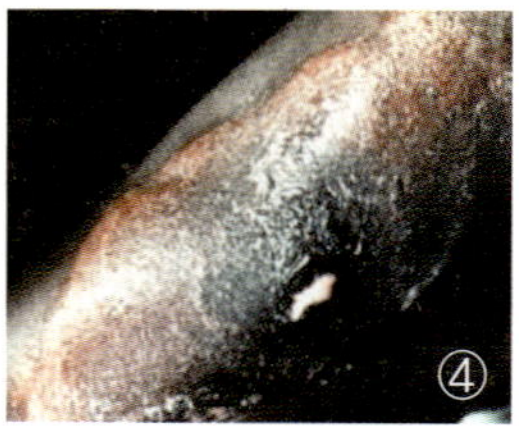

Figure 6-6(g)
Skin diseases

Leprosy

Leprosy is a chronic, intractable, infectious disease caused by *Mycobacterium leprae*. Symptoms include irregular macules and patches on the skin, loss of ability to feel pain and touch, loss of eyebrows, deformation of hands, feet and face, poor eyesight. The acidophilic bacillus attacks the skin and peripheral nerves, and can be contracted through direct contact with body fluid or blood. ④

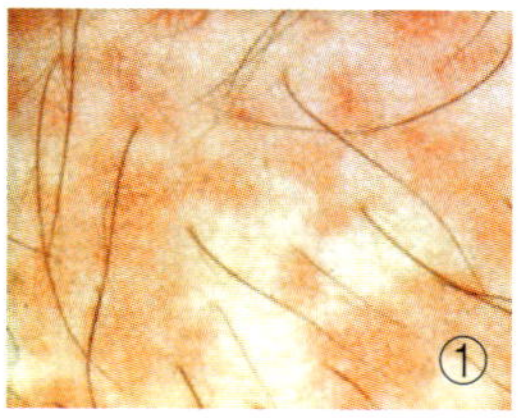

Macule

Macule is a flat, discolored lesion of size under 1 cm in diameter in blue, black and red colors. The skin color changes to brown, dark brown, etc. due to increase of pigmentation and concentration of cells carrying pigments in blood. (see Figure 6-6(h) ①)

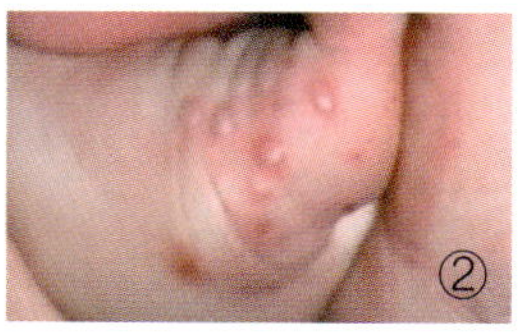

Bleb

A raised feature on the skin containing water, of size under 1 cm. It is caused by burn, allergy, dermatitis, etc. Those over 1 cm in size are called blisters. ②

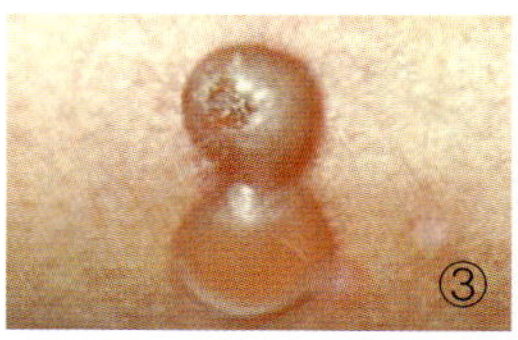

Bulla

A large blister of size over 1 cm containing clear fluid. It is usually in the shallow epidermis having thin walls and easily bursts under light force. It occurs due to delayed postburn, herpes virus infection, etc. ③

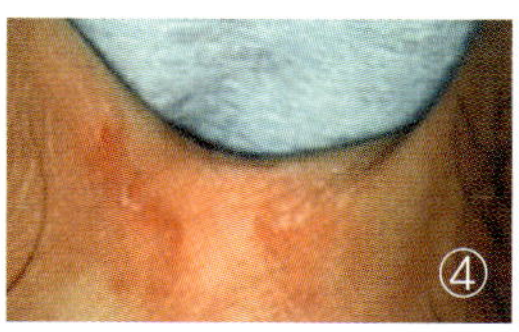

Scabies

Scabies mite as a parasite in the skin spreads the infectious disease. In scabies, the lesions that are running sores start in soft skin tissues at fingers, toes, armpits and spread all over the body, causing severe itching sensation. This condition is concentrated in people living in a group or in unsanitary living conditions. ④

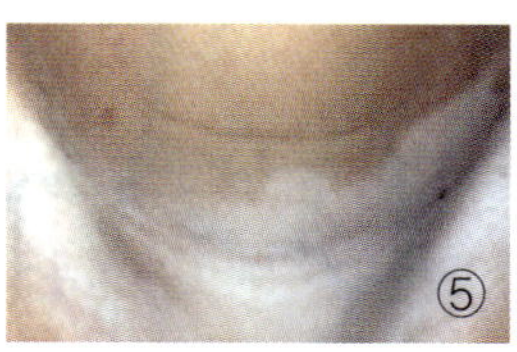

Vitiligo

In this condition, macules or patches of various sizes without melanin pigmentation on the skin appear white. ⑤

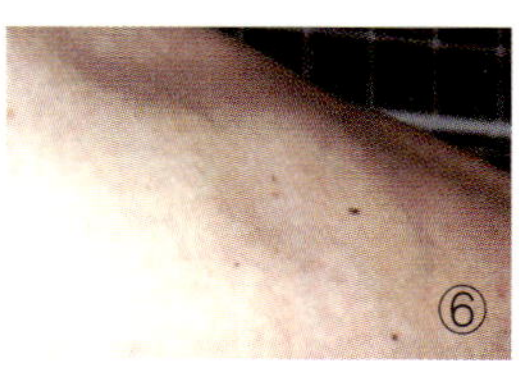

Figure 6-6(h)
Skin diseases

Systemic lupus erythematosus

This is a systemic autoimmune disease occurring more commonly in women. As a chronic inflammatory disorder it attacks skin, joints, kidney and other organs. ⑥

Lentigo

Geneally occurring in middle-aged or older people exposed to sunlight, a lentigo is a dark brown macule.

Nevus

As a congenital condition of pigmented skin spots, nevus is a colored spot classified as a benign skin tumor. Some of the variant type of cells that appear similar to the nevus cells can turn into malignant melanoma. (see Figure 6-6(i) ①)

Wart

Wart is a condition of small external skin growth caused by an infection at the most superficial layer of the skin by human papilloma virus. It is transmissible through direct contact or indirectly by touching the floor or table previously contaminated by other people, which most frequently occurs in children. ②

Kaposi's sarcoma

More frequently occurring in men than women, Kaposi's sarcoma is a malignant tumor in primitive blood vessel tissues with multiple lesions. Clinically, it is characterized by red or purple macules or nodules. It occurs more in men over 60 and AIDS patients. ③

Melanoma

Melanoma is a tumor caused by melanocytes that produce skin pigments which turned malignant. The rate of occurrence is highly related to exposure to sunlight and the depletion of ozone layer that absorb ultraviolet rays. ④

Papilloma

Papilloma refers to a benign epithelial tumor on mucosal surface growing outward in nipple-like fronds. ⑤

Adenoma

Adenoma is a benign tumor from epithelial tissue cells with glandular origin or of glandular shape or characteristics. ⑥

Squamous cell carcinoma

This is a malignant tumor of squamous epithelial cells. It is a skin cancer of non-melanoma type, and the physiological state such as the size, depth, and anatomical location of the lesion is more complex than basal cell carcoinoma. ⑦

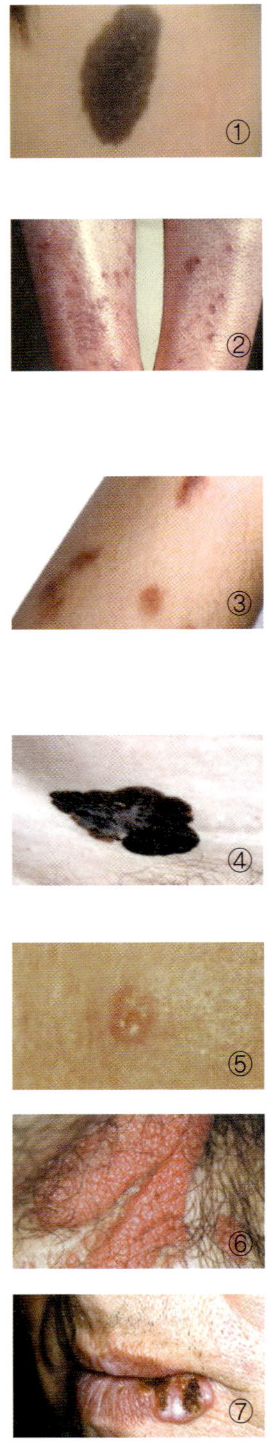

Figure 6-6(i)
Skin diseases

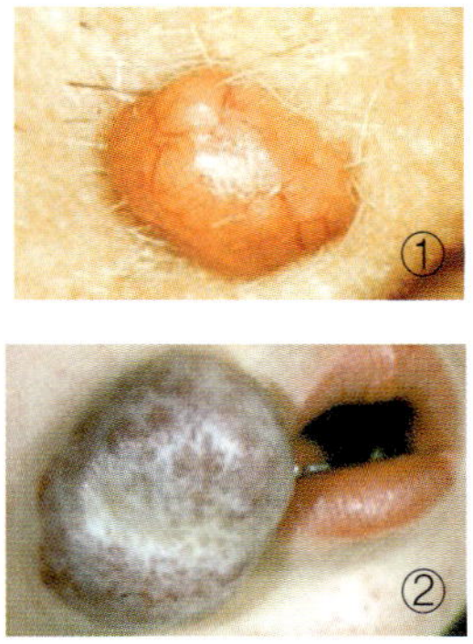

Figure 6-6(j)
Skin diseases

Basal cell carcinoma

Basal cell carcinoma is a malignant tumor originated from epidermis and the non-keratinized cells in its basal part. It has been found that long exposure to ultraviolet rays is the major factor in basal cell carcinoma cases. (see Figure 6-6(j) ①)

Hemangioma

This is a benign tumor consisting of new growth of blood vessels, and classified as a pigmented macule. ②

Terms for Surgery and Treatment

Cauterization

Cauterization is destroying of some tissue by burning it with heat energy with devices like electrocautery. This is useful in stopping hemorrhage, excising an internal organ prone to hemorrhage or endoscopic polyp excision, etc. Sometimes, laser is used in cauterizing operations.

Cryosurgery

Cryosurgery is a treatment technique of freezing cells to destroy them. When the cells are suddenly frozen, proteins and enzymes in the vicinity are also destroyed while moisture is frozen.

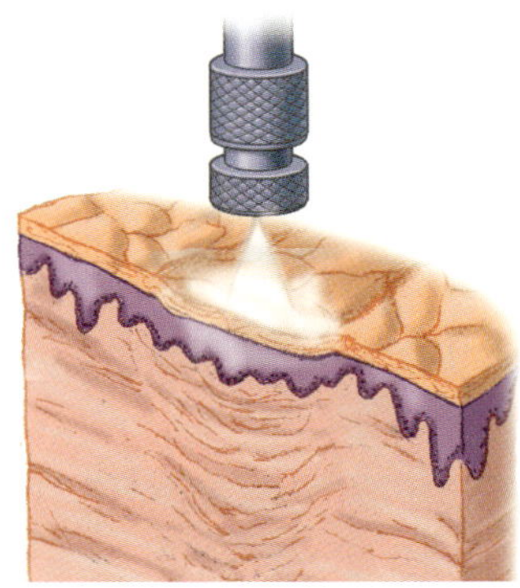

Figure 6-7 Cryosurgery

Lumpectomy

Lumpectomy is surgical excision of tumor with minimal removal of surrounding tissues.

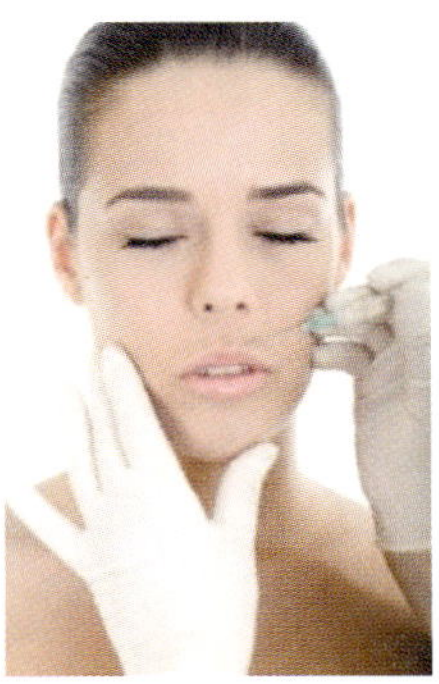

Figure 6-8
Skin treatment

Xenograft

When the patient's own tissue supply is limited, a foreign tissue may be temporarily transplanted.

Debridement

Debridement is a method of medically removing dead tissue or extraneous matter. The extraneous matter or necrotic tissue in the wound or affected lesion is removed and the area is connected to the healthy tissues in the vicinity. It is mainly used in open surgery for bone fractures.

Dermatoplasty

Dermatoplasty is a surgery to improve the skin visually and functionally on spots, hemangioma, scars (from injury, burn and surgery, etc.) and loss of skin due to previous surgery for injury, etc.

Dermabrasion

A cosmetic medical procedure using chemical or laser, in which a part of epidermis is removed. This stimulates generation of new epidermis and collagen fibers in dermis, and popularly used for treating acne, scars, wrinkles, colored spots and enlarged pores.

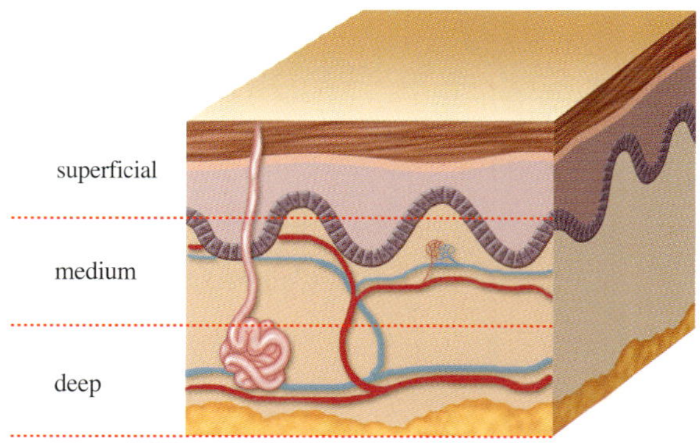

Figure 6-9 Dermabrasion

Electrodesiccation

Using high frequency electric current through needle-like electrodes, a minute skin tissue lesion is precisely heated up and dried.

Skin graft

When the skin or soft tissue is damaged, a skin tissue from other part of the body is grafted onto the damaged area. Depending on thickness of skin layer needed, split-thickness grafting and full-thickness grafting exist.

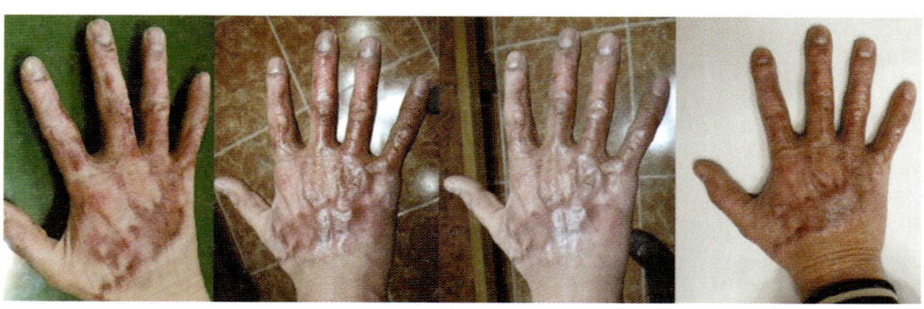

Figure 6-10 Before and after skin grafting

Terms for Test and Intervention

Intradermal test

This test is done by injecting certain amount of antigens in the dermis and evaluating how the skin responds.

Mantoux test

Mantoux test is a screening tool for tuberculosis. As the intradermal tuberculin response test devised by Mantoux, existence of tuberculosis is determined by the size of the skin lesion after intradermal injection of PPD (purified protein derivative).

Patch test

A method used to determine whether a specific substance causes allergic inflammation of the patient's skin. This is a method used to find the substance that causes skin allergy such as contact dermatitis through cutaneous responses.

Scratch test

As a method to diagnose allergic conditions, a dermic scratch is performed, a certain amount of allergen is dropped in the exposed area or injected, to see how it responds to reagin (sensitized skin antibody).

Skin test

This is the most basic skin test looking for the allergen that causes the cutaneous condition. This is a widely used method for its high sensitivity, convenience and fast test result.

Sweat test

A test to evaluate sodium and chlorides secreted from sweat glands, used for diagnosis of cystic fibrosis.

Skin biopsy

This method is to insert a hollow needle in an organ and collect a sample tissue for histopathological testing, without externally making an incision in the skin.

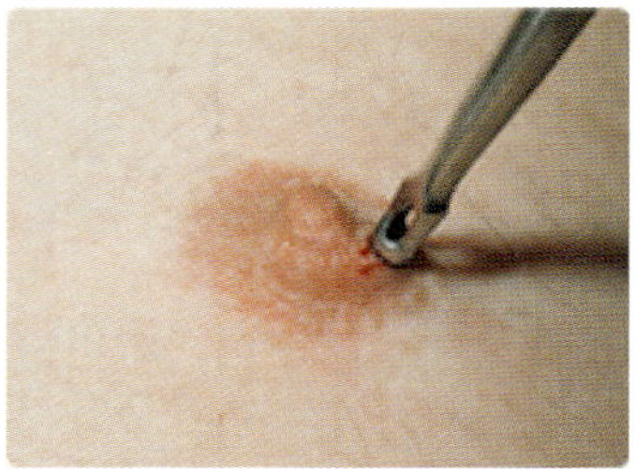

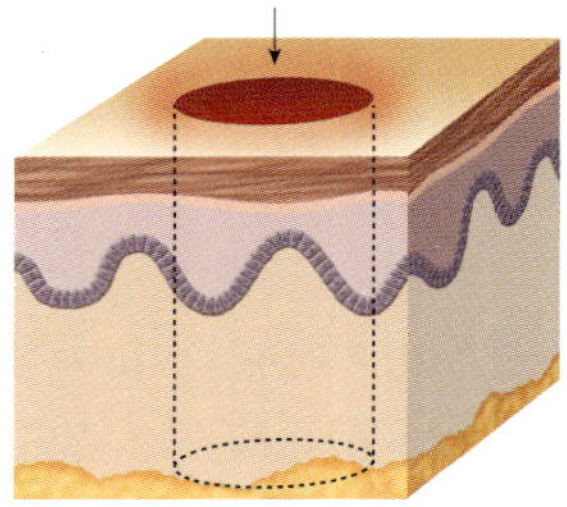

Figure 6-11 Skin biopsy

Analysis and Meaning of Key Terms

Term	Term analysis	Meaning
	albin/o	white
albinism [ǽlbənizəm]	-ism = condition	whiteness due to lack of skin pigmentation
	bi/o	life
biopsy [baiάpsi]	-opsy = vision	taking a sample tissue from living body for visual examination
	cutane/o	skin
subcutaneous [sʌ́bkjutéinjəs]	sub = under; -ous = pertaining to	under the skin
	cyan/o	blue
cyanosis [sάiənóusis]	-sis = pathological state	blue discoloration of skin due to lack of oxygen in blood
	cry/o	cold
cryosurgery [krὰiousə̀:dʒəri]	surgery = operation	surgery to destroy a bad tissue using very low temperature
	dermat/o	skin
dermatoplasty [də̀:rmətəplǽsti]	-plasty = surgical repair	plastic surgery of the skin, especially skin grafting
dermatitis [də:rmətάitis]	-itis = inflammation	inflammation of the skin

Term	Term analysis	Meaning
	-dermis	skin
epidermis [épidə:mis]	epi- = above, over	layer above the dermis
	-derma	skin
erythroderma [iríθroudə̀:rmə]	erythr/o = red	redness of the skin
xeroderma [zìroudə́rma]	xer/o = dryness	dryness of the skin
	diaphor/e	sweating
diaphoresis [dàiəfərí:sis]	-sis = condition, state	state of profuse sweating
	epitheli/o	covering
epithelium [èpiθí:ljəm]	-um = tissue, structurae	top layer(s) of the skin
	erythemat/o	redness
erythematous [eriθí:mətəs]	-ous = pertaining to	pertaining to redness of the skin
	hidr/o	sweat
hyperhidrosis [hàipərhaidróusis]	hyper-/excessive	excessive secretion of sweat
	keratin/o	hornlike
keratinocyte [kərǽtənəsait]	-cyte = cell	a cell that produces keratin
	mamm/o	breast
mammography [mæmɑ́grəfi]	-graphy = record	x-ray examination of the breasts
	melan/o	black
melanoderma [mèlənoudə̀:rmə]	-derma = skin condition	excessive amount of melanin in the skin
	myc/o	fungus
dermatomycosis [də̀rmætoumai-kóusis]	-osis = condition; dermat/o = skin	fungal infection of the skin

Term	Term analysis	Meaning
	necr/o	death
necrotic tissue [nəkrátik tíʃu]	-tic = pertaining to	tissue with dead cells
	onych/o	nail
onychia [aníkiə]	-ia = condition	inflammation or ulceration around the nail
	pil/o	hair
pilosebaceous [pàiləsibéiʃiəs]	-ous = of, seb/o = sebum	pertaining to hair and sebaceous gland
	ras/o	scrape
dermabrasion [də́:məbréiʒən]	derm/o = skin; ab- = away from	removing of top layers of the skin by abrasion
	rhytid/o	wrinkle
rhytidoplasty [rítidəplæsti]	-plasty = surgical reconstruction	surgery to reduce skin wrinkles
	seb/o, sebace/o	sebum, fat
sebaceous [sibéiʃəs]	-ous = pertaining to	relating to sebum from skin glands
	steat/o	fat
steatoma [stì:ətəmə]	-oma = mass, tumor	a cyst of mass containing fatty tissue
	ungu/o	nail
ungual [ʌ́ŋgwəl]	-al = pertaining to	relating to nail
	strat/o	layer
stratification [strætəfikéiʃən]	-tion = process of doing	process of layering (of skin tissues)
	-oma	tumor
adenoma [æ̀dinóumə]	aden/o = gland	tumor of the epithelium arising from a gland
carcinoma [kɑ̀əˑsinóumə]	carcin/o = cancer	malignant tumor of the epithelial tissue cells
hemangiofibroma [hi:mæ̀ndʒióufai-bróumə]	hem/o = blood angi/o = vessel fibr/o = fiber	benign tumor consisting of new growth of blood vessels

Term	Term analysis	Meaning
	-oma	tumor
melanoma [méləmoumə]	melan/o = black	tumor of the melanocytes turning malignant
papilloma [pæ̀pəlóumə]	paill/o = nipple-like	epithelial tumor that look like a nipple

Abbreviations

Abbreviation	Full Term	Meaning
Bx	biopsy	removing and examining living tissue for diagnostic purposes
SC	subcutaneous	below the skin
Uv	ultraviolet	ultraviolet radiation
derm	dermatology	study of the skin and its diseases
I&D	incision and drainage	surgical cutting and draining of pus
DLE	discoid lupus erythematosus	eruption of red lesions that occur locally
SLE	systemic lupus erythematosus	eruption of red lesions that affect the whole body
ung	unguent	ointment

Exercises

1. Analyze and write the meaning of the following terms :

① subcutaneous — sub- (below) + cutane/o (skin) + -ous (pertaining to)
below the skin

② hypodermic — hypo- (under) + derm/o (skin) + -ic (pertaining to)
under the skin

③ albinism — albin/o (whiteness) + -ism (condition)
lack of melanin pigmentation

④ leukodermia — leuk/o (whiteness) + derm/o (skin) + -ia (condition)
loss of skin pigmentation

⑤ hyperhidrosis — hyper- (excessive) + hidr/o (sweat) + -sis (condition)
excessive sweating

2. Write the meaning of the following suffixes :

① -oma — tumor

② -derma — skin

③ -cyte — cell

3. Write the full term of the following abbreviations :

① Bx — biopsy

② Sc — subcutaneous

③ Uv — ultraviolet

4. Connect each term in column A to corresponding onein B :

A	B
① albin/o (d)	a. sweat
② cry/o (g)	b. dry
③ hidr/o (a)	c. fungus
④ melan/o (e)	d. white
⑤ myc/o (c)	e. black
⑥ onych/o (f)	f. nail
⑦ xer/o (b)	g. cold

5. Write medical terms that mean the following :

① lack of sweat anhidrosis

② fungal infection of the nail onychomycosis

③ cell that produces melanin melanocyte

④ dry skin of a chronic nature xeroderma

6. Write terms for items in the following figure.

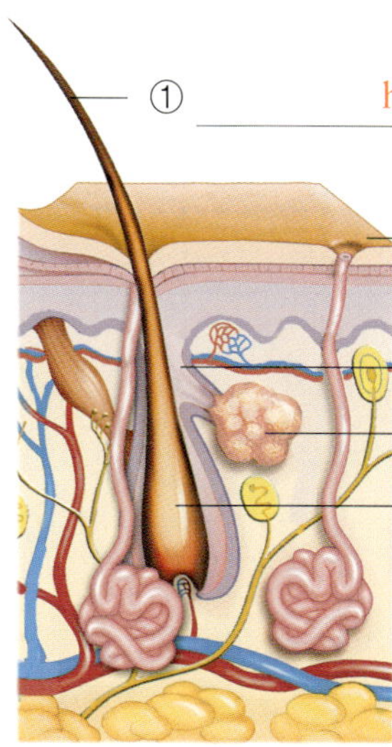

① hair

② epidermis

③ sebum

④ sebaceous gland

⑤ hair follicle

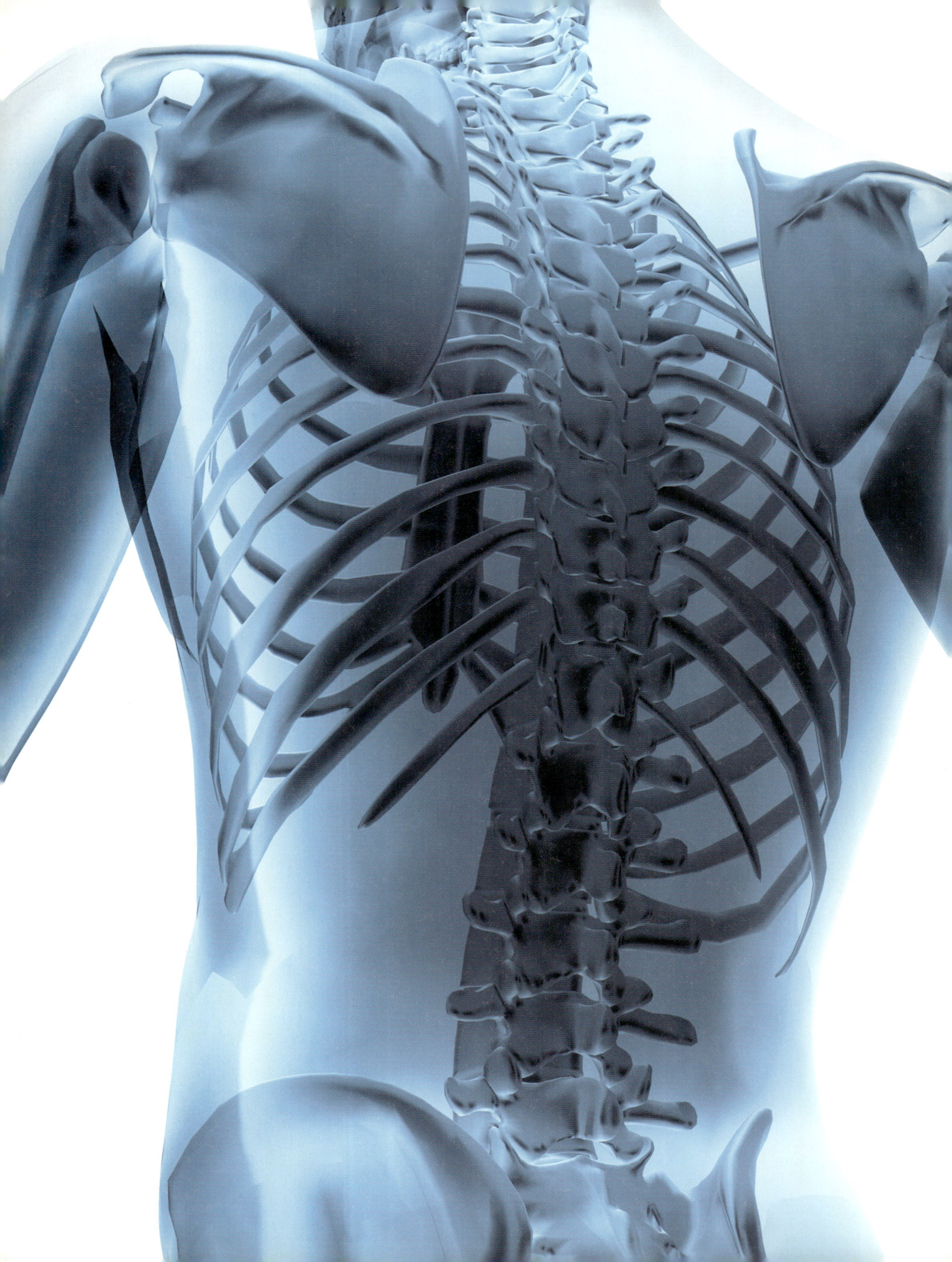

Chapter 7

Skeletal System

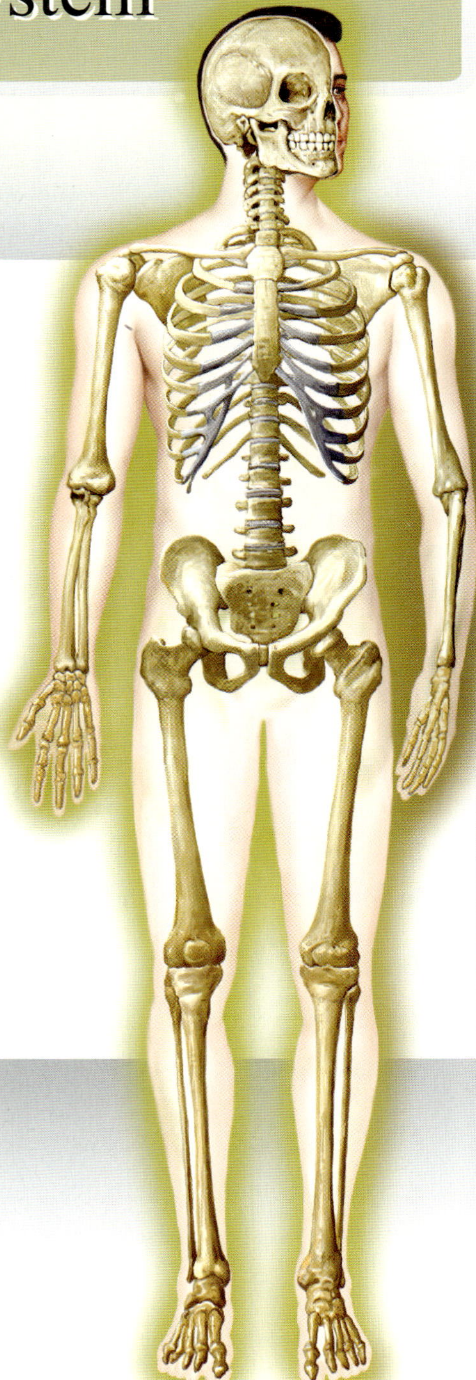

Chapter Contents

- Prolog
- Anatomical Terms
- Terms for Symptoms and Diseases
- Terms for Test and Surgery
- Analysis and Meaning of Key Terms
- Abbreviations
- Exercises

Learning Objectives

- Be familiar with names of bones and related terms.
- Name and locate bones of the body.
- Analyze and understand terms related to the skeletal system.
- Be familiar with diseases related to the skeletal system.
- Define abbreviations for the skeletal system.

Prolog

The skeletal system that integrates the human body provides five functions, i.e., support, protection, muscle attachment, blood formation and mineral storage.

The skeleton keeps the whole body in shape. It protects the internal organs that are vital to the body functions. The bones serve as attachment points for skeletal muscles, so that contractions and relaxations of the muscles can create movement of the body structure through leverage. The bone marrow, the tissue in the interior of bones, produces blood cells. The bones themselves serve as reserves for minerals such as calcium, phosphorus, sodium and magnesium.

Anatomical Terms

Bone Types

Long bone

Femur (thigh bone), tibia and fibula (lower leg bones), humerus (upper arm bone), ulna and radius (lower arm bones) are long bones that are thick, long and in hollow cylindrical shape, and contain bone marrow.

Short bone

Carpals (wrist bones) and tarsals (ankle bones) are typical bones of small and irregular shape. These bones do not have internal space for marrow.

Flat bone

Scapula (shoulder bone), ribs, ilium (pelvic bone) are typical bones of thin, flat and curved shape. These cover soft internal organs.

Irregular bone

Vertebrae, hip bones, facial bones and skull floor are typical bones of irregular shape.

Pneumatic bone

Frontal bone, maxillary bone, temporal bone, sphenoid bone and ethmoid bone belong in pneumatic bones which are mostly from bones of the skull.

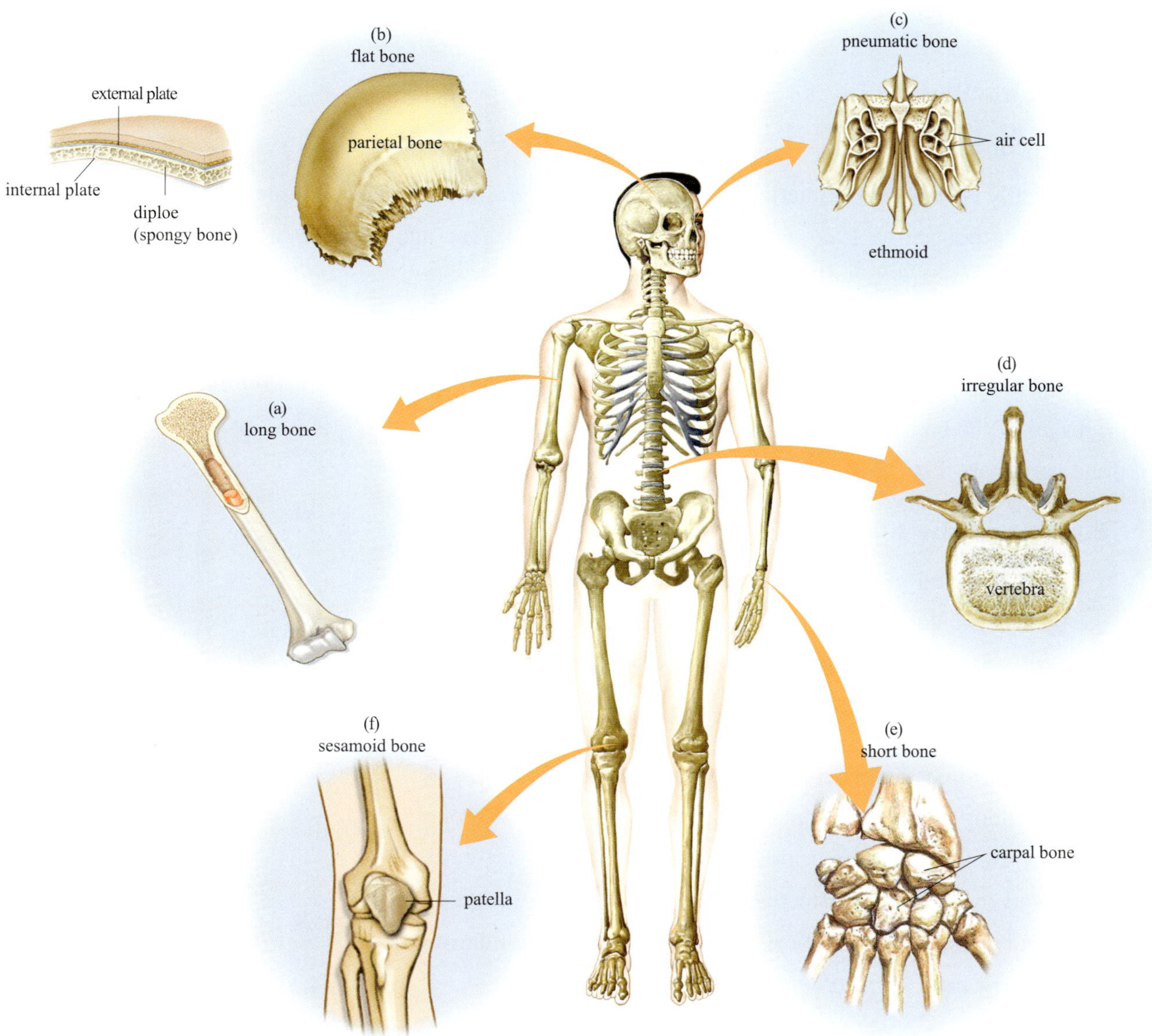

Figure 7-1 Bone shapes

Osteocytes

Osteoblast

Found when the superficial part of the bones is developing, osteoblasts are the cells that produce the bone-forming materials such as bone matrix and osteoid.

Osteoclast

As a macrophage created through fusion of a monocyte from bone marrow, an osteoclast disassembles and reabsorbs bone materials and release minerals such as magnesium and phosphorus into the blood stream.

Bone Structure

Spongy bone

Typically occupying the interior of long bones' ends, this is formed of multiple lamellae of trabeculae. It doesn't have vessels because oxygen and nutrients are supplied by capillary vessels in the bone marrow.

Compact bone

This is the hardened superficial part of a long bone which consists of the bone unit called harversian system. Blood vessels and nerves are distributed in it.

Bone membrane

Endosteum and periosteum are the two membranes that line the bones. The connective tissue layers line the inner and outer surfaces of the bone.

Bone marrow

Bone marrow is comprised of a unique type of tissue found in the medullary cavities, the interior cavities of the bones. Bone marrow consists of hematopoietic tissue cells and fat cells supported by reticular connective fibers. Red marrow produces red blood cells, white blood cells and platelets. Yellow marrow consist of fat cells, formed while at young age.

Epiphysis

Epiphysis means either end of a long bone.

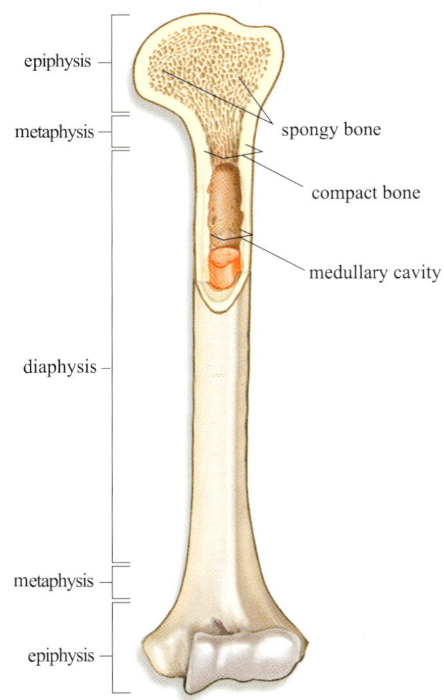

Figure 7-2 Bone structure

Metaphysis

Metaphysis is the end part of a long bone. The inner part is filled with spongy bone, and the outer surface is lined with cortical bone.

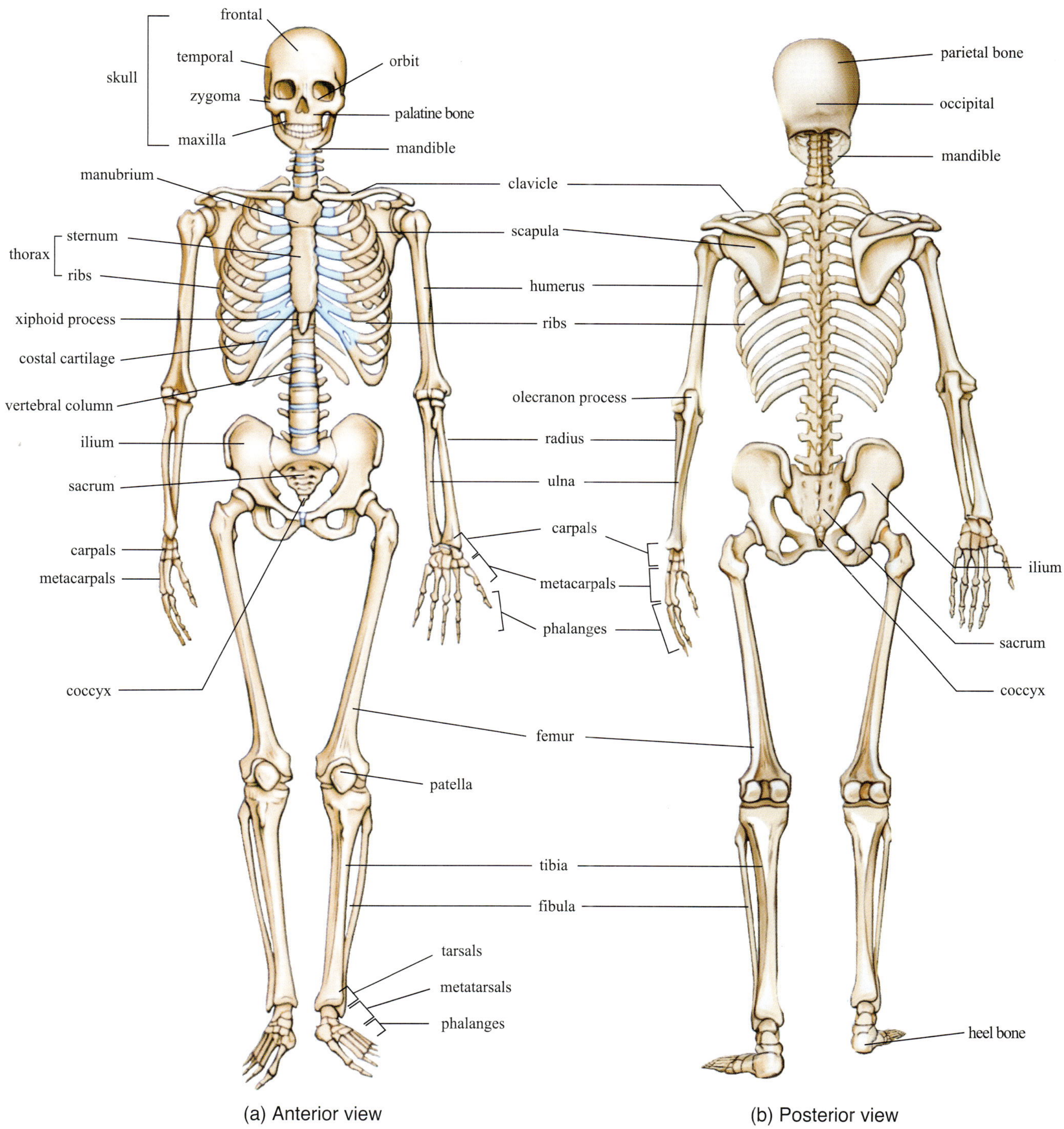

Figure 7-3 Composition of the skeleton

Diaphysis

This is the cylindrical part in the middle of a long bone.

Construction of the Skeleton

An adult human body is built with 206 bones, which are divided into axial skeleton and appendicular skeleton.

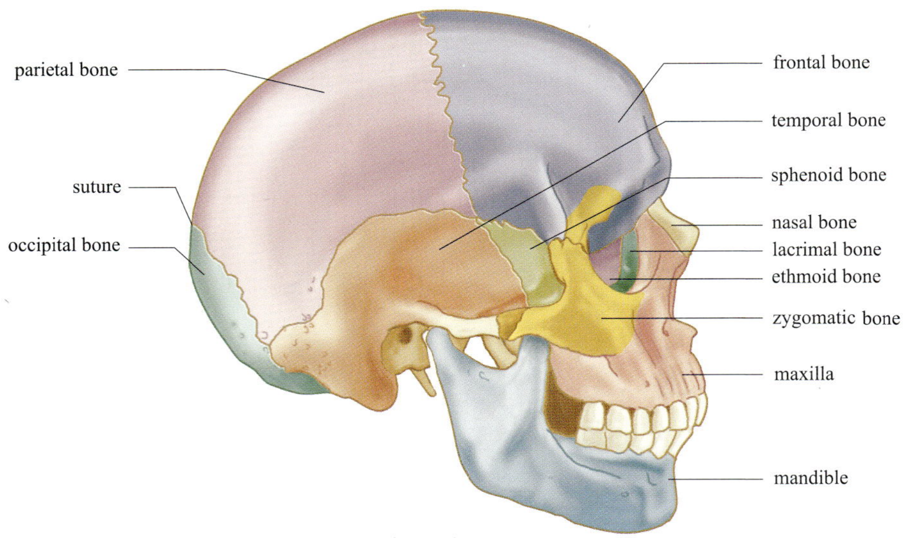

Figure 7-4 Lateral view of the skull and facial bones

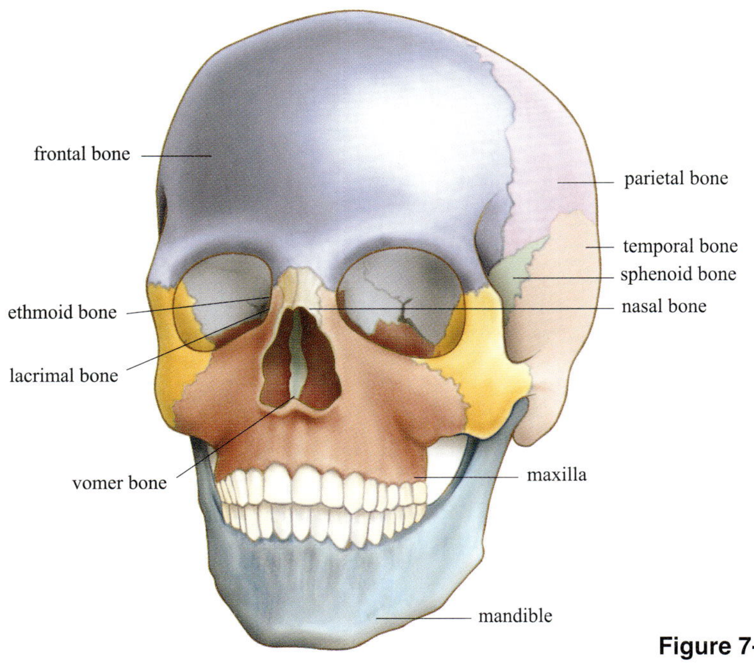

Figure 7-5 Anterior view of the skull and facial bones

Axial Skeleton

The axial skeleton comprises the skull, vertebral column, ribs and sternum.

- **Skull** (Cranial Bones)

The skull is built with the frontal bone that forms the forehead, two parietal bones that crown the head, two temporal bones that cover the sides, the occipital bone on the back, two sphenoid bones, and the ethmoid bone.

- **Facial Bones**

Nasal bone, zygomatic bone, vomer, maxilla, mandible, nasal concha and lacrimal bone make up facial bones.

- **Vertebral Column**

Thirty-three (33) bones of vertebrae make up the namesake vertebral column. Vertebrae are named by location. At the upper end, 7 cervical vertebrae support the skull. Just below in the chest area are 12 thoracic (or dorsal) vertebrae. Next are 5 lumbar vertebrae in the lower back (waist). Below them is the sacrum, which consists of 5 fused vertebral bones. At the inferior end is the tailbone (coccyx) consisting of 4 fused vertebral bones.

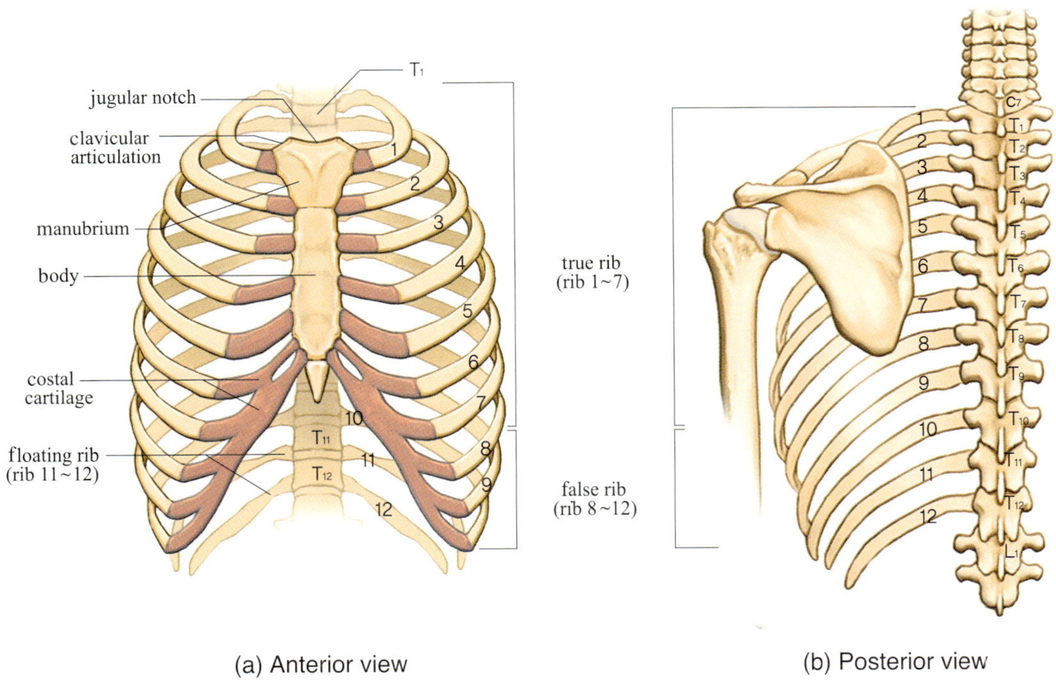

Figure 7-6 Composition of the thoracic cage

Each Vertebral bone is noted by a letter followed by a number, except for those of the coccyx. The cervical vertebrae are C_1~C_7; the thoracic are T_1~T_{12}; the lumbar are L_1~L_5; the sacral are S_1~S_5. Between the vertebrae are little round shock absorbers called intervertebral discs.

- **Thoracic Cage**

Thoracic cage includes sternum (breast bone), 12 pairs of ribs, costal cartilage and thoracic vertebrae.

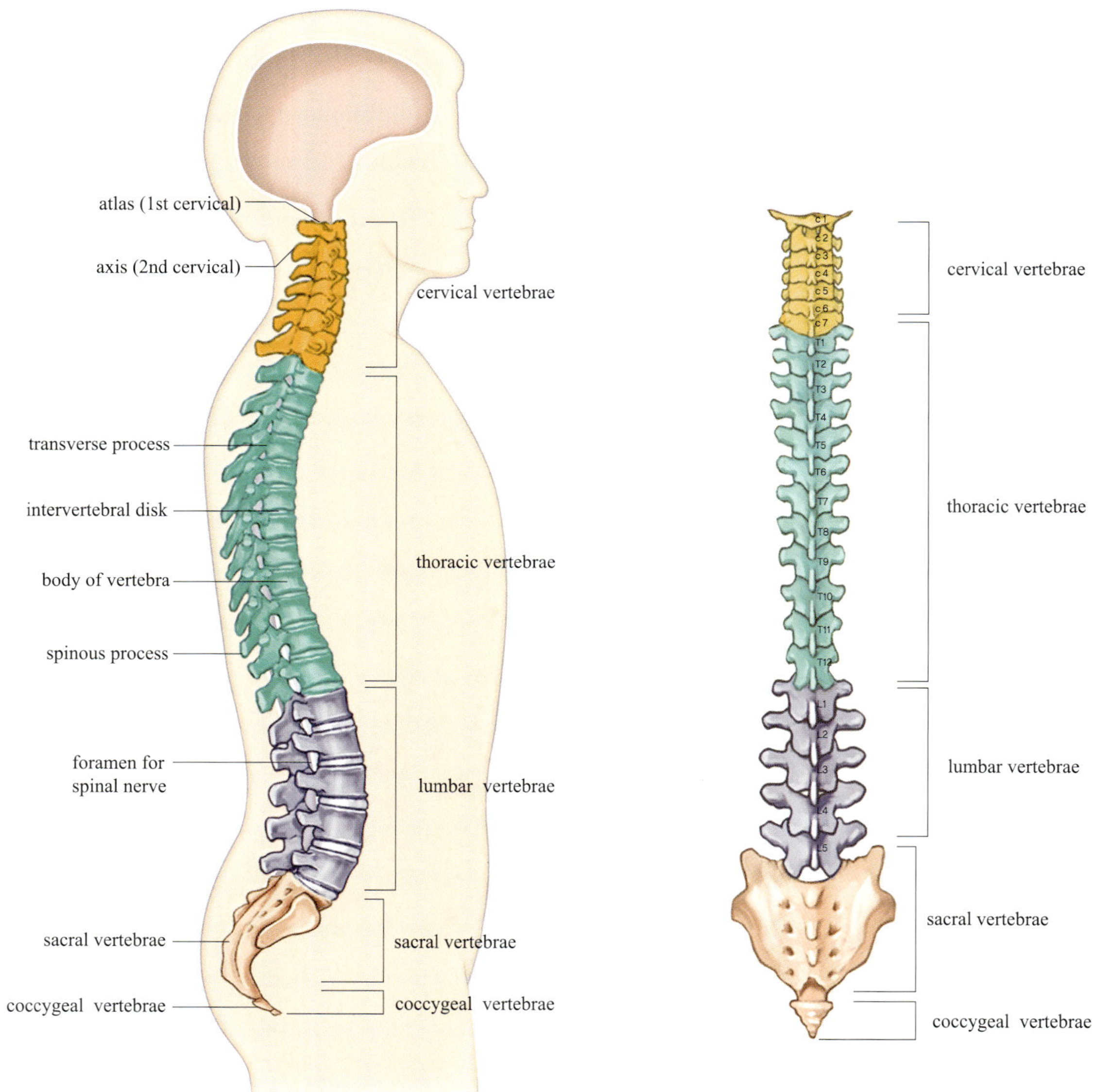

Figure 7-7 Vertebral composition

Viewed from the rear, all pairs of ribs are attached to the corresponding thoracic vertebrae. Viewed from the front, the top 10 pairs of ribs are connected to the sternum by costal cartilage. The bottom 2 pairs of ribs are not attached to the sternum and thus called floating ribs.

Appendicular Skeleton

• **Shoulder** (or Pectoral) **Girdle**

Two scapulae (shoulder blades) in the rear and 2 clavicles (collarbones) in front make up the shoulder girdle. This girdle attach the arm bones to the main body skeleton.

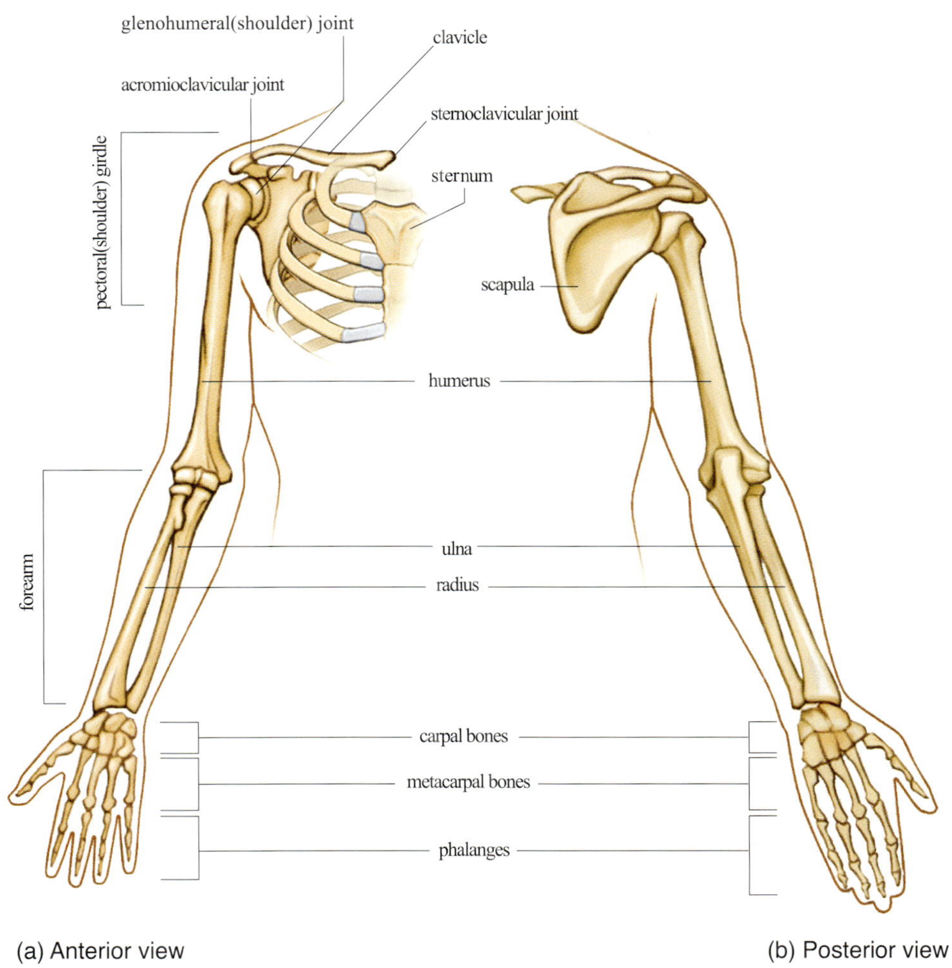

Figure 7-8 Composition of the arm bones

• **Arm Bones** (upper extremity)

The arm comprises upper arm, elbow, forearm, wrist, hand and fingers. From the shoulder girdle down, arm bones comprise humerus, radius, ulna, carpals, metacarpals and phalanges.

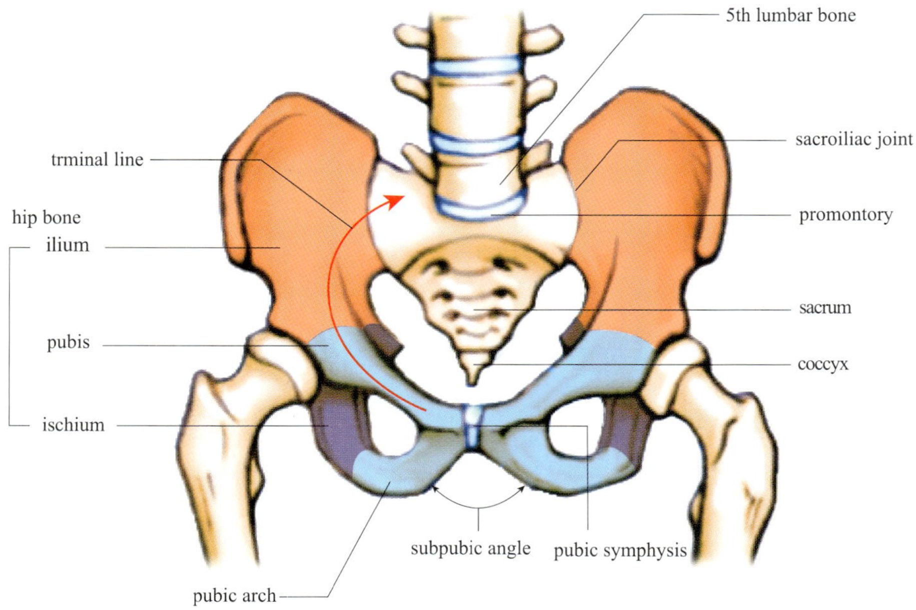

Figure 7-9 Composition of the pelvic girdle

• **Pelvic Girdle**

Pelvic girdle consists of 2 hip bones that protect the pelvic organs. Each hip bone contains 3 bones segments — the ilium, ischium and pubis bones fused together. The two hip bones meet anteriorly with the symphysis pubis and posteriorly with the sacrum to form the sacroiliac joint.

• **Leg Bones** (lower extremity)

The leg comprise thigh, knee, lower leg, ankle, foot and toes. From the pelvic girdle down, leg bones comprise femur (thigh bone), patella (knee bone), tibia (shin), fibula, talus, tarsals, metatarsals and phalanges.

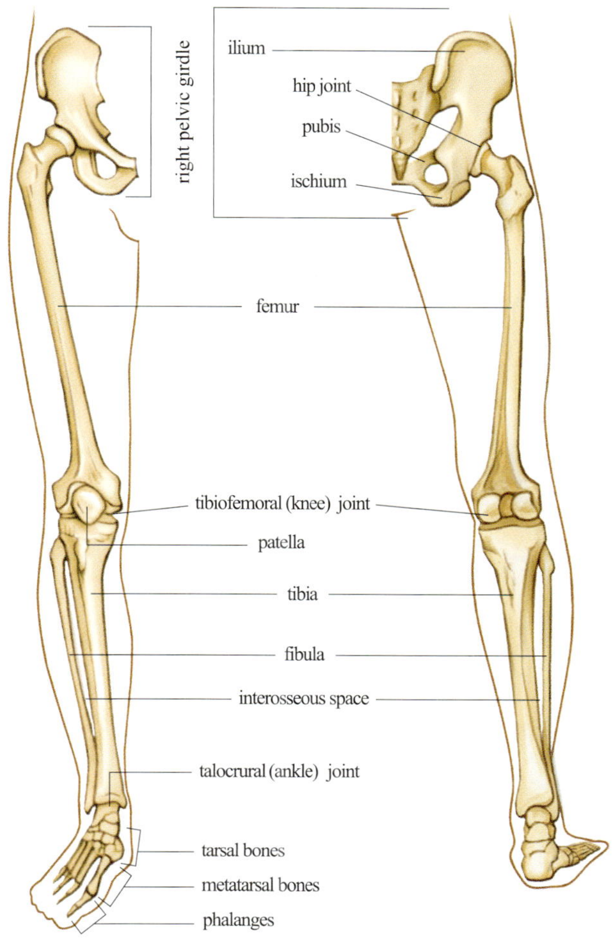

Figure 7-10 Composition of the leg bones

Joint

A joint is a place where bones meet and move relative to each other to a certain degree. Periosteum (bone surface), cartilage, ligament, tendon and muscles work together in making relative movements within a normal range.

- **Fibrous Joint**

Also called fixed or immovable joint. Due to suture, syndesmosis or gomphosis these joints have no joint cavity and there is little or no movement.

• **Synchondrosis**

As a cartilaginous joint, this type of joint is connected by hyaline cartilage. The surface of the joint can't normally move but only slightly under strong force.

• **Synovial joint**

Between the bones is a synovial cavity filled with synovial fluid, synovial membrane, joint capsule and articular cartilage. The end of the bone is covered with articular cartilage that allows various types of movements.

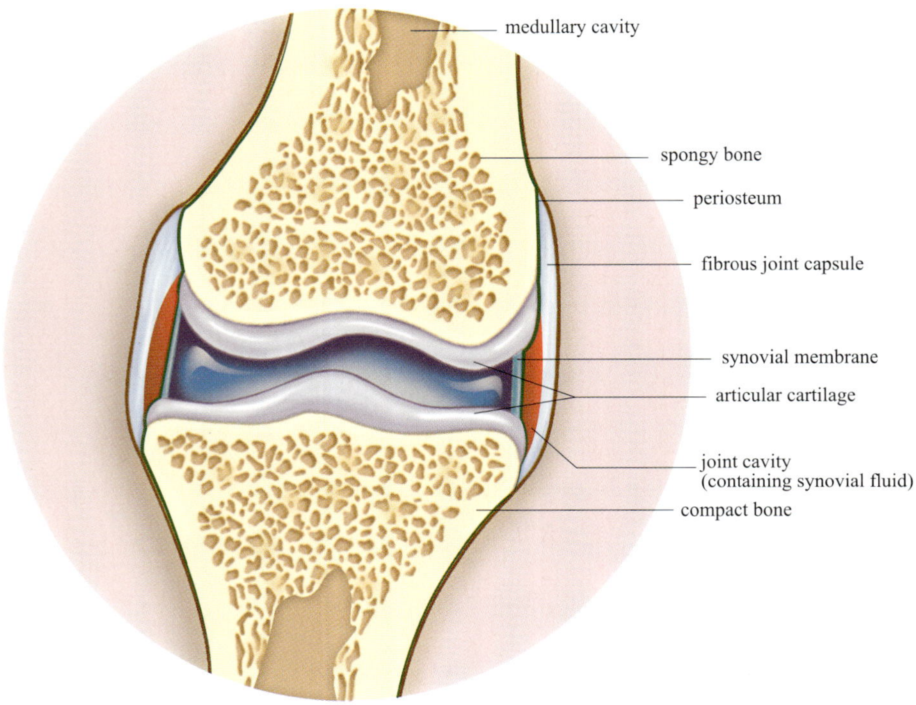

Figure 7-11 Structure of the joint

Terms for Symptoms and Diseases

Fracture

A fracture is a break or crack in a bone. Symptoms of pain, swelling, boil, spotty bleeding, petechia, deformation, related injury, shock may occur.

Congenital hip dislocation

Hip dislocation due to developmental disorder of the hip joint. It is more common in girls than in boys. The condition is accompanied by pain, growth disorder and walking difficulties.

Osteomalacia

Lack of nutrients such as vitamin D and bone minerals including calcium and phosphorus is the cause of osteomalacia. This condition may induce scoliosis, pelvic deformation, crooked legs, etc.

Osteoporosis

Lack of physical exercise, malnutrition, lack of follicular hormone, extended treatment with adrenal cortex hormone, etc. will lead to thinning of compact bones, reduced bone density, loss of spongy bones and enlarged marrow cavities. Patients with this condition are prone to frequent bone fractures.

Osteomyelitis

Osteomyelitis is inflammation of the bone and bone marrow due to pyogenic germ infection, causing necrosis and abscess in the bone.

Arthritis

As inflammation of the joint due to various reasons, arthritis may bring pain, swelling, flare and deformation to the joint.

Dislocation

External forces may sometimes dislodge a bone from the normal location. The lesion will swell and bring fever and pain. In severe cases, it may cause damage to nerves, vessels, internal organs, etc.

Subluxation

Subluxation is partial dislocation, where the joint area is connected but not accurately located. This will limit the joint movement and cause pain and swelling.

Osteosarcoma

In osteosarcoma the bone is produced by malignant tumor cells. The patient experiences pain during exercises, swelling, flares, fracture, etc.

Osteoma

This is benign tumor in the bone tissue.

Polyarthritis

Arthritis affecting multiple joints related to autoimmune disorder, affecting people at any age.

Osteoarthropathy

Pathological condition affecting bones and joints.

Tendinitis

Inflammation of the tendon that often occurs to athletes.

Tenosynovitis

Inflammation of the synovial membrane that wraps the tendon.

Bursitis

Inflammation of the synovial bursa that contains synovial fluid.

Osteochondritis

Inflammation caused by necrotic cartilaginous tissue, occurring in elbow and knee joints.

Spondylitis

Any inflammation of the vertebra (spine), infectious and non-infectious.

Dactylitis

Inflammation of the fingers or toes.

Dactylospasm

Spasm or contraction of the fingers or toes.

Podalgia

Pain in the foot due to gout or rheumatism.

Terms for Test and Surgery

Rheumatoid factor test

Diagnosis of arthritis by testing for the existence of rheumatoid factor.

Reduction

Medical procedure to restore the broken bone to the original alignment.

Internal fixation

After the broken bone is reduced in place, metal plates, rods and screws are used to fix the bone.

Arthroscopy

Using a microscopic endoscope, the internals of the joint is examined and sometimes unnecessary tissue is removed as a treatment.

Antinuclear antibody test

Testing for the existence of autoantibody to diagnose autoimmune diseases such as rheumatoid arthritis.

Arthroplasty

Arthroplasty often involves cutting off the damaged part of the joint and replacing the severed part with a prosthetic (artificial) joint. A membrane is inserted to wrap the mating part of the joint to prevent re-adhesion. This will allow renewed articulation of the joint.

Tenotomy

Tenotomy is to make an incision and reform the deformed tendon.

Condylectomy

Excision of a condyle, the protrusion of the bone, usually at the end of humerus or femur.

Chiroplasty

Plastic surgery of the hand.

Analysis and Meaning of Key Terms

Roots

Term	Term Analysis	Meaning
skelet/o :		dried body, bones and cartilage in vertebrates
skeletology [skelitolɔ:gi]	-ology = study	study of the skeleton
skeletogeny [skelitodʒeni]	-geny = generation, production	origin or formation of the skeleton
orth/o :		straightness
orthopedics [ɔ̀:rθoupí:diks]	-pedics = medical field	branch of medicine that deals with correction of disorders in bones, joints and muscles
myel/o :		bone marrow
myeloblast [máiələblæ̀st]	-blast = embryonic or immature cell	immature cell of bone marrow that develops into a myelocyte
myelocyte [máiələsàit]	-cyte = cell	bone marrow cell, to mature into granulocyte
articul/o :		joint
articulation [ɑ́:rtìkjəléiʃən]	-ation = process, condition	moveable bone coupling
condyl/o :		smooth protrusion on a bone
epicondyle [epikɑ́ndail]	epi- = above	protuberance above the condyle of a bone

Term	Term Analysis	Meaning
vertebr/a :		**backbone**
vertebral column [vǝ́:rtǝ:brǝl kɑ́lǝm]	column = pillar, vertical post	the spine composed of the vertebrae
spondyl/o :		**spine, vertebra**
spondylolysis [spɑ̀ndǝloisis]	-lysis = breakdown, separation	defect of a vertebra, mostly in the lowest (L5) of the lumbar vertebrae
rachi/o :		**spinal column**
rachiometer [rǽkiomi:tǝ(r)]	-meter = measuring device	device used for measuring spinal curvature
digit/o, dactyl/o :		**finger, toe**
dactylogram [dæktílougræ̀m]	-gram = record, drawing	fingerprint
pelv/i, pelv/o :		**hip region**
pelvimetry [pelvimǝtri]	-metry = process of measuring	assessment of the female pelvis in relation to the birth of a baby
pelviscopy [pelviskɑ:pi]	-scopy = visual examination	endoscopy of the pelvic region, esp. female reproductive organs
pub/o :		**pubis, adult, maturity**
pubic bone [pjú:bik boun]	-ic = pertaining to	part of the hipbone forming the front arch of the pelvis
suprapubic [sú:prǝpju:bik]	supra- = above	above or anterior to the pubic bone
cost/o :		**ribs**
costovertebral [kɔ:stovǝ́:rbrǝl]	-al = pertaining to	relating to the rib and vertebra
crani/o :		**skull**
cranioplasty [kréinioplæ̀sti]	-plasty = repair, restoration	surgical repair of a defect or deformity of a skull
mandibul/o :		**mandible, lower jawbone**
mandible [mǽndǝbǝl]		lower jawbone, the bone forming the skull with the cranium

Term	Term Analysis	Meaning
scapul/o :		scapula, shoulder blade
scapular [skǽpjələr]	-ar = pertaining to	pertaining to the scapula
clavicul/o :		clavicle, collar bone
clavicular [klævíkjələr]	-ar = pertaining to	pertaining to the clavicle
acromi/o :		acromion, extension of shoulder bone
acromioclavicular [ǽkroumioklæ-vikular]	clavicular = of clavicle	pertaining to the joint of acromion and clavicle
humer/o :		humerus, upper arm bone
humeroulnar [hju:mərəʌlnər]	ulnar = pertaining to the ulna	pertaining to the joint of humerus and ulna
olecran/o :		olecranon, elbow
olecranarthritis [oulecrenɑ:rθraitis]	arthritis = inflammation of the joint	inflammation of the elbow joint
uln/o :		ulna, inner forearm bone
ulnar [ʌlnər]	-ar = pertaining to	pertaining to the ulna
radi/o :		radius, outer forearm bone
radial [réidiəl]	-al = pertaining to	pertaining to the radius
carp/o :		wrist bone
carpocarpal [kɑ:rpokɑ:rpl]	carpal = relating to or near the carpus	relating to the central two rows of the carpal bones
metacarp/o :		metacarpus, the middle 5 bones articulating with the carpus
carpometacarpal [kɑ:rpometakɑ:rpl]		relating to the carpal and metacarpal bones
phalang/o :		finger or toe bones
phalange [fǽləndʒ]		the bones of fingers and toes
phalangectomy [fǽləndʒektəmi]	-ectomy = excision	excision of the finger or the toe

Term	Term Analysis	Meaning
acetabul/o :		acetabulum, the socket of the hipbone
acetabular [æsətǽbjulər]	-ar = pertaining to	pertaining to the acetabulum
ili/o :		ilium, hip bone
iliac [íliæ̀k]	-ac = pertaining to	pertaining to the ilium
iliopsoas [íliosɔɑs]	-psoas = skeletal muscle of the lumbar region	compound muscle of iliac and psoas muscles
ischi/o :		ischium, hip joint
ischium [ískiəm]	-ium = structure, tissue	part of hip bone that bears weight when sitting down
ischiadynia [ískiədinia]	-dynia = pain	nerve pain in the region of ischium
ischialgia [ískiǽldʒiə]	-algia = pain	nerve pain in the region of ischium
femor/o :		femur, thighbone
femoral [fémərəl]	-al = pertaining to	pertaining to femur
patell/o :		patella, knee cap
patellofemoral [pətələfémərəl]	-femoral = pertaining to femur	pertaining to the patella and the femur
patellapexy [pətələpexi]	-pexy = fixation	surgical fixation of the patella
tibi/o :		tibia, shinbone
tibiofibular [tíbiəfibjələr]	fibula = calf bone; -ar = pertaining to	pertaining to both tibia and fibula
tars/o :		tarsus, ankle
tarsal [tɑ́:rsəl]	-al = pertaining to	pertaining to the tarsus
tarsus [tɑ́:rsəs]		seven short ankle bones
metatars/o :		metatarsus
metatarsalgia [métətɑ:rsldʒiə]	-algia = pain	pain in the metatarsus
metatarsus [mètətɑ́:rsəs]		the part of the foot between toes and ankle

Suffixes

Term	Term Analysis	Meaning
-blast :		immature cell
osteoblast [ástiəblæ̀st]	oste/o = bone	mononucleate cell from which bone develops
-clasis :		break
osteoclasis [àstiákləsis]	oste/o = bone	surgically breaking a bone in order to correct deformity
osteoclast [ástiəkǽst]	oste/o = bone	large multinuclear cell that resorbs bone
-genesis :		generating, producing
osteogenesis [ástiədʒénəsist]	oste/o = bone	formation and development of bone
malacia :		softening
chondromalacia [kandróuməlasia]	chondr/o = cartilage	softening of cartilage, painful condition due to irritation of cartilage, often under the kneecap
-osis :		condition, disease
scoliosis [skòulióusis]	scoli/o = twist, crookedness	abnormal lateral curvature of the spine
kyphosis [kaifóusis]	kyph/o = humped back	abnormal curvature of the spine, causing hunchback
lordosis [lɔːrdóusis]	lord/o = curve, swayback	excessive curvature of the spine, causing concave anterior curve
-porosis :		porosity, condition of pores
osteoporosis [àstioupəróusis]	oste/o = bone	condition of porous bones
-sarcoma :		malignant tumor of the tissue or organ
chondrosarcoma [kandróusaːr-koumə]	chondr/o = cartilage	cartilage-based bone cancer

Abbreviations

Abbreviation	Full Term	Meaning
AE	Above the elbow	upper arm or proximal
AK	Above the knee	thigh or proximal
BE	Below the elbow	forearm or distal
BK	Below the knee	lower leg or distal
C	Cervical vertebra	vertebral part belonging in the neck
C_1	Number 1 of Cervical vertebra	the most superior of the cervical vertebrae
Co	Coccyx	tailbone
DIP	Distal interphalangeal joint	distal joint of the fingers or toes
DJD	Degenerative joint disease	osteoarthritis
Fx	Fracture	breakage or crack in the skeletal part
HNP	Herniated nucleus pulposus	(condition of) spinal disc herniation
L	Lumbar vertebra	the 5 vertebrae between the thoracic (rib) cage and the pelvis
L_1	Number 1 of Lumbar vertebra	the most superior of the lumbar vertebrae
MCP	Metacarpophalageal joint	joint between the metacarpal bones and the phalanges of the fingers
OA	Osteoarthritis	arthritis caused by chronic degeneration of the joints
Ortho	Orthopedics	study or surgery of the musculoskeletal system
PIP	Proximal interphalangeal joint	proximal joint of the fingers or toes
RA	Rheumatoid arthritis	disease of the joints due to attacks by autoimmune disease
S	Sacrum	large triangular bone located at the base of the spine connected to the pelvis
T	Thoracic vertebra	vertebral part between cervical and lumbar vertebrae
T_1	Number 1 of Thoracic vertebra	the most superior of the thoracic vertebrae
THA	Total hip arthroplasty	surgical procedure to replace the hip joint with a prosthetic implant
TKA	Total knee arthroplasty	surgical procedure to repair the knee with an artificial joint
TMJ	Temporomandibular joint	the joint of the jaw, between the temporal bone and the mandible
Tx	Traction	the act or power of pulling, adhesive friction

Exercises

1. Write the meaning of the following terms :

① femur — thighbone, between the pelvis and the knee

② humerus — the bone of the upper arm, between the shoulder and the elbow

③ ilium — the broad, upper portion of either hipbone

④ patella — kneecap, the flat movable bone at the front of the knee

⑤ tibia — shinbone, the inner and thicker of the two bones of the lower leg

⑥ forearm — the part of the arm between the elbow and the wrist

⑦ olecranon — the upper end part of the ulna beyond and behind the elbow joint

⑧ calcaneus — heel bone, the largest and quadrangular tarsal bone

⑨ carpals — wrist bone, any of the bones of the carpus

⑩ thorax — chest, the upper part of the trunk between the neck and the diaphragm

2. Write the adjective form of the following terms :

① ischium — ischial

② radius — radial

③ sacrum — sacral

④ face — facial

⑤ femur — femoral

⑥ ilium — iliac

⑦ maxilla — maxillary

⑧ clavicle — clavicular

⑨ zygoma — zygomatic

⑩ coccyx — coccygeal

3. Spell the following terms correctly :

① olecrenal — olecranal

② ileosacral — iliosacral

③ myloma — myoma, or myeloma

④ maleolus — malleolus

⑤ tibula — fibula, or tibia

⑥ thorex — thorax

⑦ calcanious — calcaneus

⑧ acetatbolum — acetabulum

⑨ vetebra — vertebra

⑩ brechial — brachial

4. Write the meaning of the following: pathological terms :

① osteoarthritis — arthritis caused by chronic degeneration of the joint

② chondroma — benign tumor of the cartilage

③ scoliosis — abnormal lateral curvature of the spine

④ osteoma — benign bone tumor

⑤ bursitis — inflammation of the synovial bursa

⑥ kyphosis — abnormal curvature of the spine, causing hunchback

⑦ lordosis — excessive curvature of the spine, causing concave anterior curve

⑧ osteomyelitis — infection and inflammation of the bone or bone marrow

⑨ polyarthritis — arthritis affecting multiple joints, often upwards of 5

⑩ tendinitis — inflammation of the tendon

5. Write the meaning of the following surgical terms :

① arthrotomy — surgical incision of a joint

② bursectomy — surgical removal of a bursa

③ osteotomy — surgical procedure of cutting a bone to modify or correct it

④ chondrectomy — surgical excision of cartilage

⑤ tenoplasty — plastic surgery to repair a tendon

⑥ tenonectomy — surgical excision of a part of a tendon

⑦ cranioplasty — surgical repair of a defect or deformity of the skull

⑧ patellapexy — surgical procedure to fix the patella for stability

⑨ arthrodesis — fusion of a joint between two bones so the joint can no longer move

⑩ chiroplasty — surgical repair of the hand

6. Fill in the blanks.

- **Using myel/o, complete the medical term that means the following :**
  ① inflammation of the bone marrow ______ osteomyelitis ______
  ② immature cell found in the marrow ______ myeloblast ______

- **Using oste/o, complete the medical term that means the following :**
  ① benign tumor of the bones ______ osteoma ______
  ② bone formation ______ osteogenesis ______
  ③ malignant tumor of the bones ______ osteosarcoma ______
  ④ condition softening of the bones ______ osteomalacia ______

- **Using arthr/o, complete the medical term that means the following :**
  ① inflammation of the multiple joints ______ polyarthritis ______
  ② incision of the joint ______ arthrotomy ______
  ③ any morbid condition of the joint ______ osteoarthropathy ______
  ④ surgical repair of the joint ______ arthroplasty ______

- **Using chondr/o, complete the medical term that means the following :**
  ① pain of the cartilage ______ chondrodynia ______
  ② inflammation of the cartilage and the bones ______ osteochondritis ______

- **Using ten/o, complete the medical term that means the following :**
  ① pain in the tendon ______ tenodynia ______
  ② inflammation of the tendon ______ tendinitis, tendonitis, tenonitis ______
  ③ incision of the tendon ______ tenotomy ______

7. Write the meaning of the following terms of skeletal structure :

① sacroiliac — pertaining to the region where the sacrum and ilium meet

② costovertebral — relating to joining a rib with the thoracic vertebra

③ occipitoparietal — relating to the occipital and parietal bones

④ sternoclavicular — relating to the clavicle and the sternum

⑤ humeroradial — relating to the humerus and the radius

⑥ carpocarpal — mediocarpal, denoting the articulation between two rows ofcarpal bones

⑦ symphysis pubis — midline cartilaginous joint located between the left and right pubic bones

⑧ iliac spine — any of the four spinal projections from the ilium

⑨ fibulocalcaneal — relating to the fibula and the calcaneus

⑩ craniofacial — relating to both the cranium and the face

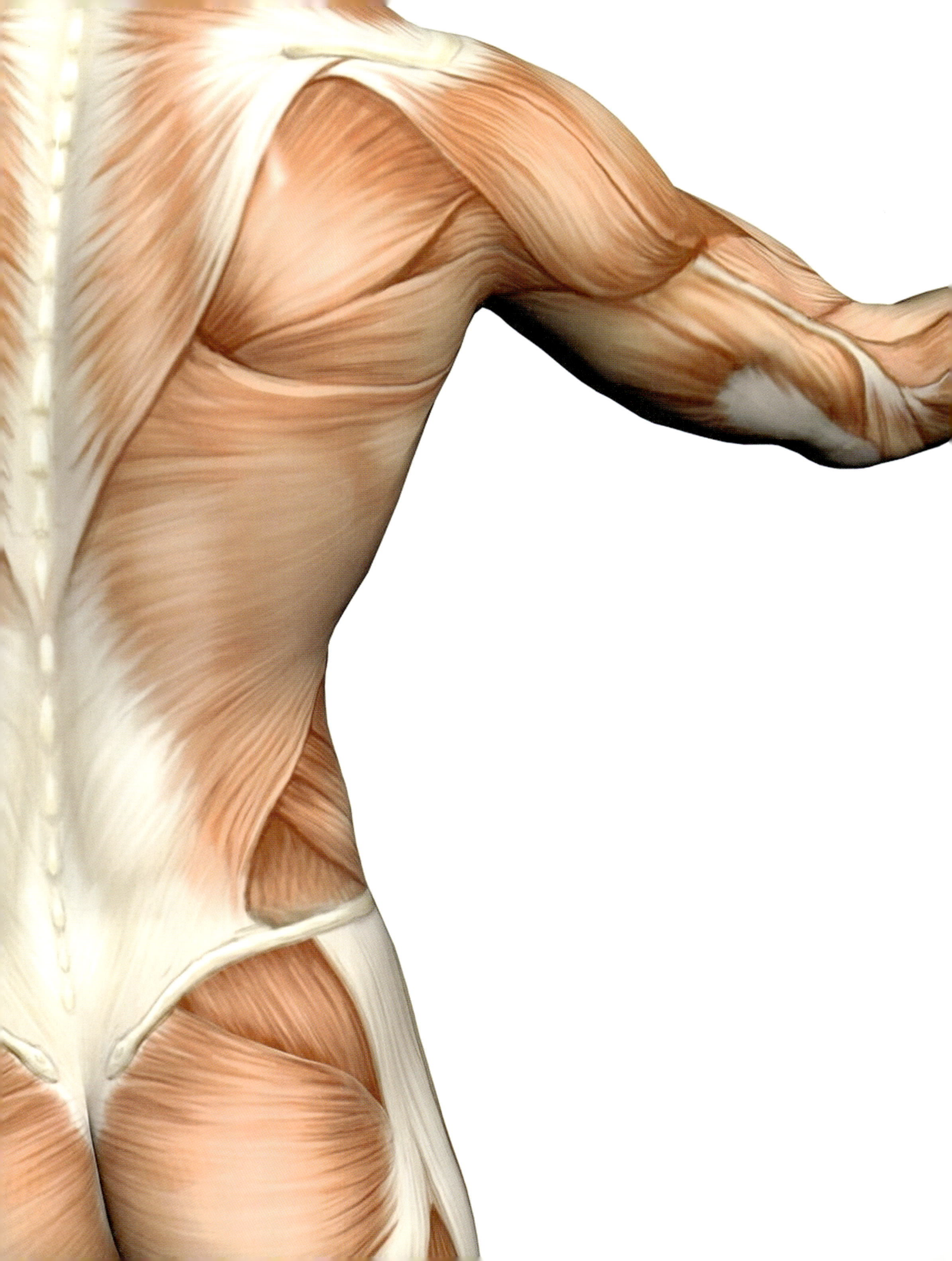

Chapter 8

Muscular System

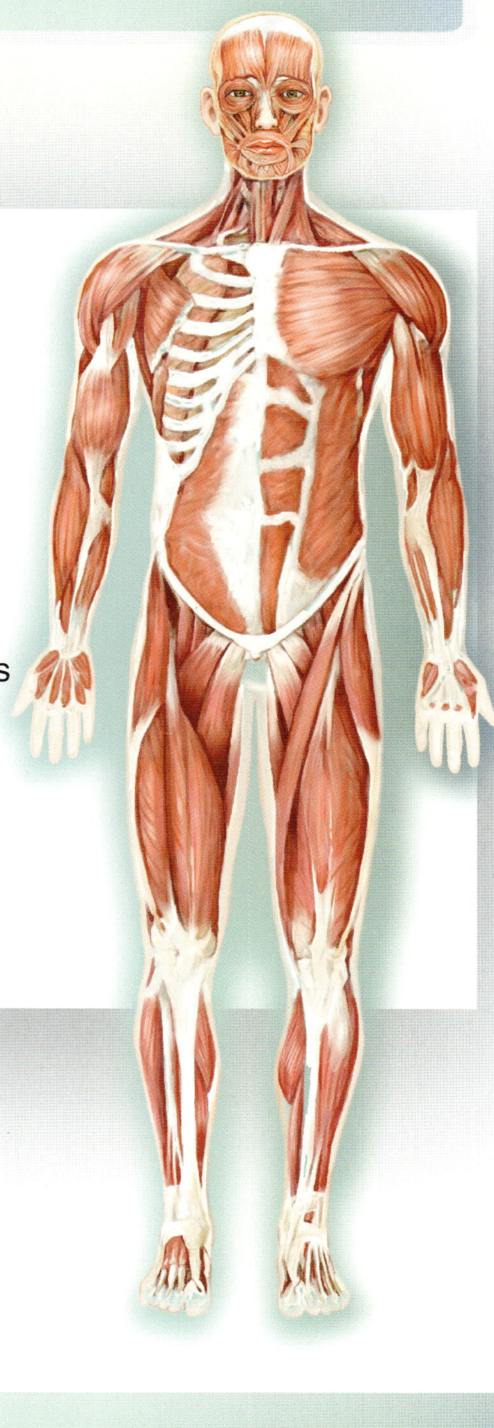

Chapter Contents

- Prolog
- Anatomical Terms
- Terms for Symptoms and Diseases
- Terms for Test and Surgery
- Analysis and Meaning of Key Terms
- Abbreviations
- Exercises

Learning Objectives

- Learn muscle types and their characteristics.
- Be familiar with skeletal muscle attachment and terms for body motions made with muscle contractions.
- Learn names, spelling and pronunciation for skeletal muscles.
- Analyze and be familiar with medical terms in muscular system.
- Be familiar with medical terms for diseases in muscular system.
- Be familiar with abbreviations used in muscular system.

Prolog

There are 600 human skeletal muscles, composed of myofilaments with specific functions that consume energy to produce power. Functions of muscles include changing the size of muscle cells by contraction in order to produce movement, generating heat and supporting the body to maintain posture. Muscles can be classified into skeletal, visceral and cardiac types. We will study the structure and functions of human body muscles and learn related medical terms.

Anatomical Terms

Attachment of Muscle

The muscle is attached to the bone via tendon or aponeurosis. Certain muscles' wing is directly attached to the bone via short fibrous connective tissue of muscle fibers. Muscles' attachment points are divided into origins and insertions. The origin of a muscle is at the bone, typically proximal and more stable than the insertion during muscle contraction. The insertion is at the bone that is typically distal and tends to move more.

Connective tissues include fascia, tendon, etc. that attach the muscle to the points where they can exert forces and maintain posture of the body.

Types of Muscles

Visceral muscles

Also called smooth muscles, they are found in the walls of organs such as stomach, intestines, vessels, salphinx, uterus, bladder, ureter. They are involuntary muscles constructed of fibers consisting of long fusiform cells.

Cardiac muscles

These are muscles that construct the wall of the heart. The muscles are striated (striped or grooved in parallel) like skeletal muscles, however, they are of involuntary type governed by autonomous nervous system.

Skeletal muscles

Being called skeletal muscles as they are attached to the skeleton, they produce various motions including flexing, chewing and facial expressions through muscle contractions. The muscles are striated in shape, meaning that the fibers are striped by light and dark belts. They are voluntary muscles controlled at will.

Structure of Muscles

When people speak of flesh and muscle, they typically mean the skeletal muscle. The constituent striated muscle fiber is made of multinucleate cells, formed through fusion of multiple cells or divisions of nuclei without the divisions of cytoplasm. The fiber of the voluntary muscle is very long and contracts fast, exerts great force but fatigues easily.

Smooth muscles are muscles that don't optically display striated muscle fibers. All muscles of internal organs except for the heart belong in this type. The involuntary muscle contracts slowly but doesn't fatigue easily, governed by autonomous nervous system. This type muscles have small but thin and long fusiform muscle fibers. The typical cell usually has an elliptical nucleus at the center, however, rarely does it have multiple nuclei.

Cardiac muscles are of involuntary type. The contractable protein filaments are arranged like striated muscles, while the constituent cells are mononucleated. However, unlike the other two muscle types, the short muscle fibers are connected and arranged in various branched and woven sections, whose contractions and relaxations produce heartbeats.

The muscles of the heart keep working without external stimulus to keep the body alive by circulating blood, even while other muscles are at rest.

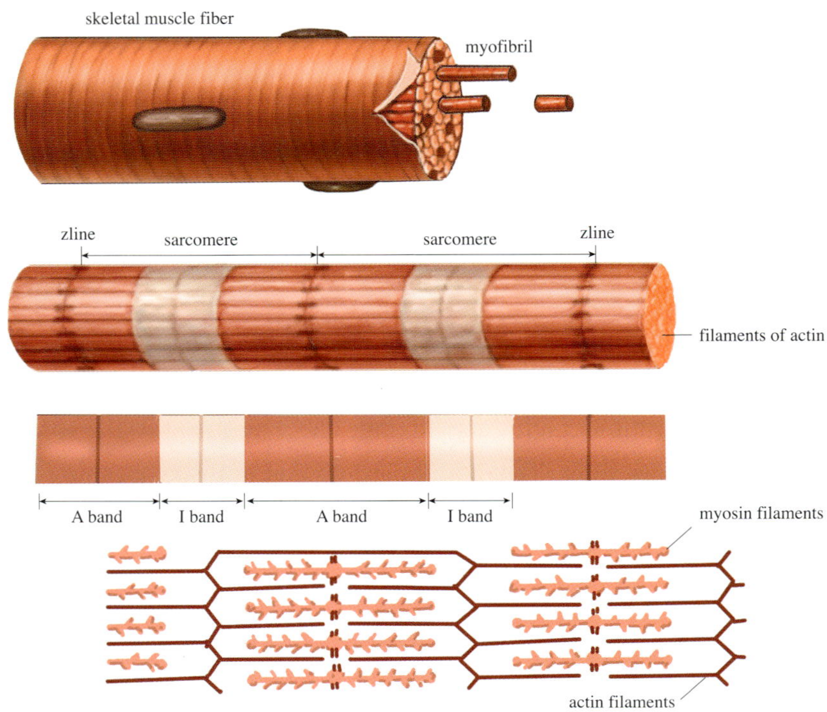

Figure 8-1 Muscle structure

Motions by Skeletal Muscles

Motion	Pronunciation	Meaning	Graphic
flexion	**fleck**-shun	decreasing the angle of the joint	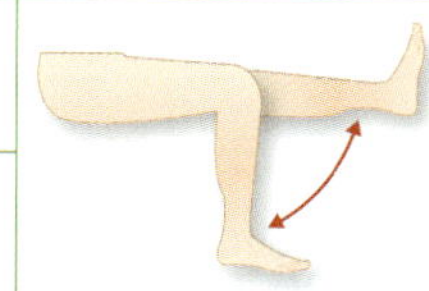
extension	eks-**ten**-shun	increasing the angle of the joint	
abduction	ab-**duck**-shun	moving away from the main body	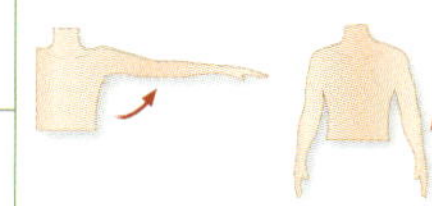
adduction	a-**duck**-shun	moving close to the main body	
rotation	roo-**ta**-shun	turning a limb about the longitudinal axis	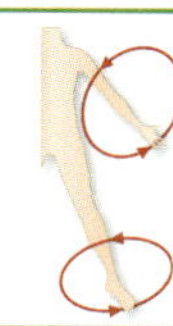
circumduc-tion	ser-kum-**duck**-shun	turning a limb conically	
pronation	pro-**na**-shuna	turning the palm forward	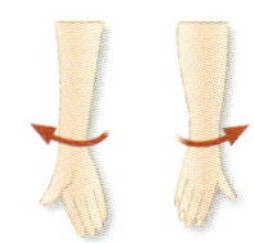
supination	su-pin-**a**-shun	turning the palm backward	
eversion	e-**ver**-zhun	turning the sole outward	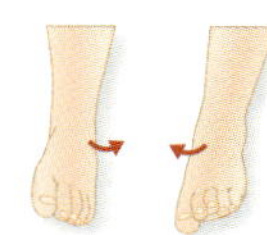
inversion	in-**ver**-zhun	turning the sole inward	
dorsiflexion	dor-si-**fleck**-shun	bending backward	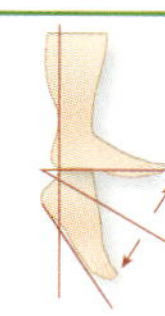
plantar flexion	plan-ta-**fleck**-shun	flexing the foot downward	

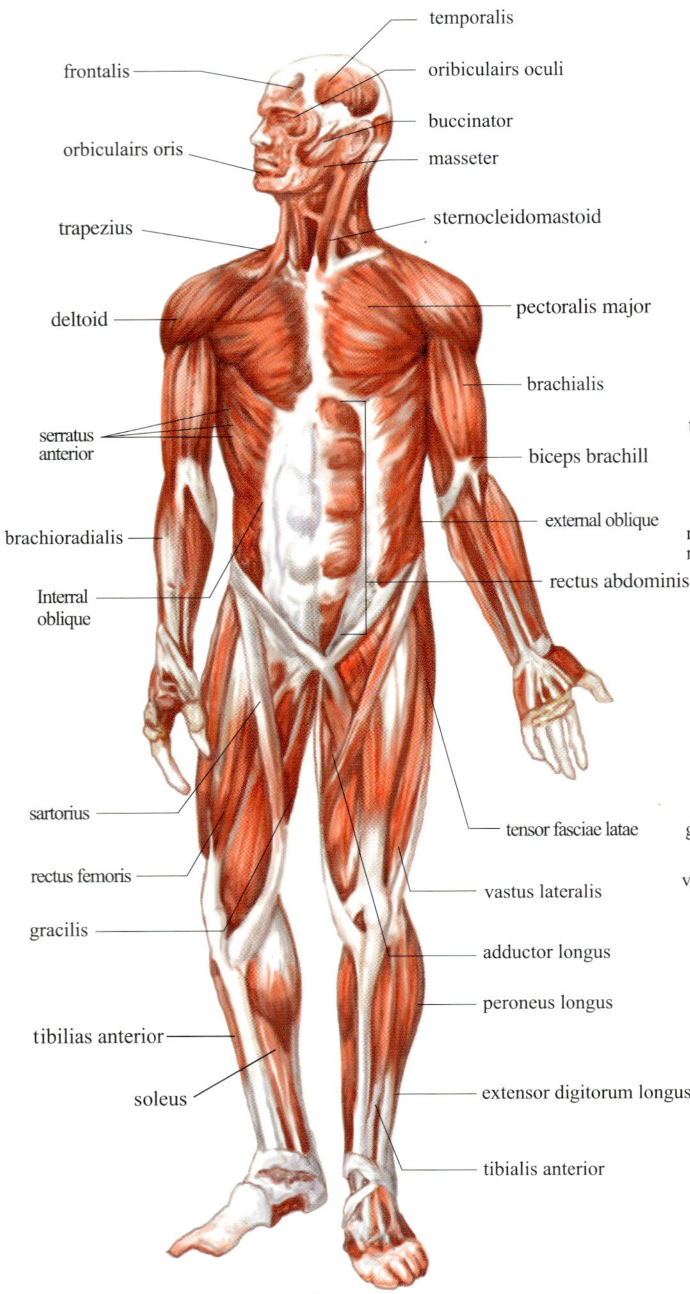

Figure 8-2 Names of skeletal muscles-anterior view

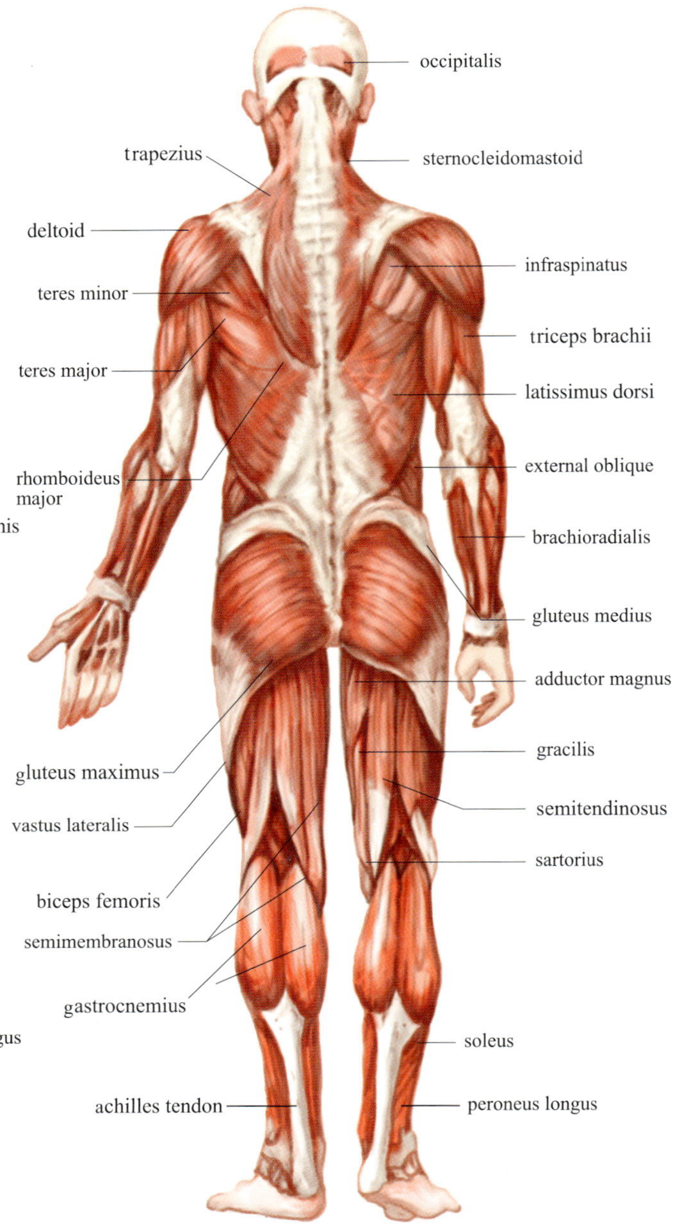

Figure 8-3 Names of skeletal muscles-posterior view

Terms for Symptoms and Diseases

Myalgia

Pain in the muscle caused by overuse or a disease.

Myofibrosis

Replacement of muscle tissue by fibrous tissue, with chronic myositis causing diffuse hyperplasia of the interstitial connective tissue pressing upon and causing atrophy of the muscular tissue.

Myopathy

A muscular disease, in which muscle fibers do not function normally due to many possible reasons. Loss of ability to walk, difficulty of breathing and dysfunction of the heart can arise due to decrease in muscle strength.

Myoma

A usually benign tumor in the smooth muscle, typically of the uterus and sometimes of the esophagus.

Dermatitis

Inflammation of the skin, caused by hormone imbalance, chemical substance or contact with foreign irritants, etc. Symptoms include swelling, discoloration, rash, etc.

Fasciitis

Inflammation of the fascia, the connective tissue surrounding muscles, blood vessels and nerves, resulting in hardening of the skin or dyskinesia. It can be caused by excessive exercise or sharp increase in weight.

Tendinitis

Inflammation of the tendon, caused by overuse of the muscle or excessive tension. The patient will experience pain, swelling or restriction of motion.

Myotonia

Congenital neuromuscular disorder characterized by the inability to relax the muscle quickly after voluntary contraction.

Dystonia

A neurological movement disorder, in which sustained muscle contractions cause twisting and repetitive movements or abnormal postures.

Muscular dystrophy

This is a group of congenital muscle diseases that weaken the musculoskeletal system and hamper locomotion. These are characterized by progressive skeletal muscle weakness, defects in muscle proteins and death of muscle cells and tissues.

Bradykinesia

Bradykinesia is marked by slow movement of the body and is linked to Parkinson's disease or other extrapyramidal disorder.

Strain

This is a condition in which the muscle or tendon is torn, twisted or overextended. The affected part will experience swelling, pain and restriction in the range of joint movement.

Sprain

A sprain is damage (tearing or stretching) to a ligament often caused by the joint being taken beyond its functional range of motion. The affected part will experience pain, swelling and restriction in the range of joint movement.

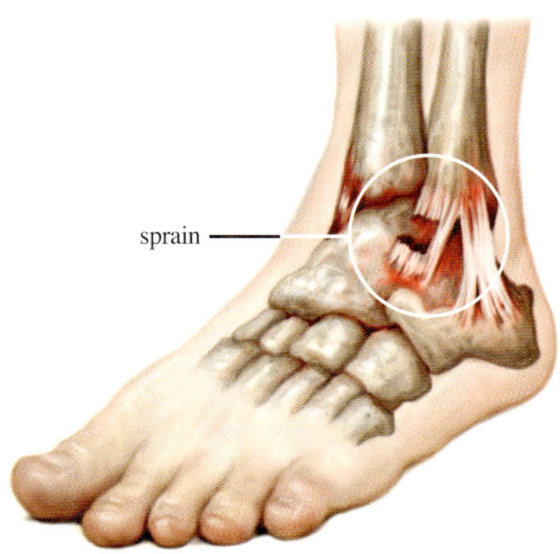

Figure 8-4 Sprain

Terms for Test and Surgery

Fasciectomy

Surgical removal of a part of the fascia.

Tenodesis

Surgical fixation or suturing of the end of the tendon to the bone.

Tenotomy

Surgical act involving an incision in a tendon.

Fasciorrhaphy

Suture of a fascia or of an aponeurosis.

Myorrhaphy

Suturing of a wound in a muscle.

Electromyography

A technique for recording and evaluating electrical activities in the peripheral nerve and the surrounding muscle.

Analysis and Meaning of Key Terms

Term	Term Analysis	Meaning
rhabdomy/o :		striated muscle
rhabdomyosarcoma [ræbdəmàiousa:r-kóumə]	-sarcoma = malignant tumor	cancerous tumor of skeletal muscle
rhabdomyoma [ræbdəmaióumə]	-oma = tumor	benign tumer of skeletal or cardiac muscle

Term	Term Analysis	Meaning
leiomy/o :		smooth muscle
leiomyosarcoma [laioumaiousa:r-kouma]	sarcoma = malignant tumor	cancerous tumor of smooth muscle
leiomyoma [làioumaióumə]	-oma = tumor	benign tumor of smooth muscle, mostly in the uterus
cutane/o :		skin
subcutaneous [sʌ̀bkju:téiniəs]	sub = under; -ous = pertaining to	under the dermis
derm/o :		skin
epidermis [èpədə́:rmis]	epi = above	superfluous layer of the skin
fibro/o :		fiber
fibrous [fáibrəs]	-ous = pertaining to	pertaining to fibre, fiber-like
fibrous connective tissue [fáibrəs kənéktiv tíʃu:]		tissue made up of fibers that attach to and support neighboring tissues
fasci/o :		fascia, membrane supporting muscles
fasciectomy	-ectomy = excision	surgical removal of part of a fascia
ton/o :		tension
atonic [ətɑ́nik]	a- = lacking; -ic = pertaining to; of condition	free of tension, lacking muscle tone
ab- :		away from
abduction [æbdʌ́kʃən]	duct/o = to lead, to carry	movjng a limb away from the main body
ad- :		toward
adduction [ədʌ́kʃən]	duct/o = to lead, to carry	bringing a limb toward the main body
dorsi- :		backward
dorsiflexion [dɔ́:rsiflekʃn]	-flexion = bending	bending backward, flexing the foot or toes upward

Term	Term Analysis	Meaning
poly- :		**many, multi**
polymyalgia [pɑːlimaiǽldʒə]	my/o = muscle; -algia = pain	pain in multiple muscles, rheumatic syndrome with pain or stiffness
ton/o :		**tension**
atonic [ətɑ́nik]	a- = lacking; -ic = pertaining to; of condition	free of tension, lacking muscle tone
-asthenia :		**weakness, loss of strength**
myasthenia [màiəsθíːniə]	my/o = muscle	muscle weakness, typically of neuromuscular type
-kinesia :		**state of movement, motion sickness**
bradykinesia [brædikinétik]	brady- = slow	slowness of body movement, due to Parkinson's disease or or other disorder
dyskinesia [dìskəníːʒiə,-kai-]	dys- = bad, abnormal	impairment of voluntary movements resulting in fragmented or jerky motions
-trophy :		**nourishment, development**
atrophy [ǽtrəfi]	a- = lacking	physiological process of reabsorption and breakdown of tissues
hypertrophy [haipə́ːrtrəfi]	hyper- = over, excessive	increase in the volume of an organ or tissue due to the enlargement of its component cells

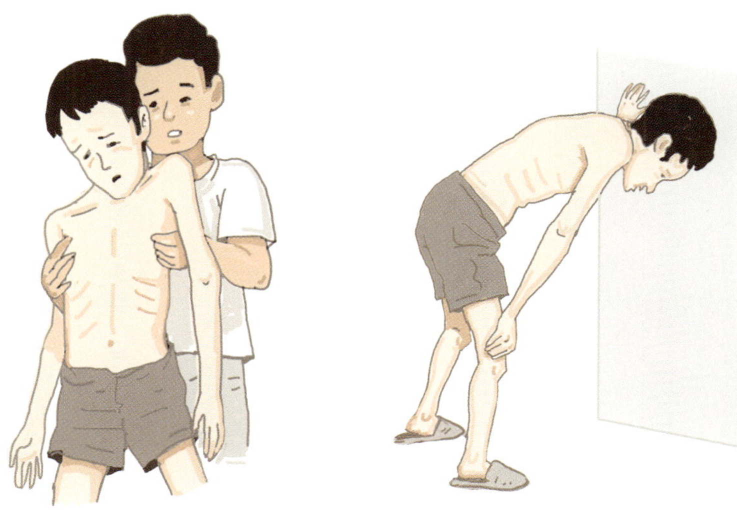

Abbreviations

Abbreviation	Full Term	Meaning
EMG	electromyography	recording and evaluating electrical activities in muscle and nerve.
IM	intramuscular	in-muscle
ROM	range of motion	angle or distance a joint can move between flexion and extension
MD	muscular dystrophy	congenital, progressive musculoskeletal weakening
MG	myasthenia gravis	muscle weakness, typically of neuromuscular type
RICE	rest, ice, compression, elevation	first-aid treatment for soft tissue injuries
SLR	straight leg raise	measuring the angle of leg flexion with the patient lying down, to determine whether the low back pain has an underlying herniated disk, often located at L_5

Exercises

1. Write the meaning of the following terms.

① myalgia — muscle pain or tenderness, due to overuse or a disease

② myosclerosis — hardening or muscle tissue

③ myoma — benign tumor of the smooth muscle, typically in the uterus

④ dermatitis — inflammation of the skin

⑤ keratosis — the condition of keratin growing on the skin or mucous membrane

⑥ onychitis — onychia, inflammation of the skin around fingernail or toenail

⑦ anhidrosis — condition of decreased or inhibited sweating

2. Write the term that means the following.

① an immature muscle cell — myoblast

② destruction of muscle tissue — necrosis

③ replacement of muscle by fibrous tissue — myofibrosis

④ a tumor containing both muscle and fibrous tissue — rhabdomyosarcoma

⑤ hardening of muscle tissue — myosclerosis

3. Find the location of each muscle from the following table.

a. head	**b**. shoulder	**c**. upper extremities	
d. lower extremities	**e**. back	**f**. abdomen	**g**. chest

① deltoid — b

② external oblique — f

③ gastrocnemius — d

④ pectoralis major — g

⑤ triceps — c

⑥ masseter — a

⑦ sartorius — d

⑧ latissimus dorsi — e

⑨ trapezius — e

⑩ rectus femoris	d
⑪ frontalis	a
⑫ gluteus maximus	d
⑬ gracilis	d
⑭ soleus	d
⑮ infraspinatus	e

4. Spell the following terms correctly.

① gastrocmemius	gastrocnemius
② external abdominal obliique	external abdominal oblique
③ infraspinates	infraspinatus
④ tensor faciae latae	tensor fasciae latae
⑤ sternosleidomestoid	sternocleidomastoid
⑥ vastos medials	vastus medialis
⑦ solius	soleus
⑧ seratus anterior	serratus anterior
⑨ terres major	teres major
⑩ abbuctor magnus	adductor magnus

5. Write the medical term for each of the following muscular movements.

① closing the angle at a joint	flexion
② movement away from the midline of the body	abduction
③ turning of a body part on its own axis	rotation
④ turning the palm backward	supination
⑤ bending backward	dorsiflexion
⑥ turning the palm forward	pronation
⑦ bending the sole of the foot	plantar flexion
⑧ turning outward	eversion
⑨ conical movement from a central point	circumduction
⑩ opening the angle at a joint	extension

Chapter 9

Nervous System

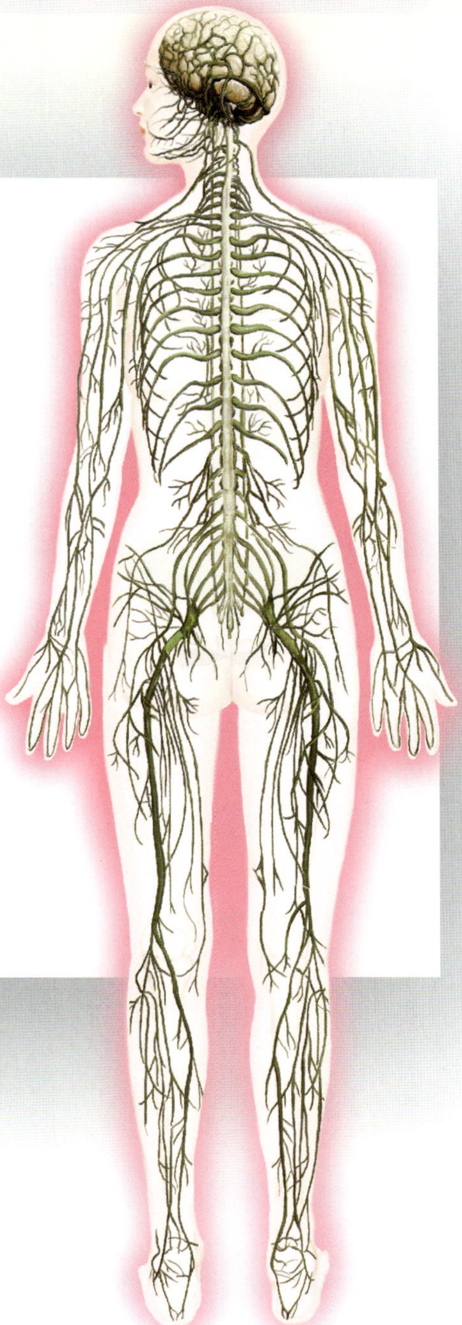

Chapter Contents

- Prolog
- Anatomical Terms
- Terms for Symptoms and Diseases
- Terms for Surgery and Treatment
- Terms for Test and Intervention
- Analysis and Meaning of Key Terms
- Abbreviations
- Exercises

Learning Objectives

- Understand the structure and divisions of the nervous system.
- Be familiar with names and locations of the parts in central and peripheral nervous systems.
- Learn structure and names of the cranial and spinal nerves.
- Analyze medical terms used in the nervous system and be familiar with them.
- Be familiar with diseases and abbreviations pertaining to the nervous system.

Prolog

The nervous system in our body is a highly specialized organization. Its functions include sensing signals and stimulations from internal and external parts of the body, and transmitting them to other part of the same system for proper response. It collects, analyzes and synthesizes various types of information, then controls other organs' activities.

In this chapter, we will learn and understand medical terms pertaining to the brain and spinal cord involved in speaking, hearing, thinking, moving, unconscious regulation of hormone secretion, detecting danger signals such as pain, etc. and the peripheral nervous system including cranial nerves, spinal nerves and autonomic nerves, etc.

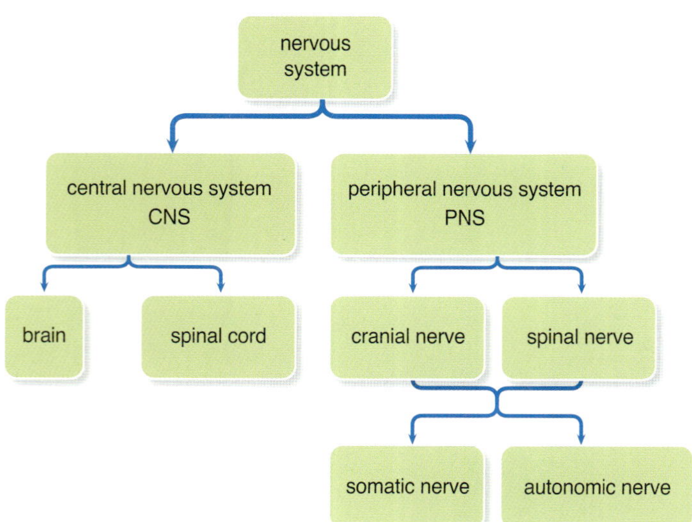

Figure 9-1 Divisions of the nervous system

Anatomically, the nervous system is divided into the central nervous system (CNS) and the peripheral nervous system (PNS). The CNS consists of the brain and the spinal cord. The PNS consists of the cranial nerves that connect to the head and the neck, and the spinal nerves that connect to the chest, the abdomen and the limbs. The PNS include autonomic nerves that transmit excitations to the involuntary muscles in the walls of the internal organs such as endocrine glands, heart, intestines, stomach and bladder.

Anatomical Terms

Central Nervous System (CNS)

The central nervous system, consisting of the brain and the spinal cord built with numerous neurons, functions as the central processing unit that collects information from the nerves, integrates them and regulates target organs.

Brain

The brain is an organ specially developed from the front end of the neural tube, and it is much larger and more structurally complex than the spinal cord. It consists of cerebrum which is the largest part, brainstem comprising midbrain, pons and medulla oblongata, and cerebellum.

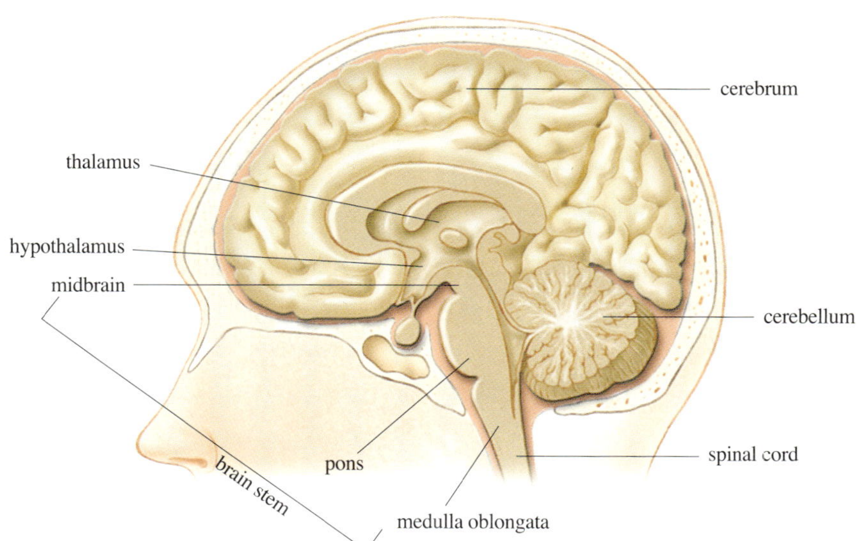

Figure 9-2 Internal structure of the brain

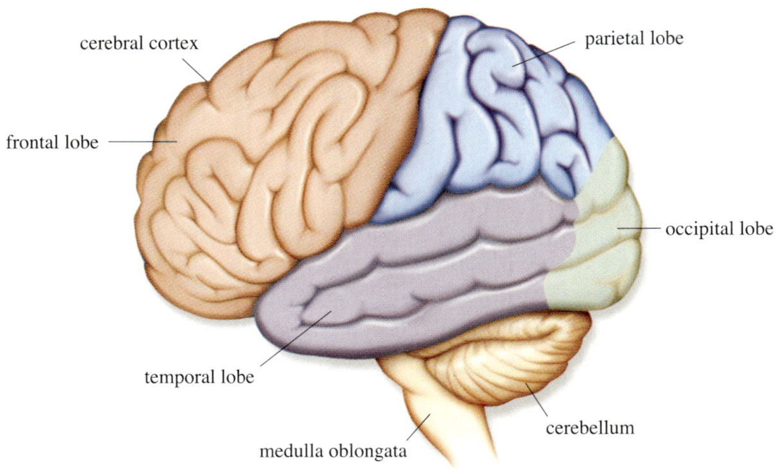

Figure 9-3 External structure of the brain

Spinal cord

Connecting the medulla oblongata, the spinal cord starts from inside the atlas (C_1) of the cerebral vertebrae down the vertebral canal to the second lumbar vertebra (L_2). The thickness of the spinal cord decreases as you go down the conus medullaris, ending with the cauda equina that connect the nerves.

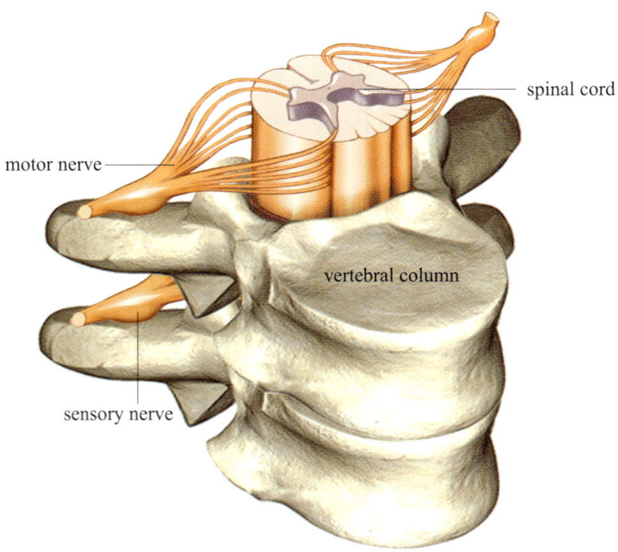

Figure 9-4 Structure of the spinal cord

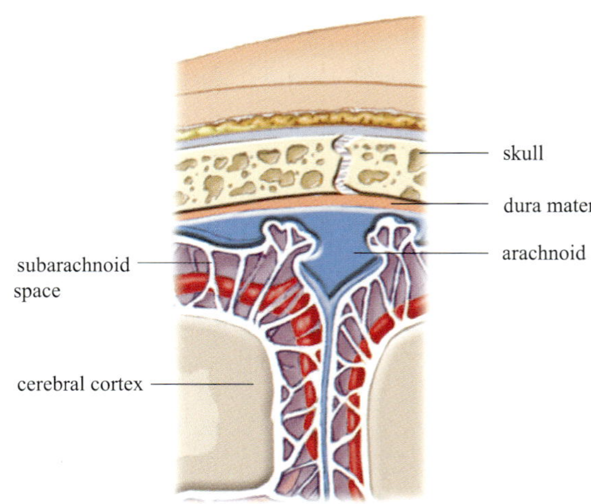

Figure 9-5 Meningeal region of the brain and spinal cord

Peripheral Nervous System (PNS)

The peripheral nervous system includes 12 pairs of cranial nerves (12 pairs) and 31 pairs of spinal nerves. It serves as the corridor for transmitting sensory and motor signals to and from the central nervous system.

Somatic nervous system

As a voluntary nervous system, the somatic nervous system consists of pairs of motor nerves and sensory nerves. Motor nerves are of efferent type in that they transmit impulses from the CNS to the peripheral organs (skeletal muscles) to induce body movements. Sensory nerves are of afferent type in that they transmit impulses from the sensory organs to the CNS.

Autonomic nervous system

The autonomic nervous system consists of the sympathetic nervous system and the parasympathetic nervous system. The sympathetic nervous system mobilizes the body in a fight-or-flight response in situations such as sudden physical attack,

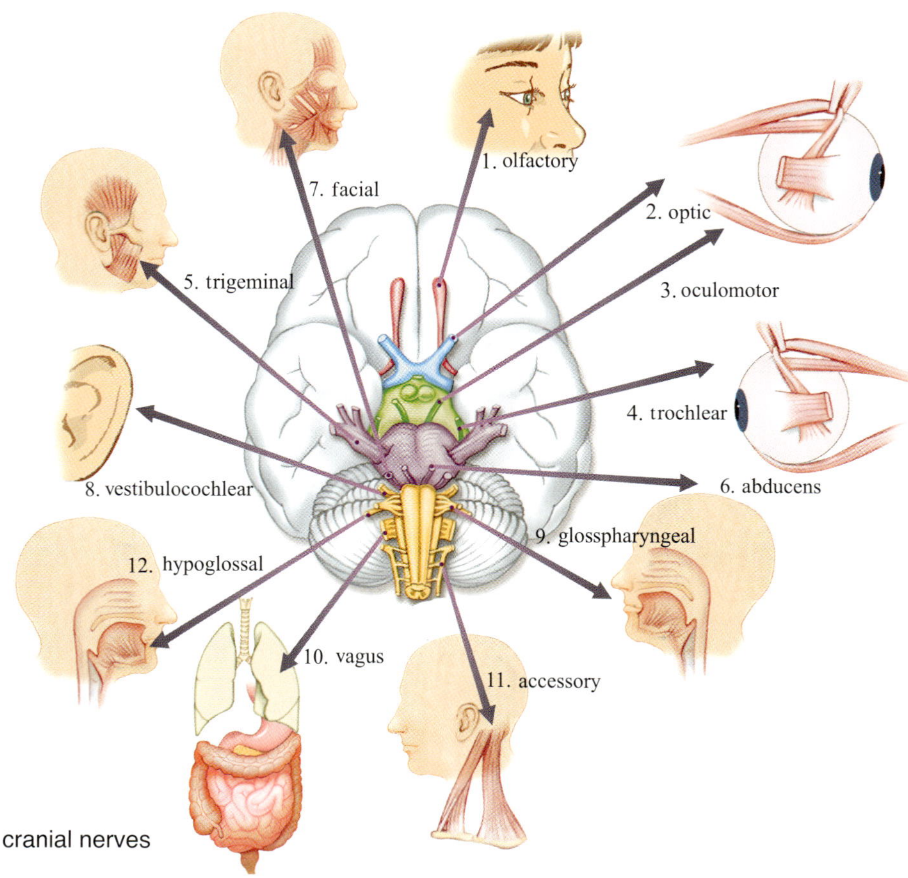

Figure 9-6 Twelve pairs of cranial nerves

fear and anger. The parasympathetic nervous system is responsible for stimulation of rest-and-digest or feed-and-breed activities such as internal organs' secretion and peristaltic motion and storing energy.

Cranial nerve

Cranial nerves emerge from the brain and are distributed throughout the head. The 12 pairs of nerves are numbered from the top and named. Cranial nerves 1, 2, 8 are of sensory type, while 3, 4, 6, 11, 12 are of motor type. Numbers 5, 7, 9, 10 are of sensory and motor types combined. Numbers 3, 7, 9, 10 include parasympathetic autonomic nerves of efferent type.

Spinal nerve

Spinal nerves branch out from the spinal cord and are distributed throughout the rest of the body. The 31 pairs of nerves are grouped and named after the

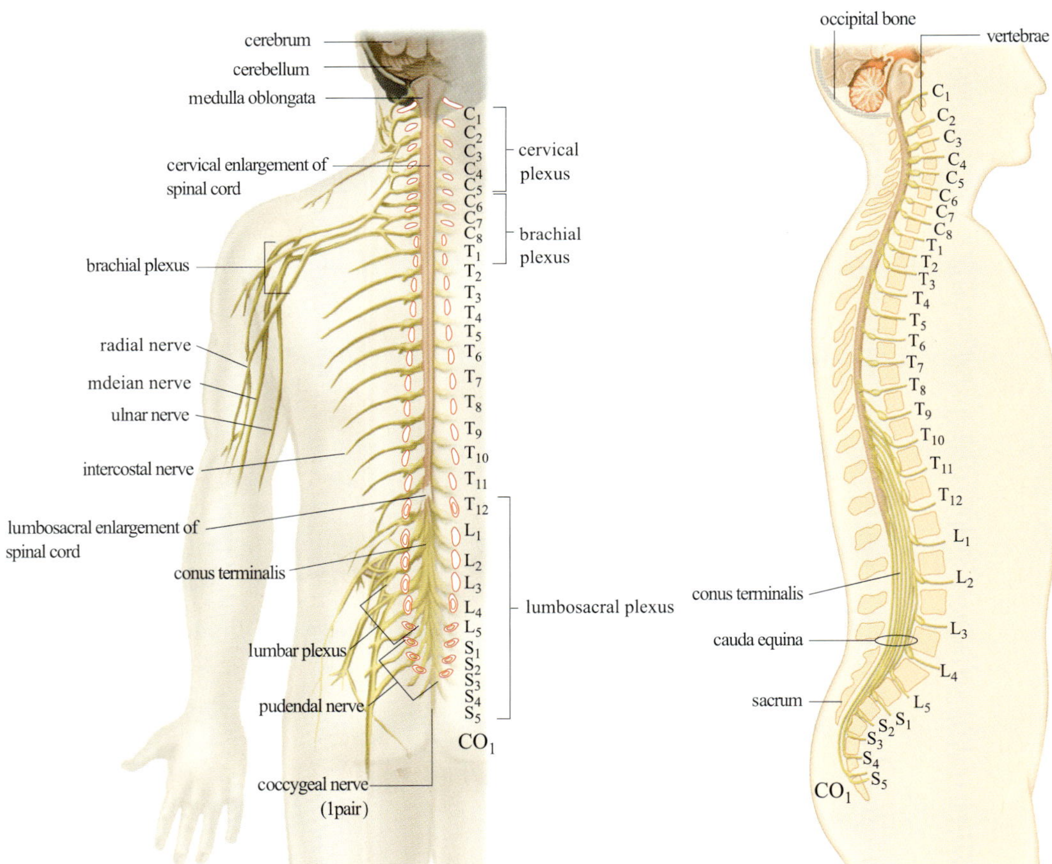

Figure 9-7 Spinal cord, spinal nerves and the spinal column

corresponding regions of the spinal column, namely cervical, thoracic, lumbar, sacral and coccygeal nerves. They are responsible for motor functions of all limbs and the functions of sensory as well as autonomic nerves of cutaneous regions except for the head.

Terms for Symptoms and Diseases

Alzheimer's disease

As known to be caused by proteopathy (anomaly of protein structures) in the brain, Alzheimer's disease affects the patient's memory, linguistic competency, temporal and spatial reasoning, performance of common everyday tasks, and even personality and behavior pattern.

Analgesia

Analgesia, the loss of the sense of pain, can be induced by drugs, accidents and chronic diseases such as diabetes which may cause anomaly in sensory nerves.

Aphasia

Cerebral dysfunction may cause loss of language skills. Broca's aphasia affects the patient's ability to speak while listening ability is intact. Wernicke's aphasia affects the ability to understand other's speech and to speak logically while being able to speak fluently.

Brain tumor

Brain tumors include tumors affecting the brain, meninges, cranial vessels and nerves. Symptoms include headache, vomiting, visual impairment, loss of hearing, tinnitus (ringing in the ear), loss of vision, etc.

Cerebral infarction

Due to disturbance in blood supply to the brain, death of some neurological tissue will occur and induce hemiplegia, facial nerve paralysis, dysarthria (motor speech disorder), sensory processing disorder, agnosia, aphasia, visual impairment, loss of consciousness, etc.

Cerebral hemorrhage

This condition is of internal bleeding due to sudden rise in blood pressure or a trauma. Symptoms include headache, vomiting, visual impairment, hemiplegia, dysarthria, sensory processing disorder, etc.

Spinal cord injury

External wound including fracture or luxation in spinal column can cause injury to the spinal cord. Flaccid paralysis, perceptual dysfunction, bladder-rectal dysfunction, bedsore, etc. may result.

Terms for Surgery and Treatment

Anesthesia

A medical technique to suppress sensation using drugs, used to induce temporary state of unconsciousness and eliminate pain.

Myelography

A radiographic examination using a contrast medium to evaluate pathological condition of the subarachnoid space and the spinal canal.

Epidural block

This is a technique to induce anesthesia to block pain by injecting substances into the epidural space.

Spinal block

This is a technique to induce local anesthesia by injecting substances into the subarachnoid space.

Regional anesthesia

The substance to induce anesthesia is applied directly to the region only.

Terms for Test and Intervention

Lumbar puncture

This is a method to extract cerebrospinal fluid directly through an inserted needle.

ANS function test

Autonomic nervous system function test is performed using deep breath and Valsalva maneuver on diabetic complications.

Electroencephalography (EEG)

The measurement and recording of electrical activities in the brain for diagnostic purposes.

Electronystagmography (ENG)

A diagnostic test to record involuntary movements of the eye caused by a condition known as nystagmus.

Caloric test

As a test of vestibulo-ocular reflex, water warmer or cooler than the body temperature is injected into the external auditory canal, to evaluate balancing and spatial orientation functions.

Deep tendon reflex (DTR)

Testing for response to external physical stimulations, this is used to determine the integrity of the spinal cord and the peripheral nervous system.

Babinski's reflex

Testing for anomaly of motor nerves in the cerebral cortex, to see if the big toe bends up and other toes fan out when the sole is rubbed in the anterior direction.

Magnetic resonance imaging (MRI)

A technique that uses nuclear magnetic resonance to form cross-sectional images of the human body, reconstructed with computer processing of differential measurements of signals from various tissues.

Computed tomography (CT)

Unlike simple X-ray imaging, CT provides tomographic (cross-sectional sliced) images of the human body using a moving cylindrical test bed and computer reconstruction.

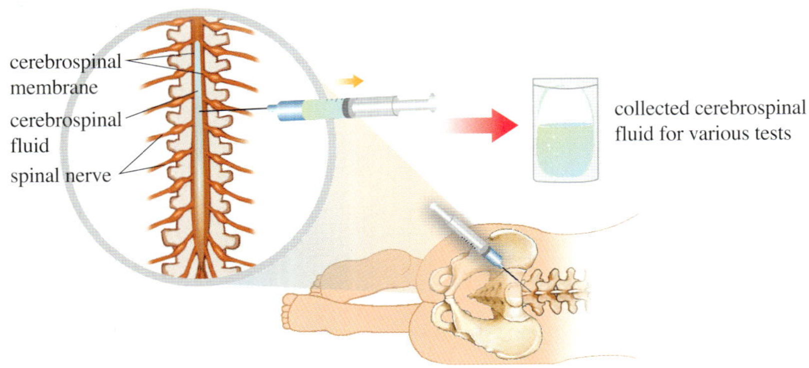

Figure 9-8 Collection of cerebrospinal fluid through lumbar puncture

Analysis and Meaning of Key Terms

Roots

Term	Term Analysis	Meaning
neur/o :		nerve
neuron [nurɑːn]	-on = unit	a cell of the nervous system that transmits signals
neuroglia [njuərɑ́gliə]	-glia = glue, supporting tissue	glial cells, non-neuronal cells that maintain homeostasis, form myelin, and provide support and protection for neurons in the brain and peripheral nervous system
neurotransmitter [nuroutrænzmi-tə(r)]	transmitter = signal relaying agent	a substance that transmits nerve impulses across a synapse

Term	Term Analysis	Meaning
gli/o :		glue, glial cell
glia [gláiə, glí:ə]		supporting tissue intermingled with the essential elements of nervous tissue especially in the brain, spinal cord, and ganglia
glioma [glaióumə]	-oma = tumor	tumor of glial cells
gangli/o :		collection of nerve cell bodies
ganglion [gæŋgliən]	-on = unit	a mass of nerve tissue containing cell bodies of neurons external to the brain or spinal cord
cerebr/o :		cerebrum
cerebrovascular [səribrouvǽskjulər]	-vascular = of blood vessels	involving cerebrum and blood vessels in it
cerebral cortex [səribrəl kɔrteks]	cortex = outer layer of an internal organ	the convoluted surface layer of gray matter of the cerebrum that functions chiefly in coordination of sensory and motor information
cerebrum [səribrəm]		the largest part of the brain in the upper part of the skull which is divided into the two cerebral hemispheres
cerebell/o :		cerebellum
cerebellum [serəbeləm]		the part of the brain between the cerebrum and midbrain
cerebellar [sèrəbélər]	-ar = pertaining to	pertaining to the cerebellum
cortic/o :		cortex, outer region
corticospinal [kɔ́:rtikouspainl]	spinal = pertaining to the spine	pertaining to the cerebral cortex and the spinal cord
cortical [kɔ́:rtikəl]	-al = pertaining to	pertaining to the cortex
thalam/o :		thalamus
thalamocortical [θǽləmokɔ́:rtikəl]	cortical = pertaining to the cortex	relating to, or connecting the thalamus and the cerebral cortex
ventricul/o :		ventricle, a small cavity
ventriculostomy [véntrikjulástɔmi]	-stomy = creating an opening	neurosurgical procedure to open the ventricle of the brain to drain cerebrospinal fluid

Term	Term Analysis	Meaning
medull/o :		medulla, soft inner part
medulla oblongata [mədʌ́ləɑ́blɔːŋɡɑ́tə]		the lower portion of the brainstem
pont/o :		bridge
pons [pɑ́nz]		a band of nerve fibers within the brainstem, between midbrain and medulla oblongata
dur/o :		dura mater
subdural [sʌbdjúrəl]	sub = under	under the dura mater layer
epidural [epidurəl]	epi = above	above the dura mater layer

Suffixes

Term	Term Analysis	Meaning
-asthenia :		weakness (especially of muscle)
myasthenia [màiəsθíːniə]	my/o = muscle	an autoimmune neuromuscular disease, with progressive weakness and fatigue of voluntary muscles
-trophy :		nourishment, development
atrophy [ætrəfi]	a- = not, lacking	physiological process of reabsorption and breakdown of tissues
-esthesia :		nervous sensation
anesthesia [æ̀nəsθíːʒə]	an- = not, lacking	loss of sensation to touch or pain, or intentional administration to induce it for surgical procedure
hypoesthesia [haipouesθíːʒə]	hypo- = below normal	partial loss of tactile sensation, numbness
hyperesthesia [haipə(r)esθíːʒə]	hyper- = excessive	unusual or pathological sensitivity of the skin or of a particular sense
paresthesia [pæ̀rəsθíːʒə, -ʒiə]	par- = abnormal	a sensation of burning, prickling, itching, or tingling of the skin, with no obvious cause

Term	Term Analysis	Meaning
-plegia :		paralysis, palsy
diplegia [daiplí:dʒə]	di- = two	paralysis that affects symmetrically opposed parts of the body
hemiplegia [hèmiplí:dʒiə]	hemi- = half	total or partial paralysis of one side of the body
monoplegia [mɑ:noupli:dʒiə]	mono- = one, single	paralysis of a single limb
paraplegia [pærəplí:dʒə]	para- = beside, abnormal, alongside of	paralysis of the lower half of the body with involvement of both legs
tetraplegia [tétrəplí:dʒiə]	tetra- = four	paralysis of all four limbs (= quadriplegia)

Abbreviations

Abbreviation	Full Term	Meaning
ALS	amyotrophic lateral sclerosis	neurodegenerative disorder inducing muscle stiffness, weakness and atrophy
TBI	traumatic brain injury	brain injury caused by external force
CVA	cerebrovascular accident	stroke, loss of brain function when blood supply to the brain is interrupted
MS	multiple sclerosis	disease of the nervous system that causes the gradual loss of muscle control
CNS	central nervous system	the part of nervous system comprising the brain, brainstem and spinal cord
PNS	peripheral nervous system	the part of nervous system which is not the central nervous system
CSF	cerebrospinal fluid	water-like fluid in and around the brain and spine, acting as a cushion
CT	computed tomography	three-dimensional radiography constructed by computer from a series of cross-sectional images
MRI	magnetic resonance imaging	computerized images of internal body tissues based on nuclear magnetic resonance
PD	Parkinson's disease	chronic neurological disorder resulting in lack of control over movement, poor balance and coordination
PET	positron emission tomography	metabolic imaging technique, detecting positron's activity from injected substances

Exercises

1. Write the meaning of the following medical terms.

① analgesia — loss of the ability to feel pain

② neuralgia — a sharp pain felt along the length of a nerve

③ anesthesia — a method or process to prevent sensation, used to eliminate pain

④ hyperesthesia — unusual or pathological sensitivity of the skin or of a particular sense

⑤ paresthesia — a sensation of burning, prickling, itching, or tingling of the skin, with no obvious cause

⑥ hemiplegia — total or partial paralysis of one side of the body due to brain damage

⑦ paraplegia — paralysis (inability to move) of the lower half of the body brain damage

⑧ epilepsy — neurological disorder causing seizures, inability to control movements and blackouts

⑨ multiple sclerosis — a disease of the nervous system that causes the gradual loss of muscle control

⑩ stroke — loss of brain function when the blood supply to the brain is suddenly interrupted

2. Write the full term for the following abbreviations.

① PET positron emission tomography

② PD Parkinson's disease

③ MRI magnetic resonance imaging

④ CT computed tomography

⑤ CSF cerebrospinal fluid

⑥ PNS peripheral nervous system

⑦ CNS central nervous system

⑧ CVA cerebrovascular accident

⑨ TBI traumatic brain injury

⑩ ALS amyotrophic lateral sclerosis (Lou Gehrig's disease)

3. Write the medical term for each of the following diseases in the nervous system.

① a condition in which abnormal amount of cerebrospinal fluid is accumulated hydrocephalus

② brain disease causing dementia in people as they grow old Alzheimer's disease

③ neurological disorder with abnormal cerebral electric signals causing convulsions epilepsy

④ damage to the insulating covers of nerve cells in the central nervous system causing disruption in nervous system's functions multiple sclerosis

⑤ inflammation of the protective membranes covering the central nervous system meningitis

⑥ abnormal growth of the brain tissue or the meninges brain tumor

⑦ temporary loss of brain function from mild traumatic brain injury, which can be recovered in 24 hours (cerebral) concussion

⑧ loss of brain function due to cerebral infarction or hemorrhage stroke

4. Spell the following medical terms correctly.

① neren	neuron
② meniingitis	meningitis
③ ancephalitis	encephalitis
④ cerebelum	cerebellum
⑤ cerebral coltex	cerebral cortex
⑥ cortikospinal	corticospinal
⑦ fons	pons
⑧ encephalemalacia	encephalomalacia
⑨ genglion	ganglion
⑩ vantricle	ventricle

5. Write terms for organ names in the following figure.

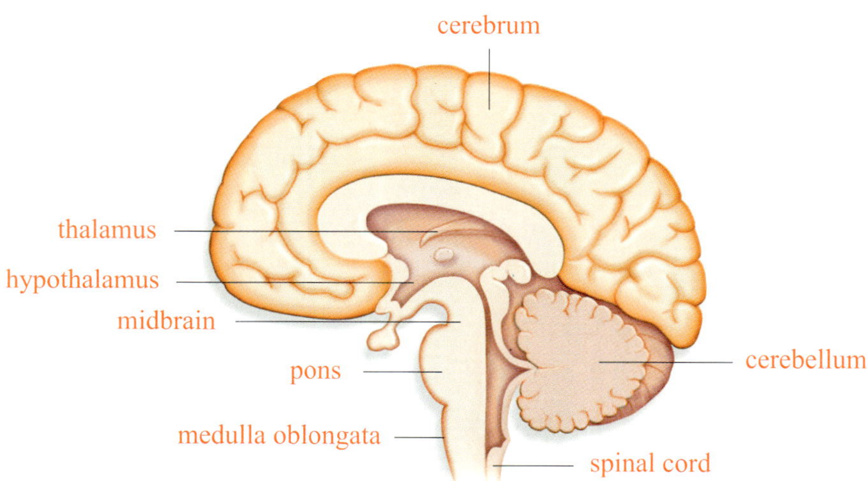

Chapter 10

Eye and Ear

Chapter Contents

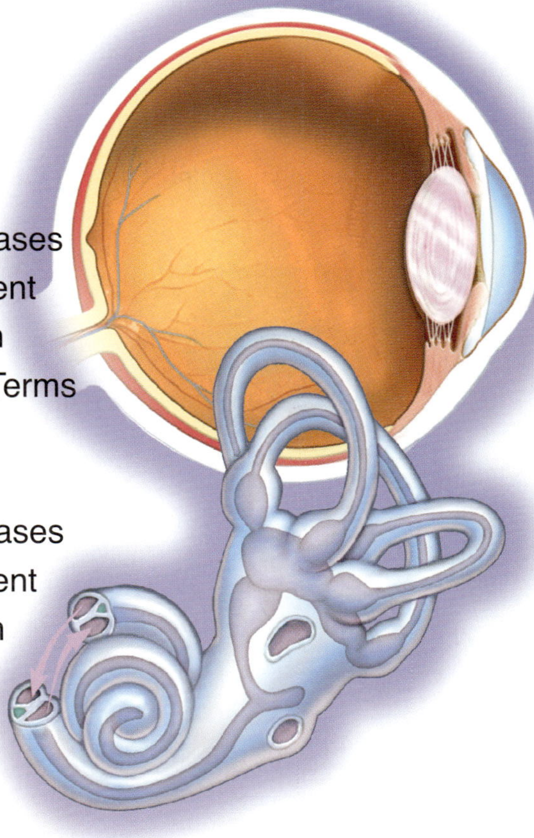

- Understanding the Eye
- Anatomical Terms
- Terms for Symptoms and Diseases
- Terms for Surgery and Treatment
- Terms for Test and Intervention
- Analysis and Meaning of Key Terms
- Understanding the Ear
- Anatomical Terms
- Terms for Symptoms and Diseases
- Terms for Surgery and Treatment
- Terms for Test and Intervention
- Analysis and Meaning of Key Terms
- Abbreviations
- Exercises

Learning Objectives

- Illustrate structure, function and location of the outer and inner parts of the eye.
- Pronounce, analyze and define medical terms related to the eye.
- Explain diagnostic and surgical terms for the eye.
- Illustrate structure and function of the ear.
- Pronounce, analyze and define medical terms related to the ear.
- Explain diagnostic and surgical terms for the ear.
- Learn abbreviations related to the eye and the ear.

Understanding the Eye

The eye as an organ refracts the incoming light to focus and collect it onto the sensitive light receptor to form an image. The receptor as a sensor of the light converts the image to nerve impulses and transmits them through the optic nerve and optic tract to the occipital lobe of the cerebral cortex for visual interpretation.

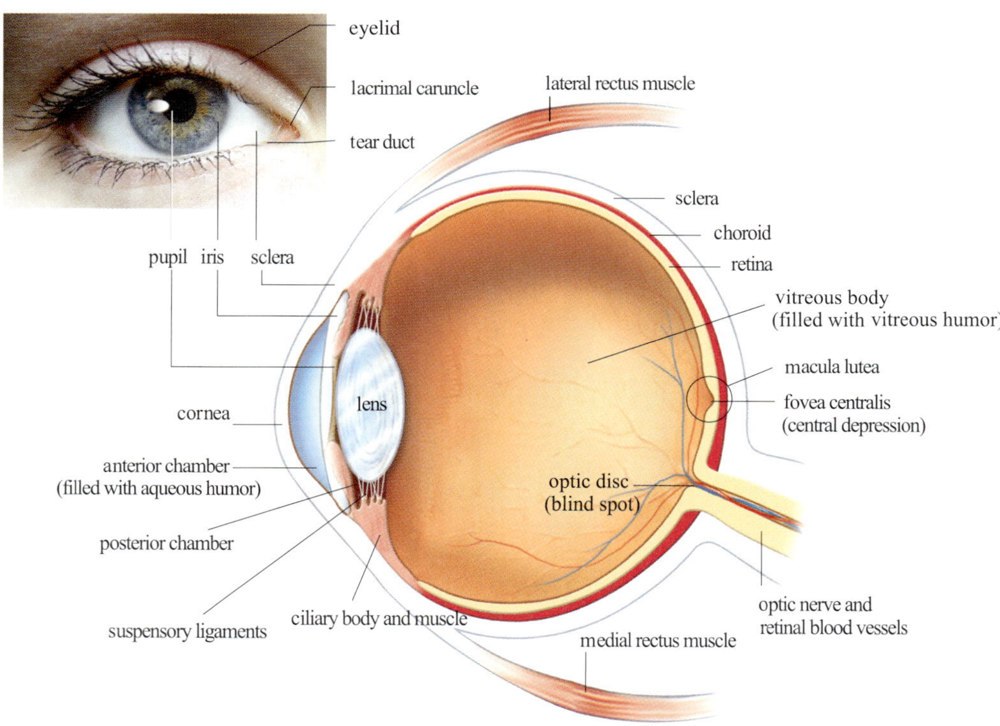

Figure 10-1
Structure of the eye

The eyes are a pair of special sensory organs governed by four cranial nerves (optic nerve, oculomotor nerve, trochlear nerve, abducens nerve) encased in an orbital fatty layer.

The eye is composed of the inner eye — the eyeball, and the outer eye — the surrounding facial structure and muscles that protect and control the eyeball. The axial length of an adult's eye is about 24 mm. The volume of the eyeball is about 6.5 cc. The wall of the eyeball is constructed with fibrous membrane in the outer layer, vascular membrane in the middle, and the inner membrane layer.

Anatomical Terms

Outer Eye

The outer eye surrounding the inner eye consists of : the orbital cavity, the hollow space that encloses and protects the eye; the six extraocular muscles attached to the sclera to control the eyeball's various movements, namely, superior rectus, inferior rectus, lateral rectus, medial rectus, superior oblique, inferior oblique; the eyelids that protect the eye from excessive light, dust and physical contact; the conjunctival membrane lining the inner surface of the eyelid; and the lacrimal apparatus which cleans and lubricates the eye. The lacrimal gland produces tear that is distributed through the lacrimal duct. The used tear is collected at the lacrimal punctum and drained through the nasolacrimal duct.

Inner Eye

The outer layer of the eyeball consists of membranes of dense fibrous connective tissues. This layer protects and keeps the contents of the eyeball in shape. The cornea, covering 1/6 of the spherical surface of the eyeball, is clear and responsible for refracting the incoming light. The sclera, covering the rest of the surface, is made of a hard connective tissue of white color.

The middle layer is called uvea which covers the inner surface of the sclera.

It contains considerable amount of melanin pigments and appear dark brown.

It consists of : the choroid which is adhered to the retinal pigmented epithelial layer and supplies nutrients to the eye; the ciliary body, located anterior to the choroid, that accommodates the lens to focus the incoming light; and the iris that represents the color of the eye and includes the pupil that control the amount of the incoming light.

The inner layer is the retina made of multi-fold nerve tissue cells, consisting of rod cells that function in dim light levels lacking color sensitivity, and cone cells responsible for central vision and color sensation in relatively bright light.

Memory key

- The eyeball consists of the outer layer (cornea, sclera), middle layer (choroid, ciliary body, iris) and inner layer (retina with rod cells and cone cells).

Orbit

The orbit is a conical bony cavity that functions as the socket for the eye.

Eyeball

The eyeball is a spherical organ responsible for vision, socketed in the orbit.

Eyelid

The eyelid is a thin fold of skin to cover and protect the anterior part of the eyeball. It consists of a connective tissue that contains a thin sheet of fibrous tissue that borders with a mucus membrane.

Canthus

Either end of the crevice between the upper and lower eyelids, namely, medial and lateral canthi.

Tarsus

The cartilaginous connective tissue plate of about 2.5 cm long, forming the basic structure of the eyelid.

Eyebrow

An eyebrow is the short hair grown on the eyelid or its edge. It grows along the protuberance of the upper part of the orbit in the frontal bone.

Eyelash

Light hair of about 10 mm long, grown in 2~3 rows on the edge of the upper and lower eyelids.

Memory key

- Eyelash hair count is 100~150 on the upper, and 70~80 on the lower eyelids. The eyelashes are so sensitive as to detect foreign particles such as dust and trigger closing both the eyelids to protect the eyeball.

Conjunctiva

A thin membrane that covers inner surface of the eyelid and the exposed area of the eyeball. There are a network of capillary blood vessels, lymphatic vessels and sensory nerve fibers.

Cornea

The cornea is the outermost wall of the eyeball, through which light passes. It is built of 5 transparent layers of fibrous tissue. The light passes the cornea and refracts itself to form image on the retina that functions as the film of the eye.

Sclera

The sclera is the outermost layer that covers 5/6 of the eyeball surface and protects the eyeball. It is made of hard and sleek white connective tissue. The sclera of a young eye appears bluish white, however, it turns yellowish with jaundice.

Uvea

Uvea is the middle layer of the eyeball that includes a thin and soft membrane comprising the iris, choroid and ciliary body.

Choroid

Choroid is the thin middle layer between the sclera that covers posterior 5/6 of the eyeball and the pigmented layer of the retina.

Iris

The iris is a round, thin membrane between the cornea and the lens, centered around the pupil. The size of the pupil is controlled by contraction or expansion of the iris to adjust the amount of incoming light. The tissue layer of the iris is rich in pigments. The color of pigmentation and the amount of blood vessels determine apparent color of the iris.

Pupil

The pupil is the round, dark area at the center of the iris, behind the cornea and anterior chamber, in front of the lens. Stimulation by light, emotional state, input from autonomous nervous system influence controlling of the muscular fiber of the iris for contraction or expansion, which changes the size of the pupil accordingly.

Ciliary body

Ciliary body exists in the space between the cornea and the lens to seal the vitreous humour, while the attached muscles control the thickness of the lens.

Crystalline lens

Directly behind the pupil, between the posterior chamber and the vitreous humour is the transparent elastic convex lens. It accommodates the angle of refraction depending on the distance from the objects in sight, and produce real image on the retina.

Retina

As a receptor of light, retina is a lining of light-sensing nerve network that generates visual impulses from the image formed on it and transmits them through the cranial nerve to the brain.

Macula

Near the center of the retina is a yellow oval spot of about 3 mm in diameter. There are concentrated layers of ganglion cells responsible for more detailed central vision than the area around it.

Anterior chamber

The space behind the cornea and in front of the iris. The space behind the iris in front of the lens is called the posterior chamber. Both chambers are filled with aqueous humour.

Aqueous humour

Aqueous humour that fills the anterior and posterior chambers helps regulate eye pressure and feed the eyeball with nutrients.

Vitreous

The space behind the lens and enclosed by the retina, filled with vitreous humour. Also called vitreous chamber or vitreous cavity.

Vitreous humour

Vitreous humour is the soft viscous liquid that fills the space behind the crystalline lens. Its transparency is essential in keeping clear vision.

Optic nerve

A pair of cranial nerves that transmits optic impulses. Nerve fibers connected to multipolar neurons in the ganglion cell layers in the retina are bundled to form a pair of optic nerves.

Optic tract

A pair of conical nerve fiber bundles that relay optic impulses from the optic chiasm to the lateral geniculate body around and behind the optic hypothalamus.

Lacrimal gland

A gland in the upper, outer portion of the orbit for each eye in the frontal bone, that secrete tear to keep the conjunctiva and cornea moist and free from infection. It is shaped and sized like an almond and connected to several lacrimal ducts running to the conjunctiva. The tear is a slightly alkaline and saline solution.

Lacrimal sac

Lacrimal sac is the upper dilated end of the nasolacrimal duct, and is lodged in a deep groove formed by the lacrimal bone and the frontal process of the maxilla. The oval shaped sac is about 13 mm long. The lower end is connected to the nasolacrimal duct. The lacrimal sac is filled with tear produced in the lacrimal gland flown through lacrimal ducts.

Lacrimal duct

A pair of ducts for the tear to flow through from the lacrimal gland to the sac.

Terms for Symptoms and Diseases

Amblyopia

Amblyopia is the condition of or a person with weak vision, while the patient may not have any underlying cause or disease.

Memory key

- There are several types of amblyopia: congenital amblyopia with no known cause; strabismic amblyopia, amblyopia due to severe refractive anomaly (near- or farsightedness, astigmatism); anisometropia (unequal refractive error between the two eyes), among others.

Aniridia

A rare congenital condition characterized by the absence of the iris, usually in both eyes and accompanied by other anomalies. The heredity is of dominant type. Symptoms include apparently large pupil, fear of sunlight, visual impairment, etc.

Aphakia

This is a condition of missing crystalline lens in the eye, in which the incoming light is refracted only by the cornea. It may be congenital or due to injury, but many are due to removal of the lens for cataract surgery.

Arcus senilis

A faint gray or whitish ring appearing in the corneal margin around the iris usually occurring in elderly people. It results from cholesterol deposits in the corneal stroma, or by hyaline degeneration (hyalinosis of the corneal stroma).

Epiphora

Tear overflow resulting from stricture of the nasolacrimal duct, or excessive tear production due to irritation.

Exophthalmos

An abnormal protrusion of the eyeball from its socket (the orbit). Major causes

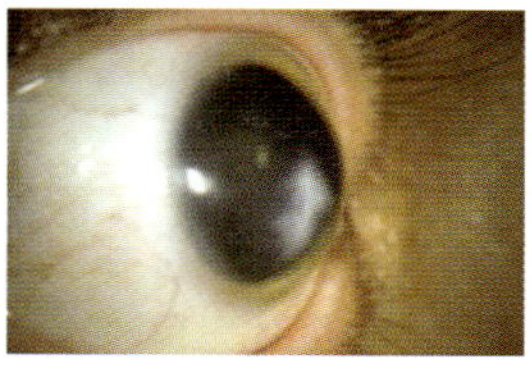

Figure 10-2
Exophthalmos

include overgrowth of thyroid or Grave's disease, endocrine dysfunction, extraocular muscle palsy, skull deformation and abnormal increase in the volume of material in the orbit. Myopia is occasionally related to this condition.

Hypopyon

A contagious disease in the cornea related to infection of the iris or ciliary body, resulting in collection of pus in the anterior chamber of the eye.

Miosis

Miosis is a term for the state of constricted pupil, down to size of 2 mm in diameter or less. Pupil size can be decreased with miotic drug or naturally by the iris sphincter muscle when gazing on a very near object or when bright light is present.

Mydriasis

Mydriasis is a state of dilated pupil resulting from iris dilator muscle contraction. The pupil becomes larger to adjust and compensate for darker incoming light.

Nyctalopia

Night blindness, the inability to see objects clearly in dim light. This is due to dysfunctional rod cells in the retina.

Memory key

- Nyctalopia can be caused by lack of vitamin A, retinal pigmentosa, chorioretinitis, vascular disorder, toxicosis, etc.

Nystagmus

A condition of unconscious and involuntary, rapid and rhythmic eye movement, which is uncontrolled and contrary to the patient's will.

Memory key

- Nystagmus is usually rapid and repeated up and down or lateral eye movement.

Papilledema

Congestion of the optic disc, which can be seen in the ocular fundus through funduscopy, can be caused by the rise in intracranial pressure, uncontrolled hypertension or thrombosis leading to central retinal vein occlusion.

Photophobia

Unusually sensitive reaction to or fear of light, especially when changing from an area of moderate lighting to a bright place. This condition is characteristic of patients with iris disorders such as glaucoma or iritis. Sometimes there is no other reason than psychological fear of bright light.

Scotoma

Loss of partial area of vision in one or both eyes, due to scintillating island of blind spot.

Xerophthalmia

A condition of dryness of the cornea and conjunctival membrane, caused by anomaly in mucus secretion by goblet cells.

Blepharitis

An eye condition characterized by chronic inflammation of the eyelid's inner skin, the meibomian cysts and glands.

Conjunctivitis

Inflammation of the conjunctiva resulting in eye congestion and discharge of unusual amount of rheum and tear. This can be caused by bacterial or viral infection, and allergic reaction due to environmental condition.

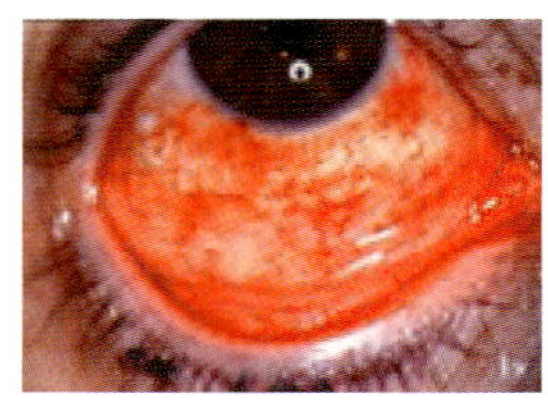

Figure 10-3
Conjunctivitis

Keratitis

Inflammation of the cornea caused by systemic infectious disease like tuberculosis and syphilis, local infectious disease like trachoma and conjunctivitis, or environmental factors like physical and chemical irritation.

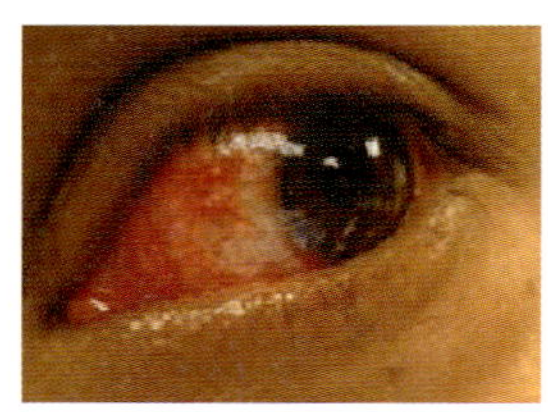

Figure 10-4 Keratitis

Choroiditis

Inflammation of the choroid which will affect the retina and the vitreous body can lead to poor eyesight. When retina inflammation accompanies it becomes chorioretinitis; when inflammation of the iris and ciliary body is accompanied it becomes uveitis. Subjective symptoms include vitreous floaters (muscae volitantes) as well as impaired eyesight. Tuberculosis, syphilis, viral infection or allergic reactions can cause this condition.

Scleritis

Inflammation of the sclera that can lead to fatal loss of eyesight.

Uveitis

The uvea, consisting of iris, ciliary body and choroid, is a set of tissues rich in blood vessels, which makes it subject to inflammations.

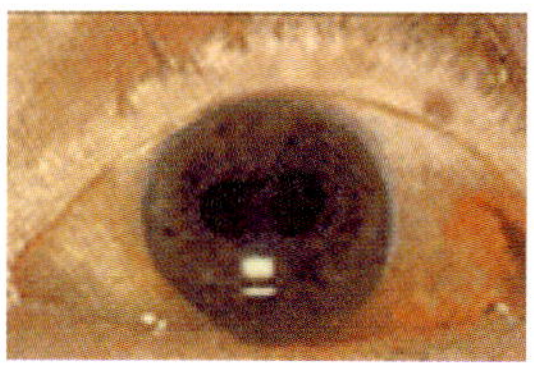

Figure 10-5 Iritis

Iritis

Inflammation of the iris will develop into iridocyclitis since the iris is near the ciliary body. Subjective symptoms include poor eyesight, photophobia, tear and pain. Objective symptoms include congestion in periphery of the cornea, turbidity of the aqueous humour, swelling of the iris, keratic precipitate and miosis.

Retinitis

Inflammation of the retina is mostly caused by systemic disease such as renal disease, diabetes, syphilis and tuberculosis, and may lead to hemorrage. Eyesight will worsen and the retinal image becomes clouded and distorted.

Dacryoadenitis

Inflammation of the lacrimal glands.

Dacryocystitis

Inflammation of the lacrimal sac, due to blockage of the lacrimal duct and bacterial infection in the stale fluid.

Optic neuritis

Inflammation of the optic nerve that may cause decline of eyesight. The affected region may start at the ganglion cells in the retina through the tract to the junction of optic nerve fibers.

Blepharoptosis

Drooping of the eyelid due to malfunctioning levator palpebrae muscle. The eyelid is spread flat with no folds. Possible causes are of congenital, nervous, muscular and injury-related.

Cataract

Visual impairment due to clouding of the crystalline lens of the eye. The iris looks hazy which can be seen through the pupil. It is painless but the eyesight becomes progressively worse depending on the location and the degree of turbidity. It is related to patient's age, exposure to radiation, systemic disease like diabetes, uveitis, long term exposure to ultraviolet rays, etc.

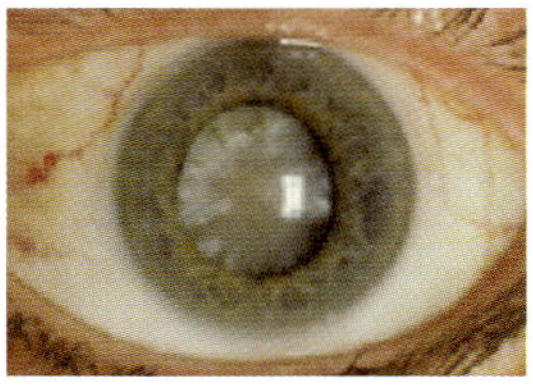

Figure 10-6 Cataract

Diabetic retinopathy

A complication arising in the retinal blood vessels following untreated chronic diabetes. The disorderly microvessels cause damage in the retina leading to loss of vision. The severity is highly related to the term length of diabetes. Microaneurysm, retinal bleeding, pus discharge, diabetic macular edema, retinal and papillary angiogenesis, desmoplasia, vitreous body bleeding, retinal detachment, etc. may result.

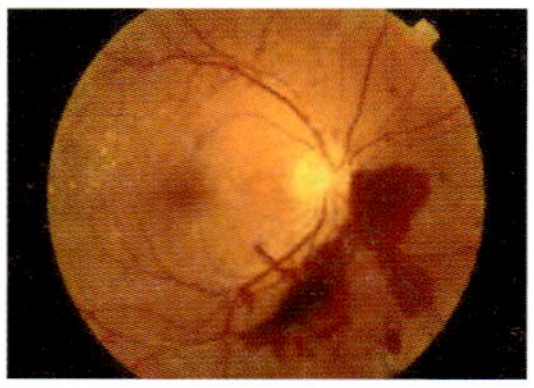

Figure 10-7 Diabetic retinopathy

Hordeolum

An acute infection of sebaceous glands of the eyelid, of external and internal types.

Glaucoma

Glaucoma is a serious eye disorder caused by excessive ocular pressure related to increased fluid pressure (aqueous humour). The high pressure induces optic nerve damage and eye pain. The fluid is a lymphatic fluid supplying nutrients to the eye tissues and must keep adequate ocular pressure by properly discharging through the anterior chamber angle. Essential glaucoma can occur with unknown cause, while secondary glaucoma can occur due to other eye diseases like iritis, intraocular bleeding etc.

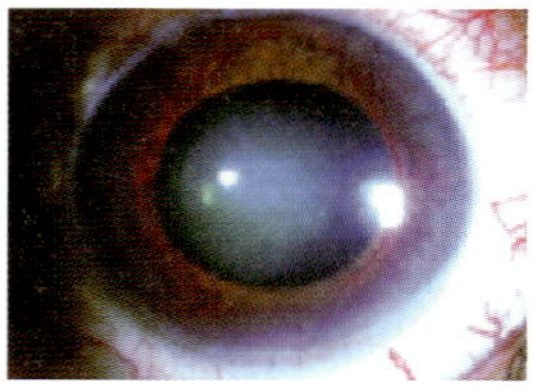

Figure 10-8 Glaucoma

Entropion

The condition in which the edge of the eyelid is folded in toward the eyeball irritating it, possibly resulting in corneal ulcer, scar, bleeding and unwanted tear discharge.

Trichiasis

The condition in which entropion of the eyelid and/or inner growth of the eyelash causes blepharitis, irritation of the cornea and conjunctiva.

Ectropion

The condition in which the edge of the eyelid is folded inside out, causing undue aging and atrophy of the conjunctival tissue of the eyelid and blockage of nasolacrimal duct.

Pterygium

An abnormal triangular mass of tissue grown on the cornea in the medial canthus of the eye obstructing vision, usually occurring in old age. Its apex connects to the cornea, and the tissue mass grows on the sclera, with the base attached to the conjunctiva.

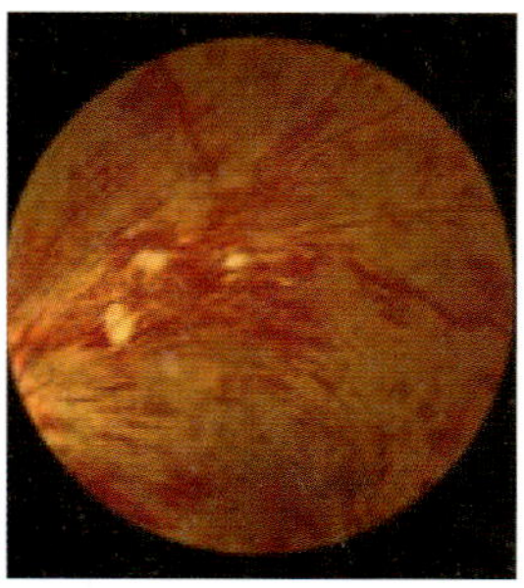

Figure 10-9
Retinal detachment

Retinal detachment

Peeling of the retina in the posterior part of the eye from the choroid, occurring with lack of vitreous humour. Retina floating in the vitreous chamber is a cause for severe vision disorder.

Retinoblastoma

A congenital, rapidly growing malignant tumor that develops from blastocytes of a retina, which may be seen as whitish growth through the pupil. It is the most common malignant tumor of the eye in children under 3 years old.

Trachoma

A chronic infection of the conjunctiva and cornea, causing photophobia, pain and excessive tear production.

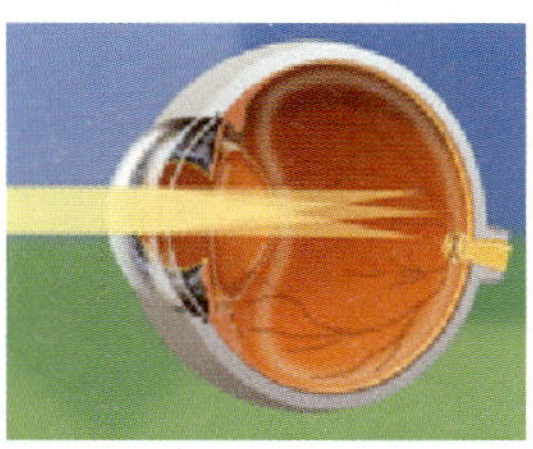

Figure 10-10
Astigmatism

Astigmatism

Blurred vision due to defect in the cornea or the lens, where incoming light rays do not meet at a focal point. If left uncorrected with eyeglasses or contact lenses, the patient will experience visual discomfort and fatigue.

Diplopia

Diplopia, commonly known as double vision, is the simultaneous perception of two images of a single object. Binocular diplopia is the result of misalignment of two eyes relative to each other due to strabismus. Monocular diplopia is double vision when viewing with only one eye, which typically indicates certain disorder in the cornea or the lens.

Hemianopsia

Blindness in half the visual field of either or both eyes, usually on one side of the vertical midline.

Emmetropia

Normal vision. Refraction of parallel light (i.e. from objects of infinite distance) without accommodation of the lens results in clear image on the central area on the retina.

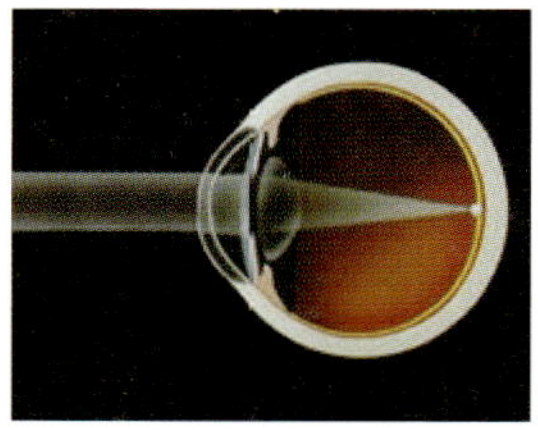

Figure 10-11
Emmetropia

Hyperopia

A disorder of vision where the eye focuses images behind the retina. Parallel light rays converge behind the retina when the lens is not accommodated. Vision is blurred when looking at a near object. This condition is due to either insufficient light refraction by the cornea and the lens or short distance between the cornea and the retina. The vision can be corrected with convex lens.

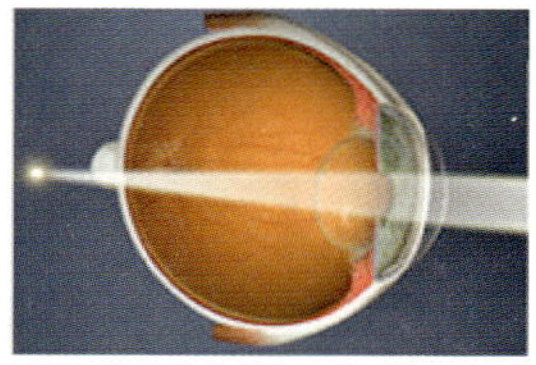

Figure 10-12
Hyperopia

Presbyopia

Presbyopia is impaired vision due to diminished flexibility of crystalline lens for people of old age. Typically, people with normal eyes start to realize this condition in the age of 40's. The lens cannot accommodate (thicken) enough to focus images at the retina. The least distance of clear vision with maximum lens accommodation is called near point distance. If near point distance exceeds 40 cm, it is presbyopia, which is similar to hyperopia.

Myopia

Without lens accommodation, parallel incoming lights focus at a point in front of the retina. Therefore, the person can have clear vision only for near objects.

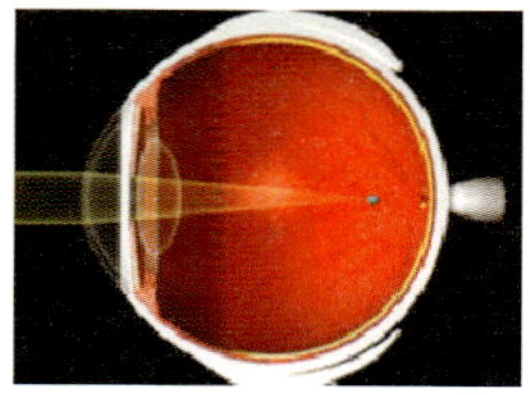

Figure 10-13 Myopia

Memory key

- Refractive myopia is attributed to the excessive refractive power of the cornea or the lens while the eye's axial length is normal. Axial myopia is attributed to excessive axial length of the eye with normal refractive power.

Strabismus

Eyes are not properly aligned with each other to focus on an object. Paretic strabismus is due to paralysis of one or more extraocular muscles, while nonparetic strabismus is due to other cause. This condition is classified according to the direction of slant as follows :

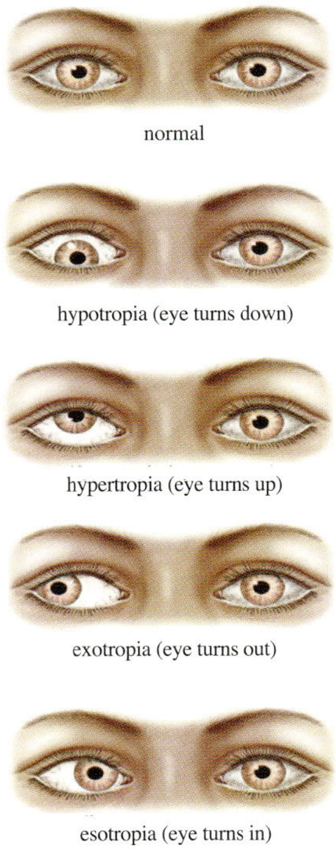

Figure 10-14
Hypertropia

Esotropia

Visual axis of one or both eyes are deviated inward. Cross-eyed condition.

Exotropia

Visual axis of one or both eyes are deviated outward.

Hypotropia

Visual axis of one eye is lower than the other, fixating eye.

Hypertropia

Visual axis of one eye is higher than the other, fixating eye.

Terms for Surgery and Treatment

Cataract surgery

When vision is impaired due to the lens that has become cloudy, the lens is replaced with an artificial intraocular lens. Currently practiced methods include phacoemulsification and extracapsular cataract extractions.

Blepharectomy

Excision of a part of the eyelid to change its appearance.

Blepharoplasty

Plastic surgery on the eyelid to restore the original shape of the eyelid and eyebrow, usually for patients with blepharoptosis.

Canthoplasty

Plastic surgery on the medial or lateral canthus.

Cyclodialysis

The creation of a passage between anterior chamber of the eye and the suprachoroidal space such that the aqueous humour may filter out and reduce pressure in cases of glaucoma.

Keratoplasty

Making incision and grafting or transplantation of the cornea in the opaque part.

Corneal transplant

Replacing the cloudy cornea with a clear one from a donor.

Dacryoadenectomy

Surgical removal or a lacrimal gland.

Dacryocystectomy

Surgical removal of a part of the lacrimal sac.

Dacryocystostomy

Surgical creation of an opening to a lacrimal sac.

Enucleation

Surgical removal of the eyeball with loss of vision to remove tumor and pain.

Iridectomy

Surgical removal of a part of the iris. It is performed frequently to reduce the intraocular pressure, to enlarge an abnormally small pupil or to treat closed-angle glaucoma.

Keratocentesis

Piercing the cornea for a special purpose.

Sclerectomy

Surgical removal of a part of the sclera.

Vitrectomy

Surgical removal of the vitreous body when the matter has become cloudy and vision is impaired.

Terms for Test and Intervention

Funduscopy (Ophthalmoscopy)

A direct or indirect funduscope (or opthalmoscope) can be used to examine the fundus or the retina of the eye. This test is also used as an aid to choose corrective eyeglasses.

Tonometry

The temporary flattening or depression of the eyeball made by some light force is measured, as an indirect way to estimate the eye tension or pressure. Two major methods are indentation tonometry and applanation tonometry.

Visual acuity

Visual acuity is the ability to discern two separate points in sight. The angle made by the two points relative to the optical center of the eye is called the visual angle. The smallest visual angle determines visual acuity of the eye.

Visual acuity test

The international visual acuity chart is used to test for the minimum size of the object the eye can tell.

Visual field test

This is performed clinically by keeping the eye's gaze fixed and testing for the area of vision.

Visual field

Visual field is the range of vision obtained with an eye's gaze fixed at an axis of vision. Due to vision blocked by the nose and the cheek, the medial vision is narrower than the lateral vision. Size of visual field varies with color — starting from white, becoming narrower with blue, orange, green (narrowest).

Diopter

Diopter is a unit of measurement of the optical power of a lens, which is equal to the reciprocal of the focal length measured in meter. An eyeglass with 1 diopter has focal length of 1 meter. Convex lenses are assigned positive diopters, and concave lenses are assigned negative diopters.

Analysis and Meaning of Key Terms

Term	Term Analysis	Meaning
choroid/o :		**choroid layer**
choroidocyclitis [kɔ̀:rɔidousai-kláitis]	-itis = inflammation; cycl/o = ciliary body	an abnormal condition characterized by inflammation of the choroid and the ciliary processes
blephar/o :		**eyelid**
blepharitis [blèfərάitis]	-itis = inflammation	inflammation of the meibomian cyst and gland in the eyelid
blepharopexy [blèfərəpeksi]	-pexy = fixation	surgical fixation of the eyelid
macroblepharia [mǽkroublefar-iάə́ʳ]	macro- = large; -ia = condition	abnormal largeness of the eyelids
aque/o :		**water**
aqueous duct [éikwiəs dʌkt]	-ous = pertaining; duct = path	a pathway for body fluid to pass through
corne/o :		**cornea**
corneal abrasion [kɔ́:rniəl əbreiʒn]	-eal = pertaining to	loss of the surface epithelial layer of the cornea
core/o :		**pupil**
anisocoria [ænaisəkóuriə]	-ia = condition; an- = lacking; is/o= equal	unequal size of the pupils of the eye
corneosclera [kɔ̀:rəsklíərə]	scler/o = sclera, white of eye	the sclera and cornea of the eye
conjunctiv/o :		**conjunctiva (lines of eyelids)**
conjunctival sac [kəndʒʌŋktivάl sæk]	-al = pertaining to	the space enclosed by the conjunctiva and the eyelid
cycl/o :		**ciliary body**
cyclitis [saikláitis]	-itis = inflammation	inflammation of the ciliary body, which may induce irritation of the sclera

Term	Term Analysis	Meaning
dacry/o :		tears
dacryocystectomy [dækriousis-téktəmi]	cyst = sac -ectomy = excision	surgical excision of the lacrimal sac
lacrim/o :		tears, tear duct
lacrimotomy [lækrimάtəmi]	-tomy = incision	surgical incision into the lacrimal duct or sac
irid/o :		iris
iridoplegia [ìridəplí:dʒiə]	-plegia = paralysis	paralysis of the sphincter of the iris
iritis [airάtis]	-itis = inflammation	inflammation of the iris
kerat/o :		cornea (of eye or skin)
keratoconjunctivitis [kèrətoukəndʒʌŋk-tivàitis]	-itis = inflammation conjunctiv/o = conjunctiva	inflammation of the cornea and the conjunctiva
keratomycosis [kerətoumáikou-sis]	myc/o = fungus -osis = disease	fungal infection of the cornea
mydr/o :		being wide
mydriatic [midriǽtik]	-iatic = pertaining to	causing or involving dilation of the pupil
mydriasis [midriósis]	-iasis = disease condition	excessive or prolonged dilation of the pupil
mi/o :		being smaller or less
miotic [maiάtik]	-tic - pertaining to	an agent that causes miosis
miosis [maióusis]	-osis = disease condition	excessive smallness or contraction of the pupil
goni/o :		angle
goniometer [gòuniάmitə]	-meter = measuring device	a device used to measure the angle
ophthalm/o :		eye
ophthalmoscope [ɑfθǽlmaskoup]	-scope = viewing instrument	instrument for examining the interior of the eye
ophthalmology [ɑfθælmάlədʒi]	-logy = study of	study of the anatomy, functions, pathology and treatment of the eye

Term	Term Analysis	Meaning
ocul/o :		eye
oculomotor [àkjuləmóutər]	-motor = pertaining to motion	pertaining to the eyeball movement
palpebr/o :		eyelid
palpebral fissure [pǽlpəbrəl fíʃər]	-al = pertaining to; fissure = crack, gap	the opening between the upper and lower eyelids
opt/o :		vision
optic disc [ɑ́ptik disk]	-ic = pertaining to	circular area of the retina where optic nerve connects to it; blind spot
optician [aptíʃən]	-ician = specialist	specialist who makes or dispenses eyeglasses and contact lenses
optic papilla [ɑ́ptik pəpilə]	papill/o = nipple	optic disc, or the papillary protrusion on it
phak/o :		lens of eye
aphakia [əféikiə]	a- = lacking	the absence of the lens of the eye
phacomalacia [fækouməláʃia]	-ia = disease condition; -malacia = softening	softening of the eye lens due to soft cataract
pupill/o :		pupil
pupilloplegia [pəpíləriplíːdʒiə]	-plegia = paralysis	slowness or inability of the pupil react to light changes
retin/o :		retina
retinopathy [rètinɑ́pəθi]	-pathy = disease	disorder of the retina, non-inflammatory
retinopexy [rètinəpeksi]	-pexy = fixation	surgical correction of a detachment of the retina by forming chorioretinal adhesions
retinal [rètinəl]	-al = pertaining to	pertaining to the retina
retinal detachment [rètinəl ditǽtʃmənt]	detach- = separate	separation of the retina from the choroid
scler/o :		sclera (white of eye)
scleritis [sklìːrɑ́itis]	-it is = inflammation	inflammation of the sclera
vitre/o :		glass
vitreous cavity [vítriəs kǽvəti]	-ous = pertaining to	the space behind the lens filled with vitreous humour, the clear gel-like liquid
vitrectomy [vitréktəmi]	-ectomy = excision	surgical removal of some or all of the vitreous humour from the eye

Term	Term Analysis	Meaning
ton/o :		tension, pressure
tonometer [tounámitər]	-meter = measuring device	the instrument used to measure eyeball pressure
tonography [tounágrəfi]	-graphy = process or recording	measurement of the eyeball pressure
phot/o :		light
photosensitivity [fòutəsènsitíviti]		unusually high sensitivity or response to light, such as allergic reaction in the presence of sunlight
photocoagulation [fòutoukouæ̀gjul-èiʃən]	coagul/o = clotting; -ation = process	surgical procedure in which a diseased retinal tissue is treated using laser
photoallergy [fòutouǽlrdʒi]		allergy activated by light, such as photodermatitis
-opia :		vision condition
emmetropia [èmətróupiə]	emmetr/o = in due measure	normal eyesight
hyperopia [háipəróupiə]	hyper- = above, excessive	image is focused behind the retina; distant objects are seen better than the near
myopia [maiápiə]	my- = closing	image is focused in front of the retina; distant objects appear blurred and near objects are seen more clearly
amblyopia [æ̀mblióupiə]	ambly/o = dim, dull, blunt	dim or blurred vision in one or both eyes
diplopia [diplóupiə]	dipl/o = double	double vision, where one perceives two images for the same object
hemiopia [hèmióupiə]	hemi- = half	decreased vision or blindness in half the visual field in one or both eyes; hemianopsia
presbyopia [prèzbióupiə]	presby/o = old age	inability to focus on nearby objects due to ageing
-tropia :		state of turn
esotropia [èsətróupiə]	eso- = inward	strabismus in which one or both eyes deviate inwards
exotropia [èksoutróupiə]	exo- = outward	strabismus in which one or both eyes deviate outwards

Term	Term Analysis	Meaning
-tropia :		state of turn
hypertropia [háipətróupiə]	hyper- = above, excessive	strabismus in which one eye points upward
hypotropia [hàipətróupiə]	hypo- = below, deficient	strabismus in which one eye points downward
-tropion :		state of turn
entropion [entrάupiən]	en- = in, within	a condition in which of the eyelid folds inward
ectropion [ektrάpiən]	ec- = out, outside	a condition in which of the lower eyelid turns outward

Understanding the Ear

The ear is an organ that detects and processes sound. It also aids in physical balancing of the body. The ear can be divided into outer, middle and inner parts. It accepts auditory input, transforms it into nerve impulses and transmits them to the temporal lobe of the brain. Body balancing is detected by the labyrinth in the conic bone structure inside the temporal bone.

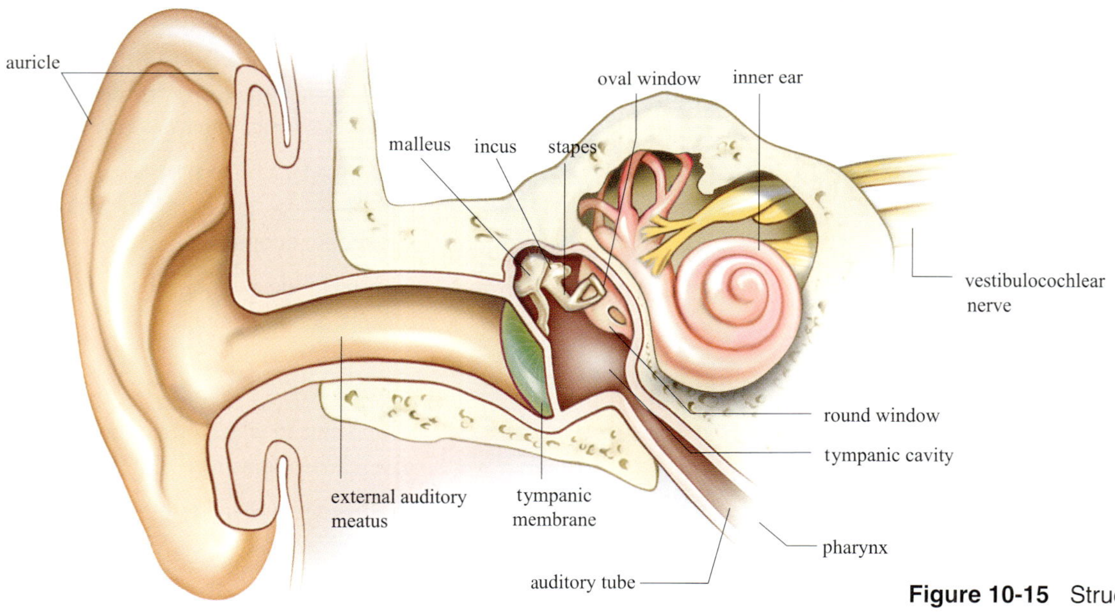

Figure 10-15 Structure of the ear

Anatomical Terms

Outer Ear

The outer ear gathers the sound waves and transmits them to the middle ear. It consists of the auricle (pinna), the external auditory meatus (ear canal) and the tympanic membrane (eardrum) which separates them from the middle ear. The tympanic membrane vibrates when the sound waves hit it, and the vibration is transmitted through the middle ear to the inner ear.

Memory key

- The outer ear consists of the auricle, the external auditory meatus and the tympanic membrane.

Auricle

The auricle is the part of the ear external to the head that gathers sound. It is grown out of the outer end of the auditory meatus, whose clamshell shape is maintained by a thin plate of elastic cartilage. The earlobe is filled with fatty tissue.

Cerumen

Cerumen (earwax) is a mixture of secretions from sweat glands, sebaceous glands and corneous separations from the epidermis.

Middle Ear

The middle ear is constructed with auditory ossicles including 3 little bones (malleus, incus, stapes) and elastic cartilage which cooperate in transforming sound waves received from the tympanic membrane to vibration of proper level and transmitting them to the inner ear.

The stapes in the middle ear vibrates the oval window between the middle ear and the inner ear, which in turn converts the vibration to electrical impulses recognized and interpreted by the brain. The air pressure differential caused by vibration of the tympanic membrane is moderated through air passage in the eustachian tube that connects the middle ear and the pharynx.

When infectious germs from the pharynx invades the eustachian tube, otitis media may occur which is a common threat to young children.

Memory key

- The middle ear consists of malleus, incus and stapes.

Tympanic cavity

Between the outer ear and the inner ear is the tympanic cavity, a part of the middle ear inside of the tympanic membrane. It is surrounded by the cranial bone and mucous membranes, and connected through the eustachian tube to the mucous membrane of the phayngeal lateral wall. In the cavity are a set of auditory ossicles, namely, malleus, incus and stapes.

Tympanic membrane

Commonly known as eardrum, the tympanic cavity is a thin, oval, translucent membrane located between the outer ear and the middle ear, at the inner end of the external auditory meatus. Its function is to transform sound waves to vibration, and transmit it through auditory ossicles to the inner ear.

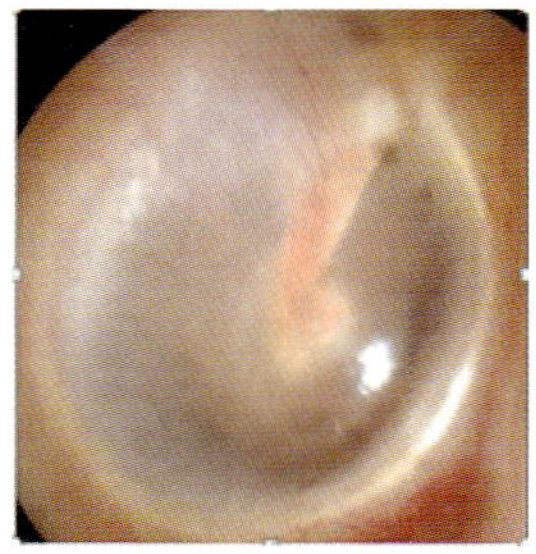

Figure 10-16
Tympanic membrane

Auditory ossicle

Auditory ossicles are a set of three tiny bones connected through joints in the middle ear : incus, stapes malleus.

Malleus

One of the three ossicles in the middle ear, shaped like a mallet (hammer). It is attached to the tympanic membrane and transmits sound vibration to the incus.

Incus

As the second bone of the ossicles in the middle ear, the incus relays sound vibration from the malleus to the stapes.

Stapes

As the third bone of the ossicles in the middle ear, the stapes relays sound vibration from the incus to the inner ear through the oval window.

Oval window

This is an oval opening in the wall surrounding the middle ear that is seen from the inner ear. The footplate of the stapes vibrates the oval window to transmit the sound vibration to the cochlea in the inner ear. The window directly faces the cochlear duct, where the resonance causes vibration of the lymphatic fluid in the cochlea, which in turn is recognized as sound input by the nervous system.

Round window

This is a round opening located inferior to and slightly larger than the oval window in the wall surrounding the middle ear.

Auditory tube (eustachian tube)

This is the canal connecting the middle ear and the rhinopharynx, composed of bone and cartilage, and lined with mucous membrane. The tympanic cavity is ventilated through this tube which equalizes the cavity air pressure.

Inner Ear

The inner ear, the innermost part of the ear, is the sensory organ responsible for sensing sound and physical balance of the body. It consists of the labyrinth, a hollow cavity in the temporal bone of the skull with a system of passages. The organ of Corti in the cochlear duct has sensitive hairy cells whose movements stimulate nerve cell fibers to generate auditory nerve impulses that in turn are transmitted to the temporal lobe of the brain. The semicircular canals are responsible for sensing body rotation, while the vestibular part senses transverse motion.

Memory key

- The inner ear consists of bony labyrinth and membranous labyrinth. The bony labyrinth contains perilymph (fluid) and include vestibule, semicircular canals and cochlea. The membranous labyrinth contains endolymph (fluid) and includes utricle, saccule, semicircular canals and cochlear duct.

Vestibule

The vestibule of the inner ear is the central part of the bony labyrinth as a small entrance cavity for the semicircular canals and the cochlea.

Labyrinth

Ducts and sacs in the inner ear enclosed by the temporal bone is the bony labyrinth containing perilymph. The membranous labyrinth contains endolymph and is suspended inside the bony labyrinth having similar shape but thicker. The membranous labyrinth is especially important as a sensory component, where the auditory nerve fibers are distributed. At the center of the bony labyrinth is the space called vestibule.

Bony labyrinth

The bony cochlear duct and semicircular canals containing perilymph in the conical otocyst in the temporal bone of the inner ear. Membranous labyrinth containing endolymph is suspended in the bony labyrinth.

Membranous labyrinth

The membranous semicircular canals, filled with endolymph, are responsible for sense of balance and are suspended in the bony canals.

Cochlea

The spiral, bony tunnel containing the cochlear duct that converts sonic vibrations to electrical impulse transmitted through the auditory nerve to the brain.

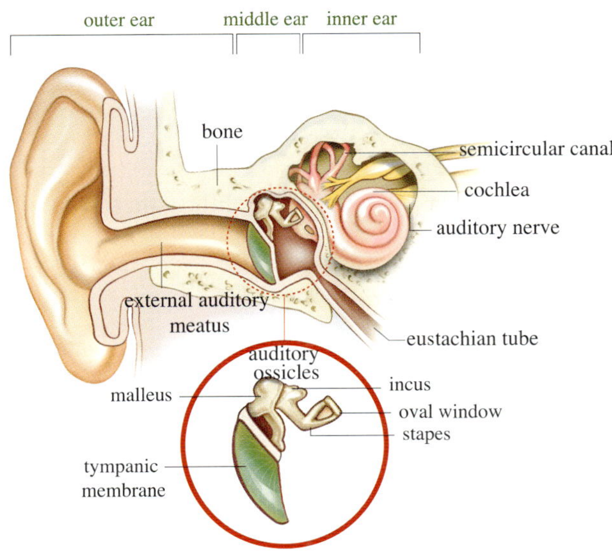

Figure 10-17 Auditory ossicles

Semicircular canal

The three semicircular canals in the bony labyrinth are responsible for sensing physical balance of the body. The membranous semicircular canals are a part of equilibrium sensors, while the bony semicircular canals are like-shaped containers for the former with 4~5 times the thickness. When the body rotates and the endolymph in the bony labyrinth flows through the canals, the flow stimulates the sensory epithelium. The vestibular chamber has five openings for the fluid to move through the passages, plus the utricle and the saccule.

Utricle

The utricle is the larger one of the two otolith organs belonging in the membranous labyrinth, located inferior to the semicircular canals. The sac-shaped sensory organ senses linear motion and balance of the body.

Cochlear duct

The snail-shaped spiral tunnel in the inner ear, divided into three chambers, each filled with lymph, relays auditory signals received from the middle ear to the auditory nerves.

Terms for Symptoms and Diseases

Otalgia

Pain in the ear. Its primary cause is inflammation of the external auditory meatus. The disease responsible for the pain in the middle ear is acute otitis media, with symptoms of fever, tinnitus, hearing impairment, sensation of ear blockage, etc.

Dizziness

The sensation of being unstable and feeling unable to maintain bodily balance when standing up or sitting down.

Vertigo

A type of dizziness, due to disorder of the semicircular canal or vestibular cells of the brain stem. The patient has the perception that the surrounding objects are rotating relative to him/her.

Otorrhea

A condition in which pus is discharged due to chronic otitis media.

Tinnitus

Pathological condition having sensation of ringing in the ear when there is no such sound.

Anotia

This is a congenital condition where one or both auricles are missing.

Macrotia

Macrotia is a congenital condition of unusually large auricles.

Microtia

Microtia is a congenital condition of unusually small auricles.

Otitis externa

This is an acute inflammation caused by pyogenic bacterial attack in the sebaceous glands of the external auditory meatus. Pain, fever, hearing difficulty, tinnitus may result.

Cholesteatoma

A destructive and expanding growth consisting of keratinizing squamous epithelium that occur in the meninges, central nervous system, the cranium and most frequently in the middle ear. It may lead to chronic suppurative otitis media with symptoms like ear drainage and hearing difficulty as well as complications such as dizziness and facial paralysis.

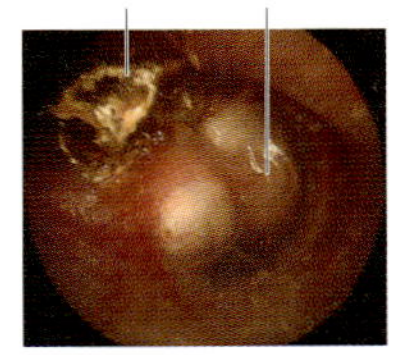

Figure 10-18
Cholesteatoma

Mastoiditis

Mastoiditis is inflammation of the mastoid as a further development of otitis media. Air contained in the mastoid process can be seen with radiography.

Myringitis

Myringitis is inflammation of the tympanic membrane. It accompanies acute otitis externa or acute otitis media. Acute myringitis can come with an external wound, eczema, exposure to cold air or influenza.

Otitis media

As an inflammation in the middle ear derived from acute infectious disease, cold, pneumonia, disease in nose or throat, external wound in tympanic membrane, etc., the patient will experience symptoms like fever, acute pain and tinnitus.

Syringitis

Inflammation of the syrinx (eustachian tube), which is susceptible to viral infection similar to common cold. This condition can also be caused by air pressure differential during mountain trekking or air trips.

Labyrinthitis

Inflammation of the inner ear, which typically occur after the otitis media. Cerebrospinal meningitis, syphilis, ear injury can also cause this condition. Symptoms include hearing difficulty, tinnitus, dizziness, nausea, vomiting, etc.

Otosclerosis

As a pathological condition in the bony labyrinth of the ear, this may cause conductive hearing loss.

Deafness

Disorders in the auditory path will cause hearing difficulties.

Presbycusis

This is a progressive bilateral symmetrical age-related sensorineural hearing difficulty.

Congenital word deafness

A congenital linguistic communication disorder of auditory comprehension type. The patient can hear the words normally but cannot effectively write to dictation, while he/she otherwise has normal ability to speak, read or write.

Acoustic neuroma

Acoustic neuroma, the most frequently occuring type of schwannoma, is a benign primary intracranial tumor of the myelin-forming cells of the vestibulocochear nerve.

Otomycosis

As fungal ear infection in the external auditory meatus, this condition is characteristic of itching sensation and exudative inflammation.

Terms for Surgery and Treatment

Otoplasty

Plastic surgery to correct deformation or deficiency of the ear.

Myringotomy

A surgical procedure of making tiny incision in the eardrum, to relieve pressure caused by excessive buildup of fluid, or to drain pus from the middle ear.

Tympanotomy

Surgical incision of the tympanic cavity.

Tympanoplasty

A reconstructive surgery to restore the auditory function of the middle ear by rebuilding the tympanic membrane and protecting the round window from excessive sound pressure.

Myringoplasty

Plastic surgery of the tympanic membrane by grafting and closing of the perforation.

Mastoidectomy

Removing some of the mastoid process is performed behind the ear or through the auditory tube.

Ossiculectomy

Surgical excision of one or more of the ossicles (malleus, incus, stapes) of the middle ear.

Stapedectomy

Surgical removal and prosthetic replacement of part or all of the stapes to relieve deafness due to otosclerosis.

Terms for Test and Intervention

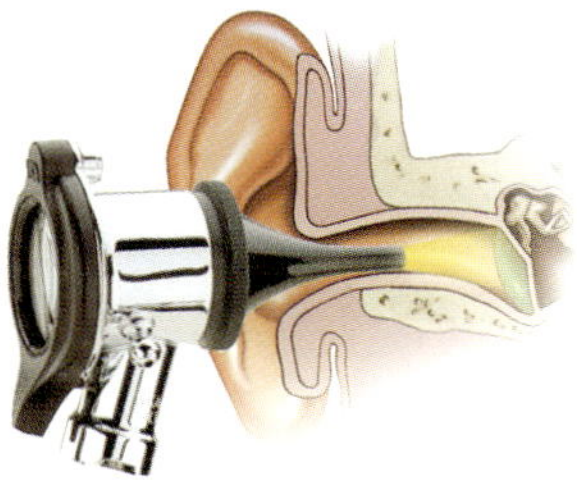

Figure 10-19
Otoscopy

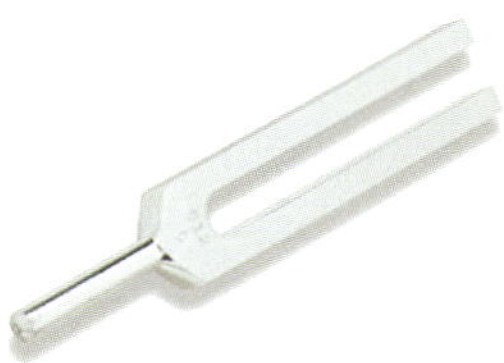

Figure 10-20
Tuning fork

Otoscopy

Visual examination of the outer ear and the tympanic membrane. A normal eardrum is a translucent membrane of clean pearly light gray or pale rose color.

Audiometry

Audiometry is measurement of hearing acuity for variations in sound intensity and pitch as well as ability for distinguishing speech from background noise.

Tympanometry

A test for the condition of the middle ear and function of the tympanic membrane and the conduction bones by creating variations of air pressure in the ear canal.

Tuning fork test

This is a test to determine whether the patient's hearing loss is of conductive or sensorineural type.

Analysis and Meaning of Key Terms

Term	Term Analysis	Meaning
audit/o, audi/o :		hearing
auditory meatus [ɔ́:dito:ri miéitəs]	-ory = pertaining to meatus = tubular passage	ear canal
audible [ɔ́:dəbl]	-ible = able	able to hear
audiometer [ɔ:diɑ́:mitɚ]	-meter = measuring device	instrument used to determine hearing ability
aur/o, aur/i :		ear
aural [ɔ́:rəl]	-al = pertaining to	pertaining to the ear
aural rehabilitation [ɔ́:rəl rihəbìlitéiʃən]	rehab = restoration	rehabilitation for people with hearing disability

Term	Term Analysis	Meaning
cochle/o :		**cochlea**
cochlear canal [kákliə kənǽl]	-ar = pertaining to canal = duct	spirally coiled cavity of the inner ear as a passage for sound to be transmitted to the nerve
electrocochleog-raphy [iléktroukákliəg-rəfi]	electr/o = electricity -graphy = recording	measurement of the electrical signal in the cochlea generated by sound
labyrinth/o :		**labyrinth**
labyrinthectomy [læ̀bərinθéktəmi]	-ectomy = surgical	removalsurgical removal of the labyrinth
ot/o :		**ear**
otalgia [outǽldʒiə]	-algia = pain	earache, usually originating from inside the ear
otitis [outáitis]	-itis = inflammation	inflammation or infection of the ear
otitis externa [outáitis ikstə́:rnə]	externa = external	inflammation of the ear canal or the auricle
otitis media [outáitis midiə]	media = middle	inflammation of the middle ear
-acusis, -cusis :		**hearing condition**
diplacusis [dípləkú:sis]	dipl/o = double	a condition in which a single sound is perceived as two separate sounds
hyperacusis [hàipərəkú:sis]	hyper- = excessive	condition of over-sensitivity to some frequency
presbycusis [prèzbikú:sis]	presby- = old age	hearing difficulty due to old age
-phonia :		**sound, voice**
aphonia [eifóunjə]	a- = lacking	loss of voice, inability to speak, mostly due to dysfunctional laryngeal nerve
myring/o :		**tympanic membrane, eardrum**
myringotomy [àiriŋgátəmi]	-tomy = process of cutting, incision	surgical incision into the eardrum to drain fluid

Term	Term Analysis	Meaning
ossicul/o :		ossicles, middle ear bones
ossiculoplasty [ɑsikulóplæ̀sti]	-plasty = surgical repair or reconstruction	surgical reconstruction of the ossicles
staped/o :		stapes
stapedectomy [stèipidéktəmi]	-ectomy = excision, surgical removal	remoral of the stapes
tympan/o :		tympanic membrane, eardrum
tympanoplasty [tìmpənouplǽsti]	-plasty = surgical repair or reconstruction	surgical reconstruction of the eardrum

Abbreviations

Abbreviation	Full Term	Meaning
accom	accommodation	adjustment of the eye for seeing at different distances
OD	oculus dextra	right eye
OS	oculus sinister	left eye
OU	oculus unitas	both eyes
PERLA	Pupils equal, react to light and accommodation	examination of pupils for equal size, reactivity to light and accommodation
PERRLA	Pupils equal, round, regular, react to light and accommodation	examination of pupils for equal size, regular shape, reactivity to light and accommodation
IOL	Intraocular lens	artificial lens implanted in the eye to treat cataracts of myopia
IOP	Intraocular pressure (=IOT)	fluid pressue inside the eye measured with tonometer
EOM	Extraocular movement	examination of the function of the eye muscles
VF	Visual field	horizontal and vertical angular limits of view with both eyes fixed, measured by perimetry
VA	Visual acuity	acuteness or clearness of vision, test usually done with 20/20 chart
XT	Exotropia(=ES)	strabismus in which the eye turns outwards
AC	Air conduction	transmission of sound waves through the ear canal
AD	auris dextra	right ear
AS	auris sinistra	left ear
AU	auris unitas	both ears
BC	Bone conduction	conduction of sound to the inner ear through the bones of the skull
EENT	Eyes, ears, nose, throat	
ENT	Ears, nose, throat	
HD	Hearing distance	
NIHL	Noise-induced hearing loss	hearing loss due to continuous exposure to loud sound
TM	Tympanic membrane	eardrum

Exercises

1. Analyze the following terms into prefix, root, suffix and write the meaning.

① blepharoplasty — blephar/o + -plasty
plastic surgery of the eyelid

② keratomycosis — kerat/o + myc/o + -sis
inflammation of the cornea due to fungal infection

③ presbyopia — presby/o + -opia
inability of the eye to focus due to old age

④ ossiculoplasty — ossicul/o + -plasty
surgery to repair the tiny bones of hearing in middle ear

⑤ tympanoplasty — tympan/o + -plasty
surgery to repair the eardrum improve hearing

⑥ presbycusis — presby/o + -cusis
inability of the ear to tune to sound due to old age

2. Write the medical term that means the following.

① eye disease that damages the optic nerve and impairs vision — glaucoma

② infection of a sebaceous gland of the eyelid — hordeolum

③ double vision — diplopia

④ weakness of eyesight — amblyopia

⑤ spirally coiled, tapered cavity of the inner ear — cochlear duct

⑥ small hammer-shaped bone in the middle ear — malleus

⑦ small anvil-shaped bone in the middle ear — incus

⑧ small stirrup-shaped bone in the middle ear — stapes

3. Write the full term for the following abbreviations.

① OD oculus dextra

② VA visual acuity

③ AD auris dextra

④ IOP intraocular pressure

⑤ OS oculus sinister

⑥ EOM extraocular movement, extraocular muscle

⑦ AS auris sinistra

⑧ TM tympanic membrane

⑨ OU oculus unitas

⑩ AU auris unitas

4. Connect each term in column A to corresponding one in B.

A		B
① glauc/o	(b)	a. ear
② presby/o	(d)	b. gray
③ ot/o	(a)	c. hearing
④ tympan/o	(f)	d. old age
⑤ audi/o	(c)	e. tear
⑥ lacrim/o	(e)	f. eardrum
⑦ irid/o	(h)	g. pupil
⑧ core/o	(g)	h. iris

5. Write the medical term for each item in the following figure.

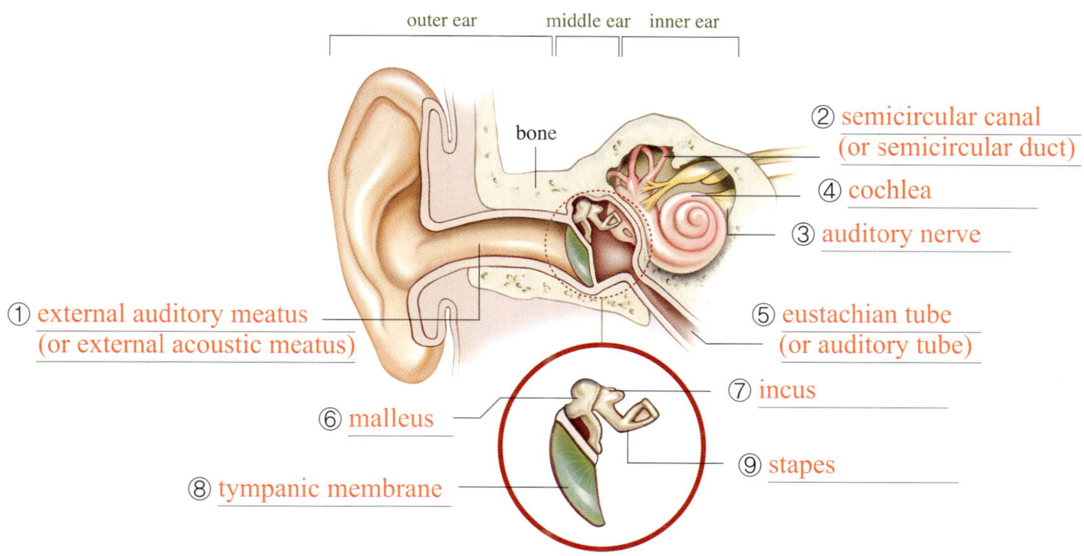

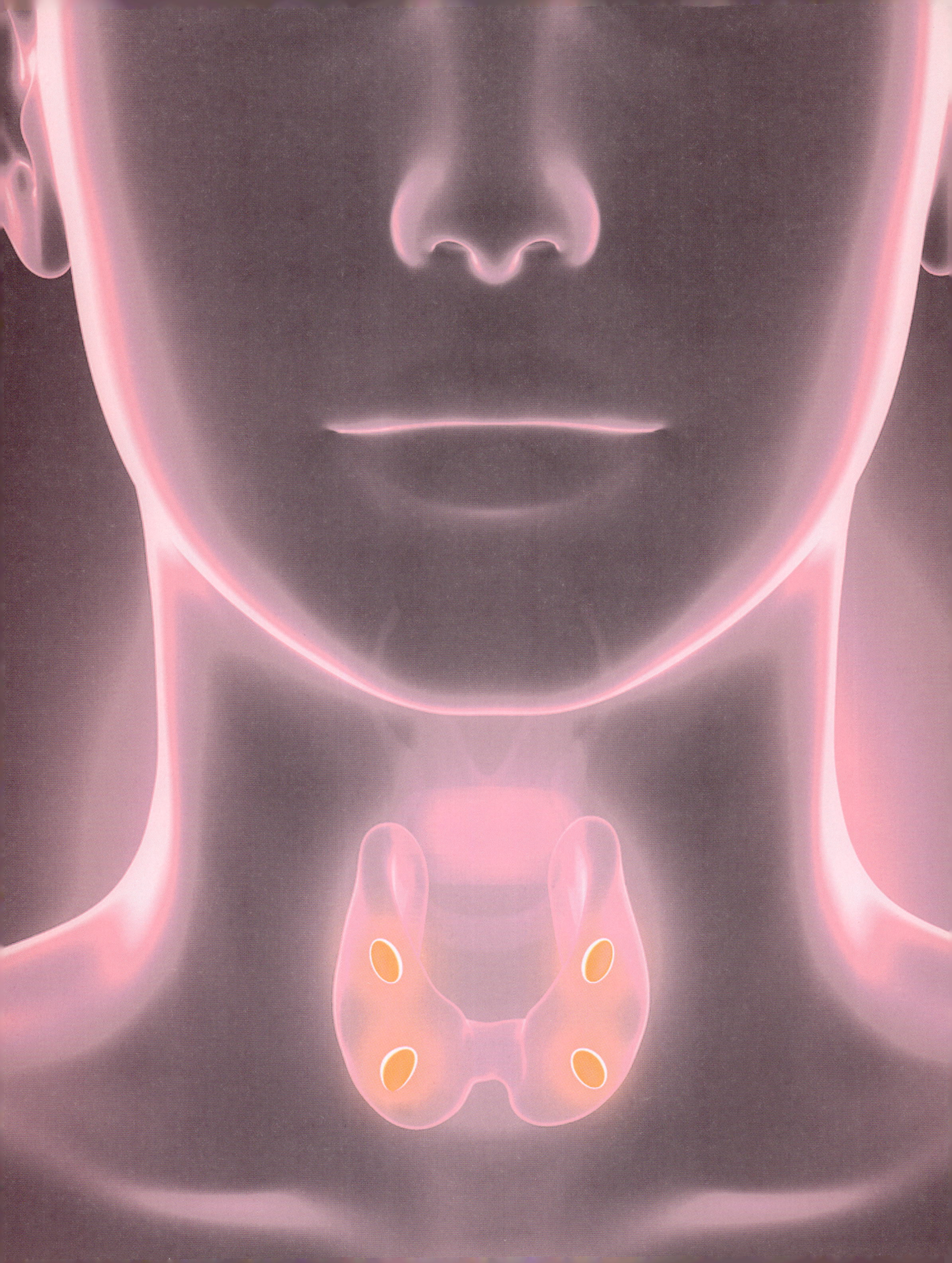

Chapter 11

Endocrine System

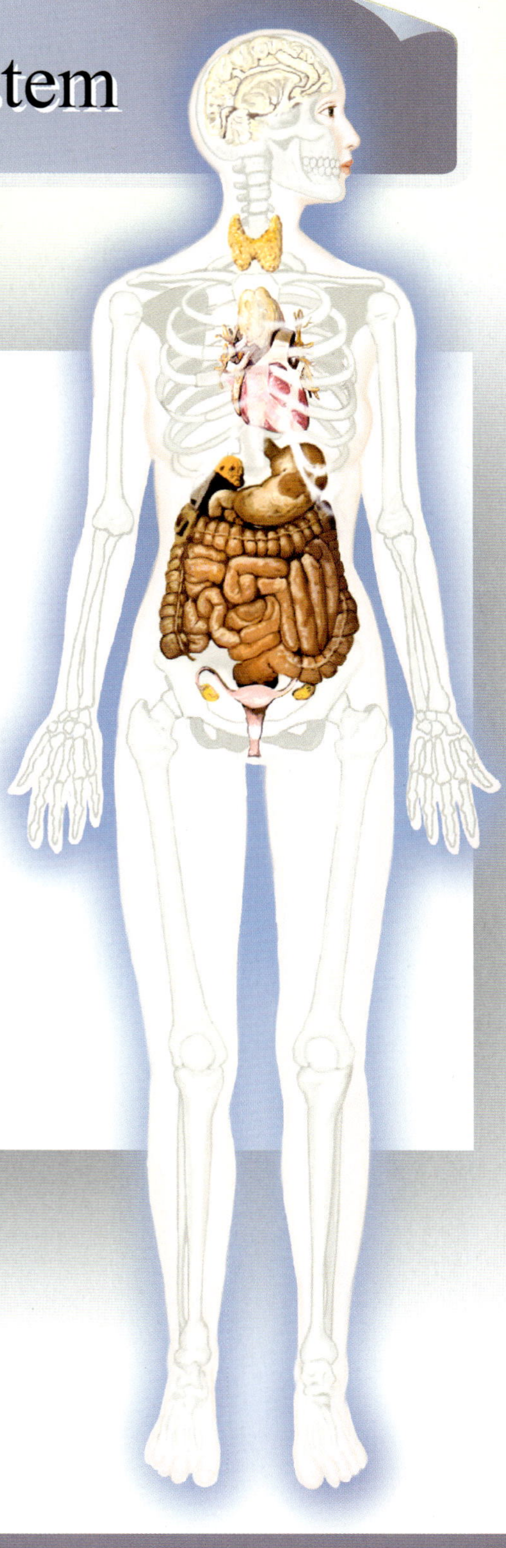

Chapter Contents

- Prolog
- Anatomical Terms
- Terms for Symptoms and Diseases
- Terms for Surgery and Treatment
- Terms for Test and Intervention
- Analysis and Meaning of Key Terms
- Abbreviations
- Exercises

Learning Objectives

- Define hormone and homeostasis.
- Tell difference between exocrine and endocrine glands.
- Understand central and peripheral endocrine glands.
- Learn functions of hormones produced by anterior and posterior pituitary glands.
- Learn functions of hormones produced in pancreas, thyroid, parathyroid, pineal and adrenal glands.
- Pronounce, analyze and define medical terms related to the endocrine system.
- Learn abbreviations related to the endocrine system.

Prolog

The endocrine system is involved in regulating development, growth and metabolic activities, and maintaining homeostasis of the body. Endocrine glands include hypothalamus, hypophysis (pituitary gland), pineal body, thyroid, parathyroid, thymus, adrenal gland, pancreas, ovary, testis, etc.

The endocrine system refers to a collection of glands that secrete hormones directly into the circulatory system to be carried towards distant target organs. This is in contrast to the exocrine system including sweat glands, lacrimal glands, salivary glands, mammary glands and liver, which secrete substances using their own ducts. However, the pancreas is a dual-feature gland, having features of both endocrine and exocrine glands.

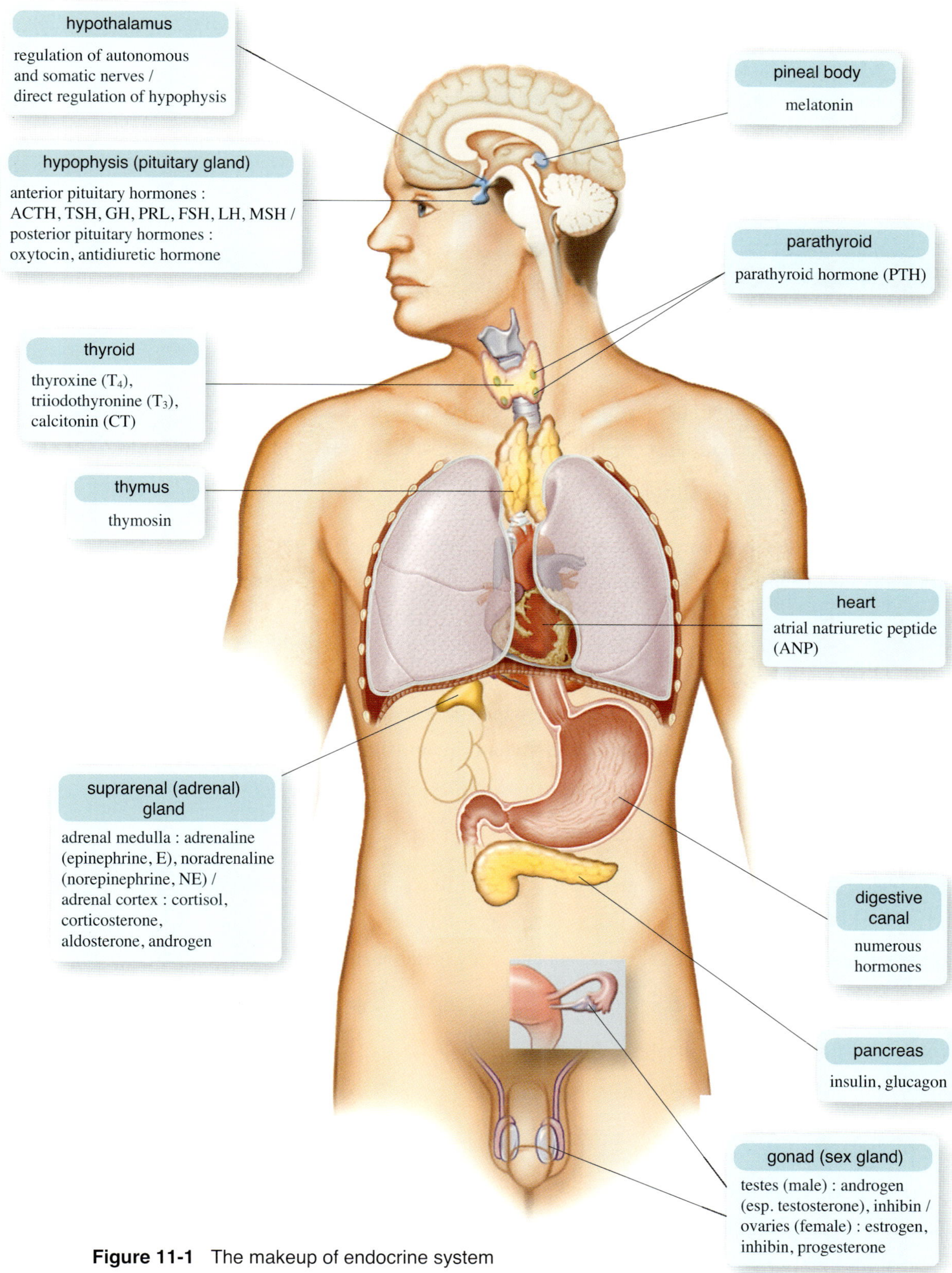

Figure 11-1 The makeup of endocrine system

Memory key

- Endocrine glands: glands that don't have their own ducts but secrete hormones into blood stream.
- Exocrine glands: glands that have their own ducts through which to deliver the secretion to the destination.

Anatomical Terms

Hypothalamus

Located below the thalamus, just above the brainstem, it secretes hormones that regulate the secretion of hormones by the pituitary gland (hypophysis).

Hypophysis

This is the pituitary gland about the size of a pea, at the bottom of the hypothalamus at the base of the brain. It is composed of anterior and posterior lobes that secrete hormones that regulate many physiological processes.

Pineal body

At near center of the brain is the gland shaped like a tiny pine cone that secretes melatonin, a hormone that affects circadian rhythm and modulates sleep patterns.

Thyroid gland

As one of the largest endocrine glands, it is shaped like a butterfly, situated in the neck just below the thyroid cartilage. Its left and right lobes produce thyroid hormones such as thyroxine that regulate general body metabolism.

Parathyroid gland

Two pairs of grain-sized glands on the back of the thyroid gland that produce parathyroid hormone, which regulates the calcium level in the blood.

Thymus gland

The thymus is a lymphatic gland located at the center of the thoracic cavity. It secretes hormones called thymosin and thymopoietin that stimulate T-cells essential for immune functions.

Pancreas

Located behind the stomach, it secretes digestive enzyme-containing pancreatic juice. It also produces two hormones of opposing duties regarding regulation of blood sugar level - insulin that lowers it and glucagon that raises the same.

Adrenal gland

The adrenal gland is located superior to both of the kidneys. The adrenal cortex secretes cortisol and aldosterone, while the adrenal medulla secretes epinephrine (adrenalin), norepinephrine (noradrenalin) and dopamine.

Ovary

A pair of ovaries are located in the female pelvic region. They produce ovum, secrete estrogen that is responsible for the development of secondary female characteristics, and progesterone that promotes and maintains pregnancy.

Testis

A pair of small egg-shaped testes are in the scrotums. They produce testosterone, the male hormone that is responsible for the development of secondary male characteristics and stimulates sperm production and release.

Table 11-1 Endocrine hormone functions

Hypophysis		Functions
Adenohypophysis (anterior pituitary)	Adrenocorticotropic hormone (ACTH)	• stimulates synthesis and release of corticosteroid (aldosterone and cortisol) by adrenocortical cells (adrenal cortex)
	Follicle stimulating hormone (FSH)	• stimulates secretion of estrogen and progesterone • stimulates maturation of ovarian follicles or spermatogenesis
	Thyroid-stimulating hormone (TSH)	• stimulates synthesis and release of thyroxine (T_4) and triiodothyronine (T_3) and iodine absorption by thyroid gland
	Growth hormone (GH)	• stimulates growth and cell reproduction of bones and tissues • stimulates release of somatomedin from liver

Hypophysis		Functions
Adenohypophysis (anterior pituitary)	Luteinizing hormone (Luteal hormone, LH)	• stimulates ovulation • stimulates testosterone synthesis
	Prolactin (PRL)	• does not function as stimulant for other hormones • stimulates growth of mammary glands and lactation
	Melanocyte-stimulating hormone (MSH)	• does not function as stimulant for other hormones • controls coloration of skin cells
	Melatonin	• reduces coloration of skin cells
	Serotonin	• stimulates gastrointestinal movement, helps capillary vessel constriction and hemostasis
Neurohypophysis (posterior pituitary)	Antidiuretic hormone (ADH)	• stimulates water reabsorption by renal capillaries • controls urine accumulation
	Oxytocin	• stimulates uterine contraction during labor and delivery • stimulates lactation

Thyroid gland	Functions
Thyroxine (T_4)	• regulates cell metabolism
Triiodothyronine (T_3)	• stimulates growth
Calcitonin	• reduces calcium level in blood

Parathyroid gland	Functions
Parathormone (PTH)	• raises calcium level in blood

Thymus gland	Functions
Thymosin	• maintains basal metabolism, metabolizes carbohydrates, proteins and lipids • stimulates growth, maturation and nervous functions

Pancreas	Functions
Glucagon	• breaks down glucose from glycogen and raises blood sugar level
Insulin	• stores glucose into glycogen and lowers blood sugar level

Adrenal gland		Functions
Adrenal cortex	Cortisol	• a glucocorticoid that increase blood sugar level • released in response to antibody formation and stress
	Corticosteroid	• an adrenal cortex hormone
	Mineralocorticoid	• controls water and electrolyte in the body, increases sodium reabsorption
	Androgen	• stimulates development of secondary male characteristics
	Estrogen	• stimulates development of secondary female characteristics
Adrenal medulla	Epinephrine (= adrenaline)	• sympathetic nerve-activated elevation of heartbeat, vasodilatation, rise of blood sugar level
	Norepinephrine (= noradrenaline)	• sympathetic nerve-activated vasoconstriction to raise blood pressure level

Ovary	Functions
Estradiol	• stimulates development of ovum and secondary female characteristics
Progesterone	• prepares the uterus for implantation of a fertilized ovum and maintains pregnancy

Testis	Functions
Testosterone	• stimulates sperm generation and development of secondary male characteristics

Terms for Symptoms and Diseases

Addison's disease

Disease caused by lack of adrenocortical hormone, characterized by hypoglycemia, hyponatremia, weight loss, lowered blood pressure, darkening of the skin, extreme fatigue, pernicious anemia, etc.

Aldosteronism

Excessive secretion of aldosterone (hyperaldosteronism) may lead to imbalance of electrolytes that cause this medical condition. Weakness, temporary paralysis, personality changes, hyperglycemia, diabetes, hypertension, metabolic alkalosis, etc.

Cretinism

A condition of stunted physical and mental development due to lack of thyroid hormones (hypothyroidism), including mental deficiency, obesity, dwarfism, macroglossia (enlargement of the tongue), etc.

Cushing's syndrome

Excessive secretion of glucocorticoid by the adrenal cortex may cause Cushing's syndrome. Symptoms include obesity in the face, neck and trunk, kyphosis, hypertension, amenorrhea, hirsutism, fertility disorder, hyperglycemia, purpura, plethora and myasthenia.

Diabetes insipidus

Decreased amount of antidiuretic hormone from posterior hypophysis will cause diabetes insipidus, characterized by excessive thirst and excretion of large amount of highly diluted urine, because of the lack of ability for the renal tubule to reabsorb water and salt.

Diabetes mellitus

Common diabetes due to dysfunctional carbohydrate metabolism related to lack of insulin. This disease can be divided into type 1 DM, insulin-dependent diabetes that requires insulin injection to control blood sugar level, and type 2 DM, non-insulin-dependent (insulin-resistant) diabetes related to obesity and lack of exercise.

Dwarfism

Abnormal shortness in stature typically due to congenital lack of growth hormone from the hypophysis. Dwarfism is occasionally defined when the adult standing height is under 1 meter.

Exophthalmos

An abnormal protrusion of the eyeball from its socket, due to several causes including hyperthyroidism.

Gigantism

Also known as giantism, gigantism is a condition characterized by excessive growth and height significantly above average, typically caused by overproduction of growth hormone.

Goiter

Goiter is a swelling of the neck or larynx resulting from enlargement of the thyroid gland, typically caused by iodine deficiency.

Graves' disease

A symptom of hyperthyroidism characterized by exophthalmos.

Hirsutism

Hirsutism is the excessive hairness on women, in those parts of the body where terminal hair does not normally occur or is minimal. Typically the cause is unknown but symptoms are manifest with the physiological state in adolescence, pregnancy, menopause, etc. The condition can also be observed with diseases including tumor in gonads that secrete androgens.

Hyperparathyroidism

Excessive secretion of hormones from the parathyroid may cause hypercalcemia, abdominal pain, excessive thirst, poor appetite, fatigue, arthralgia, pruritus, etc.

Hyperthyroidism

Hyperactivity of the thyroid may cause excessive secretion of hormones and the accompanying symptoms and diseases like restlessness, emotional instability, decreased body weight, exophthalmos, goiter, etc.

Often, women in the 20's through 50's experience being overly sensitive to ambient temperature due to basal hypermetabolism.

Hypoparathyroidism

Lack of parathyroid hormone may cause low calcium level in blood.

Hypothyroidism

Lack of thyroid hormones causes decreased basal metabolism characterized by fatigue, weakness, weight gain, etc. The patient may reveal symptoms of absentminded facial expression, hoarse voice, slowness of speech, facial edema, fear of cold weather, drooping eyelids, rough hair and skin, thickened tongue and paresthesia.

Myxedema

Myxedema is often synonymous with severe hypothyroidism (esp. lack of thyroxin), focused on dermatological changes. Symptoms include swelling of the hands and face, rough and hard skin, macroglossia, slowness of speech, anemia, etc.

Obesity

Obesity is a medical condition in which excess body fat has accumulated to the extent that it may have negative effect on health. The simple obesity is due to overeating and lack of exercise. Another kind of obesity is related to metabolic anomaly due to dysfunctional endocrine system, heredity, etc.

Pheochromocytoma

A neuroendocrine vascular tumor of the adrenal medulla, causing prolonged or intermittent hypertension, spasmodic headache, palpitation, anxiety, dithering, paleness or flushing of face, emesis, pain in the chest and abdomen, paresthesia in the limbs, etc.

Simmonds' disease

A disease characterized by panhypopituitarism that causes asthenia, progressive emaciation (loss of weight and body hair), arterial hypotension, atrophy of the thyroid, adrenal cortex and gonads, etc.

Tetany

A condition characterized by muscular spasm and deformation of hands and arms, caused by hypocalcemia, often associated with deficient parathyroid secretion.

Virillism

The appearance of secondary male characteristics owing to increased production of androgen in the female, typically arising from physiological anomaly of adrenal virillism.

Terms for Surgery and Treatment

Adrenalectomy

Surgical removal of one or both adrenal glands.

Hypophysectomy

Surgical removal of a part or the whole hypophysis (pituitary gland).

Oophorectomy

Surgical removal of one or both of the ovaries.

Orchiectomy

Surgical removal of one or both of the testes.

Parathyroidectomy

Surgical removal of one or more of the parathyroid glands.

Pinealectomy

Surgical removal of the pineal gland.

Thyroidectomy

Surgical removal of a part or the whole thyroid gland.

Thyroidotomy

Surgical incision into the thyroid cartilage, or biopsy of the thyroid gland.

Terms for Test and Intervention

Fasting blood sugar (FBS)

Blood sugar level test after fasting except for water for several hours.

Radioactive iodine uptake (RAIU)

Test for thyroid function, using radioactive iodine capsule swallowed by the patient and scanning for the level of absorption by the thyroid.

Thyroid function test

A blood test for thyroid panel, including TSH, T_3, T_4 levels.

Thyroid scan

Test for thyroid function, using radioactive iodine injection and scanning for the thyroid's location, size, shape, nodule, etc.

Thyroid stimulating hormone measurement

Blood test for level of thyroid stimulating hormone to help detect, monitor and treat hyperthyroidism and hypothyroidism.

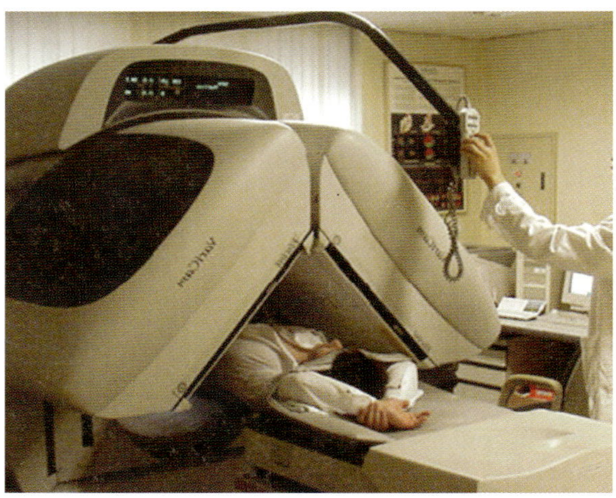

Figure 11-2 Thyroid scan

Analysis and Meaning of Key Terms

Terms for diseases

Term	Term Analysis	Meaning
acr/o :		extremity, top
acromegaly [ækrouméɡəli]	-megaly = enlargement	a disease characterized by enlargement of the extremity, due to excessive secretion of growth hormone by the pituitary gland
aden/o :		gland
adenoma [ædənóumə]	-oma = tumor; mass	benign tumor of a gland
calc/o :		calcium
hypercalcemia [hàipərkælsí:miə]	-emia = blood condition; hyper- = excessive	unusually high concentration of calcium in the blood
gonad/o :		gonads, sex glands (testes and ovaries)
hypergonadism [hàipərɡónadizm]	-ism = condition, state; hyper- = excessive	abnormally high activity of the sex organs (testes or ovary)
gynec/o :		woman
gynecomastia [dʒìnikoumǽstiə]	-ia = condition; mast/o = breast	excessive development of male breasts, resembling women's
insulin/o :		insulin
hypoinsulinism [hàipərinsəlinizm]	-ism = condition, state; hypo- = deficient	the state of insufficient insulin production by the pancreas, leading to diabetes
kal/o :		potassium
hyperkalemia [hàipərkəlí:miə]	-emia = blood condition; hyper- = excessive	unusually high concentration of potassium in the blood
natr/o :		sodium
hyponatremia [hàiponatremiə]	-emia = blood condition; hypo- = deficient	unusually low concentration of sodium in the blood
parathyroid/o :		parathyroid gland
hyper-parathyroidism [hàipər-pærəθáirɔidìzm]	-ism = condition, state; hyper- = excessive	overactivity of the parathyroid glands resulting in excess production of parathyroid hormone, leading to hypercalcemia and calcium loss in the bones

Term	Term Analysis	Meaning
pituitar/o :		pituitary gland
panhypopituitarism [panhípopitóitərizm]	-ism = condition, state; pan- = all; hypo- = deficient	hypopituitarism producing below normal amount of most pituitary hormones, causing pituitary dwarfism, underdevelopment of secondary sex characteristics, etc.
thyr/o, thyroid/o :		thyroid gland, shield
euthyroid [ju:θɑiroid]	-oid = resembling; eu- = normal, good	thyroid functioning normally
hyperthyroidism [hàipəθairɔidizəm]	-oid = resembling; ism = condition, state; hyper- = excessive	state of overactive thyroid, causing pathological condition such as goiter and exophthalmos
thyroiditis [θàiərɔidáitis]	-itis = inflammation	inflammation of the thyroid
thyrotomy [θàiərotahmi]	-tomy = to cut	surgical incision into the thyroid cartilage

Other terms

Term	Term Analysis	Meaning
adrenal/o, adren/o :		adrenal gland
adrenalectomy [ədrénəlektəmi]	-ectomy = excision	surgical removal of one or both adrenal glands
andr/o :		male
androgen [ændrəʒdən]	-gen = producer of something	male sex hormone that stimulates masculine characteristics
crin/o :		secretion
endocrinologist [endoukrənɑ:lədʒist]	-logist = specialist; endo- = within	specialist in endocrine systems
endocrinology [endoukrənɑ:lədʒi]	-logy = study of; endo- = within	study of endocrine glands, hormones and related physiology
estr/o :		female
estrogen [éstrədʒən]	-gen = producer of something	female sex hormone that stimulates feminine characteristics

Term	Term Analysis	Meaning
gluc/o :		glucose, sugar
glucogenesis [glù:koʒénisis]	-genesis = production	breaking down glycogen to produce glucose
gluconeogenesis [glù:kounì:ənisis]	-genesis = production; neo- = new	metabolic process of producing glucose from noncarbohydrate sources such as protein and lipids
glyc/o :		sugar
glycolysis [glaikáləsis]	-lysis = breakdown; -emia = blood condition	metabolic pathway of converting glucose into energy or other forms
hyperglycemia [hàipərglaisí:miə]	hyper- = excessive; -emia = blood condition	state of excessively high blood sugar level
glycogen/o :		glycogen (storage form of sugar)
glycogenolysis [glikojenolìsis]	-lysis = breakdown, separation	production of glucose by breaking down glycogen
home/o :		sameness
homeostasis [hòumioustéisis]	-stasis = standing stable, stopping, controlling	state of maintaining stable physiological balance
pancreat/o :		pancreas
pancreatogenic [pæ̀ŋkriətóudʒenik]	-genic = produced by	produced by or related to pancreas
ure/o :		urea (end product of protein breakdown, found in urine)
antidiuretic hormone [æ̀ntidàiərétik hɔ́:rmoun]	-tic = pertaining to; anti- = against	hormone that limits accumulation of dilute urine

Suffixes and prefixes

Term	Term Analysis	Meaning
-assay :		analysis of a mixture to identify its contents
radioimmuno-assay(RIA) [rèidiouìmjənou-ǽsei]	radi/o = radioactive; immun/o = protection	measurement of antigens using radioactive substance in antibody

Term	Term Analysis	Meaning
-crine :		**secrete, separate**
endocrine hormone [éndəkrin hɔ́:rmoun]	endo- = within	hormones released into the blood stream
exocrine gland [eksəkrin glænd]	exo- = outside, outward	a gland that delivers secretions through a specific duct
-dipsia :		**thirst**
polydipsia [pàlidípsiə]	poly- = many, much	excessive thirst often due to a disease
-physis :		**to grow**
adenohypophysis [adə́nóhipofísis]	aden/o = gland; -hypo- = below, under	glandular anterior lobe of hypophysis
neurohypophysis [njùərouhaipɑ́fəsis]	neur/o = nerve; hypo- = below; under	posterior lobe of hypophysis, consisting of maily neuronal projections (axons)
-trophic :		**pertaining to nourishment**
gonadotrophic hormone [gounǽdoutrɑ́fik hɔ́:rmoun]	gonad/o = gonads, sex glands (ovaries, testes)	hormone secreted by the anterior pituitary that stimulates the gonads and controls reproductive activities
somatotrophic hormone [səmǽtətrɑ́fik hɔ́:rmoun]	somat/o = body	hormone secreted by the anterior pituitary that promotes growth
-tropic :		**turning, changing, affecting**
adrenocorticotropic hormone (ACTH) [ədri:noukɔ́:rtikou trɑ́fik hɔ́:rmoun]	adren/o = adrenal gland; cortic/o = cortex, outer layer	anterior pituitary hormone that stimulates the production of steroids from the adrenal cortex
oxy- :		**sharp, quick**
oxytocin [ɑ̀ksətóusin]	-tocin = labor, birth	post pituitary hormone that stimulates contraction of the uterus to induce labor

Abbreviations

Abbreviation	Full Term	Meaning
ACTH	Adrenocorticotropic hormone	corticotropin; a peptide hormone from the pituitary gland that regulates the secretion of glucocorticoids
ADH	Antidiuretic hormone	vasopressin; a hormone secreted by the posterior pituitary gland that regulates retention of water
DM	Diabetes mellitus	diabetes; a medical disorder characterized by hyperglycemia
FBS	Fasting blood sugar	blood sugar level test after fasting except for water for several hours
FSH	Follicle stimulating hormone	a pituitary hormone that stimulates ovarian follicles or spermatogenesis
GH	Growth hormone	a pituitary hormone that promotes growth and regulates metabolism
LH	Luteinizing hormone	a pituitary hormone that stimulates ovulation or production of androgen
MSH	Melanocyte-stimulating hormone	pituitary gland hormone that regulates production of melanin
OT	Oxytocin	hormone that stimulates contractions during labor and production of milk
PRL	Prolactin	pituitary gland hormone that stimulates growth of mammary glands and lactation
PTH	Parathyroid hormone	parathyroid gland hormone that helps raise the levels of calcium ions in the blood
RAIU	Radioactive iodine uptake	a thyroid gland function test by using a radioactive tracer and a special probe to measure iodine absorption
TFT	Thyroid function test	a term for blood test to check thyroid hormone productions, including TSH, T_4, T_3, etc.
TSH	Thyroid-stimulating hormone	thyrotropin; a pituitary hormone that stimulates thyroid hormone production
RIA	Radioimmunoassay	measurement of antigens using radioactive substance in antibody
T_3	Triiodothyronine	a thyroid hormone affecting growth, development, metabolism, body temperature, heart rate etc.

Abbreviation	Full Term	Meaning
T_4	Thyroxine	a thyroid hormone, prohormone for T_3
TRH	Thyrotropin-releasing hormone	a hypothalamus-produced hormone that stimulates anterior pituitary release of hormones that again stimulates hormone production from the thyroid gland

Exercises

1. Analyze the following terms and write the meaning.

① hyponatremia

hypo- (below) + natr/o (sodium) + -emia (blood condition)

lower than normal sodium (or salt) level in blood

② hyperparathyroidism

hyper- (above) + para- (beyond, beside) + thyr/o (thyroid) + -ism (condition)

abnormally high parathyroid gland activity

2. Write the meaning of the following medical terms.

① unusually high level of calcium in the blood — hypercalcemia

② abnormally low level of insulin in the blood — hypoinsulinemia, hupoinsulinism

③ male breasts grown large like women's — gynecomastia

④ hyperfunction of the gonads (high levels of sex hormones) — hypergonadism

3. Write the functions of the following hormones.

① parathyroid hormone

raises calcium level in the blood

② insulin

breaks down glucose and lowers blood sugar level

③ aldosterone

regulates the balance of sodium and potassium level in the blood

④ norepinephrine

increase the heart rate to raise blood pressure level

⑤ adrenocorticotropic hormone

stimulates synthesis and release of corticosteroid (aldosterone and cortisol) by adrenal cortex

4. Write the full name of the following abbreviations.

① FSH follicle stimulating hormone

② ACTH adrenocorticotropic hormone

③ TSH thyroid stimulating hormone

5. Write the medical term that means the following.

① Production of sugar from fats and proteins : gluconeogenesis

② Breakdown of glycogen to form glucose : glycogenolysis

③ A disease characterized by enlargement of the extremity. It is caused by excessive secretion of growth hormone by the pituitary gland : acromegaly

④ Abnormal enlargement of the male breast : gynecomastia

⑤ Benign tumor of a gland : adenoma

6. Find the endocrine gland from A that secretes the hormones in B.

A	B
1. anterior pituitary	A. cortisol : (5)
2. posterior pituitary	B. glucagon : (8)
3. thyroid gland	C. antidiuretic hormone : (2)
4. parathyroid	D. follicle stimulating hormone : (1)
5. adrenal cortex	E. adrenocorticotropic hormone : (1)
6. adrenal medulla	F. androgen : (5)
7. pineal gland	G. progesterone : (5)
8. pancreas	H. parathormone : (4)
	I. growth hormone : (1)
	J. luteal hormone : (1)
	K. oxytocin : (2)
	L. melanocyte stimulating hormone : (1)
	M. epinephrine : (6)
	N. calcitonin : (3)

Chapter 12

Circulatory, Cardiovascular System

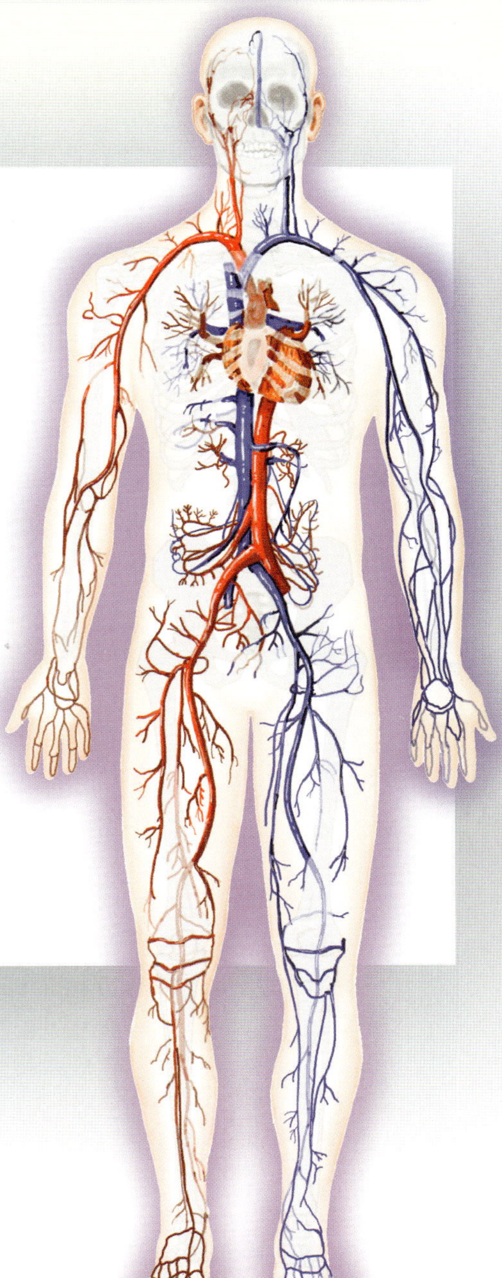

Chapter Contents

- Prolog
- Anatomical Terms
- Terms for Symptoms and Diseases
- Terms for Surgery and Treatment
- Terms for Test and Intervention
- Analysis and Meaning of Key Terms
- Abbreviations
- Exercises

Learning Objectives

- Learn structure, names of the organs and their locations in the cardio-vascular system.
- Analyze and understand terms relating to the cardiovascular system.
- Pronounce and define anatomical terms relating to the cardiovascular system.
- Pronounce and define symptomatic terms relating to the cardiovascular system.
- Pronounce and define surgical terms relating to the cardiovascular system.
- Define abbreviations commonly used in the cardiovascular system.

Prolog

The heart is responsible for circulating blood to the whole body through blood vessels by continuous cycles of contraction and expansion. It is the fist-sized organ located between the sternum and the lungs. The system continuously delivers nutrients and oxygen to and removes waste materials from all body tissues through the lungs and the kidneys. In this chapter we will learn the structure, functions and the terms relating to the cardiovascular system.

Anatomical Terms

Heart

Interior of the heart

- **Atrium**

  The word atrium comes from a Latin word meaning a small chamber. Atria are chambers with thin walls holding blood, ready to flow into ventricles.

- **Right atrium**

  The right atrium receives deoxygenated blood from all over the body through superior and inferior vena cavae.

• **Left atrium**

The left atrium receives oxygenated blood from the lungs through the pulmonary veins.

• **Ventricle**

Ventricles are blood-pumping chambers with thick muscular walls, that receive blood from the atria.

• **Right ventricle**

At the lower right part of the heart is the right ventricle that receives blood from the right atrium and pumps it out to the lung through the pulmonary arteries.

• **Left ventricle**

At the lower left part of the heart is the left ventricle that receives blood from the left atrium and pumps it out to the whole body through the aorta and arteries.

• **Cardiac valve**

The four chambers of the heart are separated by four cardiac valves to prevent blood from flowing backward.

• **Atrioventricular valve**

These two valves separate the atria and the ventricles. They open to fill the

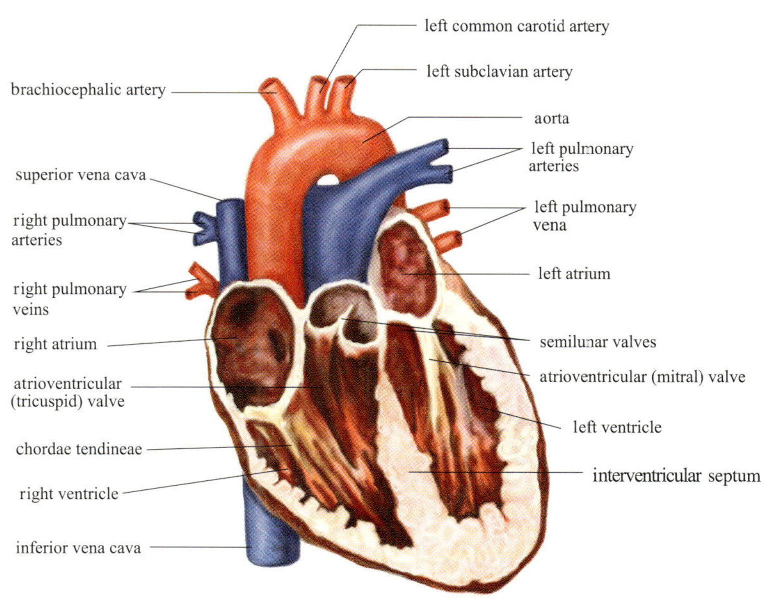

Figure 12-1 Structure of the heart

ventricles during the relaxing period of the heart, and close to prevent backflow during the contracting period.

- **Tricuspid valve**

This is an atrioventricular valve between the right atrium and the right ventricle.

- **Mitral valve**

This is an atrioventricular valve between the left atrium and the left ventricle.

- **Semilunar valve**

These two valves are located between ventricles and pulmonary arteries or aorta. Each has three cusps of semilunar shape.

- **Pulmonary valve**

This is a semilunar valve to prevent backflow between the right ventricle and pulmonary arteries.

- **Aortic valve**

This is a semilunar valve to prevent backflow between the left ventricle and the aorta. It opens during the contracting period of the heart to allow blood outflow.

Memory key

- There are four chambers in the heart - right atrium, right ventricle, left atrium, and left ventricle.
- There are four valves in the heart. The two atrioventricular valves separate the atria and the ventricles. The right atrioventricular valve is the tricuspid valve, and the left atrioventricular valve is the mitral valve.
- The two semilunar valves are between the ventricles and the arteries. The one for the right ventricle is the pulmonary valve, and the one for the left ventricle is the aortic valve.

Walls of the heart

- **Heart wall**

The wall of the heart is made up of three layers : endocardium, myocardium and epicardium.

- **Endocardium**

The innermost layer in the heart wall, made of thin layer of connective tissue.

- **Myocardium**

The middle and thickest layer made largely of cardiac muscle cells. The contraction of this layer results in pumping blood into the major arteries.

- **Epicardium**

The outermost layer of the heart wall, made of thin epithelial connective tissue.

- **Pericardium**

The pericardium is a double-walled sac containing the heart. It holds the heart in place and lubricates it to prevent friction during pumping activities. It consists of parietal and visceral pericardia.

- **Parietal pericardium**

This layer is fused to the fibrous pericardium.

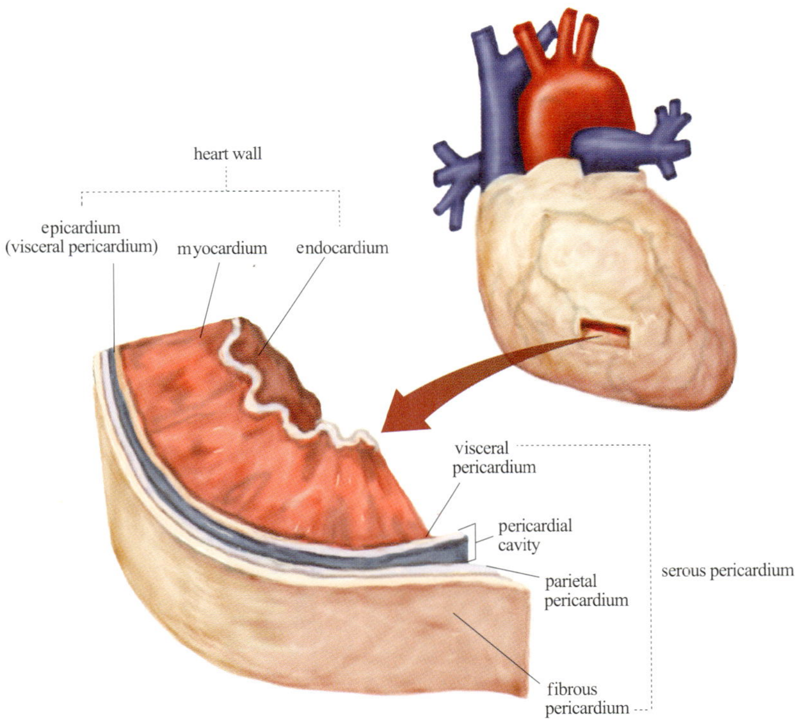

Figure 12-2 Wall of the heart

- **Visceral pericardium**

  This layer is a part of the epicardium.

- **Pericardial fluid**

  In between the parietal and visceral pericardial layers is a small pericardial cavity that contains a supply of pericardial fluid that functions as lubricant for the heart movement.

Memory key

- The heart wall consists of endocardium, myocardium and epicardium.
- The endocardium is the innermost layer in the heart, made of thin layer of connective tissue.
- The myocardium is the middle and thickest layer made of cardiac muscle.
- The epicardium is the outermost layer of the heart made of thin epithelial connective tissue.

Coronary arteries

- **Coronary artery**

  Coronary artery supplies blood to the myocardium and other constituents of the heart. It comes out of the aorta after it arises from the left ventricle, and is distributed on the walls of the heart, being branched into two portions.

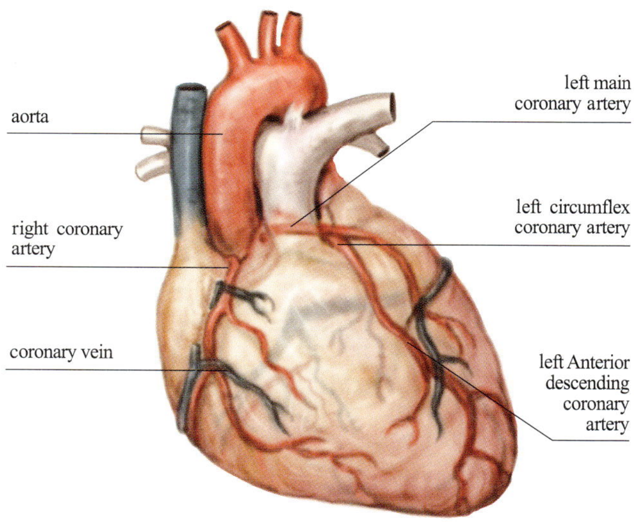

Figure 12-3 Coronary arteries

- **Left coronary artery**

  The left coronary artery supplies blood to the walls of the left heart, and can be divided into left circumflex coronary artery and left anterior descending coronary artery.

- **Right coronary artery**

  The right coronary artery supplies blood to the walls of the right heart.

Conduction system of the heart

The heart muscles (myocardia) contract and relax rhythmically and periodically upon stimulation by the electric impulses specifically ordered and coordinated to move the heart. The myocardia are special fibrous muscle tissues that conduct electrical impulses.

- **Sinoatrial node, SA node**

  The sinoatrial node is the impulse-generating (pacemaker) tissue located on the wall of the right atrium, at the synapse near the superior vena cava. It is the electrical device that supplies electrical impulses to control muscle contractions for pumping activities of the atria and ventricles.

- **Atrioventricular node, AV node**

  The atrioventricular node is a small node of specialized tissue located in the inner wall dividing the left and right atria and ventricles. Its function is to coordinate the time interval of contraction between the atria and ventricles.

- **Atrioventricular bundle, AV bundle, bundle of His**

  This is a collection of heart muscle cells specialized for electrical conduction that ties inner atrial and ventricular walls, and transmits impulses from the atria to the ventricles.

- **Left and right bundle branches**

  The atrioventricular bundle branches into the left and right bundle branches which run along the interventricular septum. These distribute the impulses to the ventricular muscles through Purkinje fibers.

- **Purkinje fibers**

  Located in the inner ventricular walls, Purkinje fibers consist of specialized cardiomyocytes extended from the bundle branches, and distribute impulses to the ventricular muscles.

Electrocardiogram

The instrument that records the electrical activity of the heart shows the wave pattern of heart's impulses. It picks up depolarization and repolarization of the heart muscle cells of the atria and ventricles. From the waveform the examiner can tell the direction and magnitude of the electrical current that are useful in the diagnosis.

- **P-R interval**

  The time interval P-R indicates the time it takes for the impulse to travel from the atria to the ventricles.

- **P wave**

  The waveform at the P indicates the electrical activity when the atria contract.

- **QRS wave**

  The waveform at the QRS indicates the electrical activity when the ventricles contract.

- **T wave**

  The waveform at the T indicates the electrical activity when the ventricles repolarize.

Memory key

- In the conduction system of the heart, the transmission starts at the sinoatrial node and passes through atrioventricular node, atrioventricular bundle, left and right bundle branches, to Purkinje fibers.
- The electrical activities of the heart muscles are recorded as electrocardiogram.

Blood vessels

- **Blood vessels**

  Tubular component of the circulatory system that carries blood, such as artery, vein or capillary.

- **Arteries**

  Arteries are blood vessels that convey blood away from the heart. They are made mainly of thick walls with elastic smooth muscle cells, which expand and contract per the heartbeat.

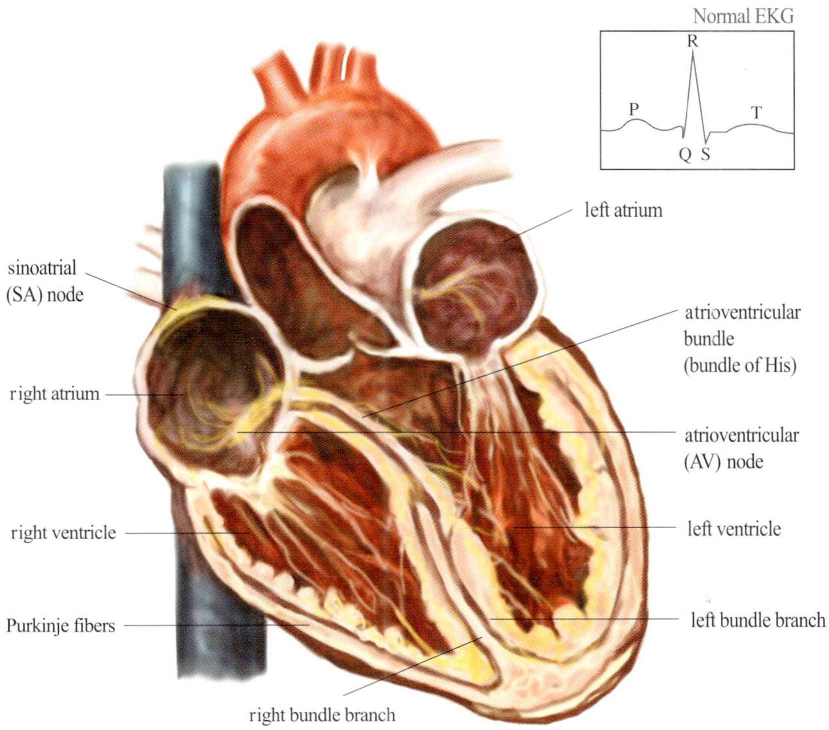

Figure 12-4 Conduction system of the heart

• **Arterioles**

Smallest of arteries that connect to the capillaries.

• **Aorta**

Aorta is the root systemic artery that receives blood directly from the left ventricle of the heart via the aortic valve, and this is the largest artery. It can be divided, depending on the direction or target location, into ascending, descending, thoracic or abdominal aortas.

• **Veins**

Veins are blood vessels that carry blood toward the heart. They are less elastic and less muscular than the arteries.

• **Venules**

Smallest of veins that receive blood from the capillaries.

• **Vena cavae**

The largest veins that carry blood collected from smaller veins all over the body into the right atrium. There are superior and inferior vena cavae.

• **Capillaries**

The most numerous and smallest of the body's blood vessels. The thin-walled capillary vessels supply oxygen and nutrients to tissues and take away carbon dioxide.

Memory key

• The complete cycle of blood circulation include : (superior and inferior) vena cavae > right atrium > tricuspid valve > right ventricle > pulmonary valve > pulmonary arteries > lungs > pulmonary veins > left atrium > mitral valve > left ventricle > aortic valve > aorta > arteries > arterioles > capillaries > venules > veins > (back to) vena cavae

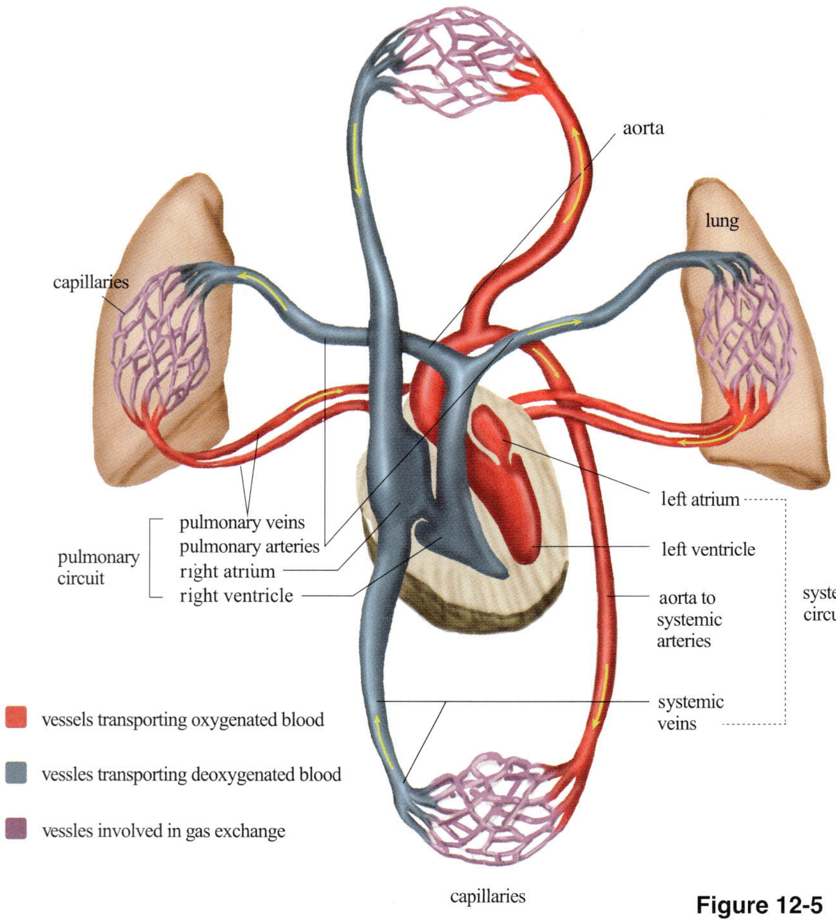

Figure 12-5 Systemic and pulmonary circulation

Terms for Symptoms and Diseases

Angina pectoris

A disease accompanied by chest pain caused by myocardial ischemia due to temporary blockage of the coronary artery.

Angiospasm

A condition in which a blood vessel's spasm leads to vasoconstriction.

Aortic insufficiency (aortic regurgitation)

Leaking of the aortic valve of the heart that causes blood to flow backward during ventricular diastole. This condition may lead to left ventricular hypertrophy and lung congestion.

Aortic stenosis

This is a disease of the heart valve in which the opening of the aortic valve is narrowed, causing heightened pressure in the left ventricle.

Arrhythmia

A condition of heartbeat in which the electrical stimulation is not optimally tuned (irregular, too fast or too slow).

Arteriosclerosis

Hardening, narrowing or loss of resiliency in arteries usually due to cholesterol deposits in the arterial walls.

Atherosclerosis

Narrowed condition of the elastic artery such as aorta caused by plaques (accumulation of fatty deposits, usually cholesterol, atheroma or fibroma).

Cardiac arrest

Also known as heart attack, a state of sudden cessation of heartbeat resulting in the loss of blood circulation.

Cardiac tamponade

A condition in which fluid accumulates in the pericardium resulting in external compression of the heart.

Cardiomegaly

An abnormally enlarged heart (as either cardiac dilation or cardiac hypertrophy).

Cardiomyopathy

Deterioration of or a disease in the myocardium.

Chest pain

Chest pain may be caused by cardiovascular dysfunction, or other causes of respiratory, gastrointestinal, psychological nature, etc.

Coarctation of aorta

A congenital condition in which the aorta is narrowed in the area in contact with other large vessels nearby.

Congestive heart faillure

A disease marked by shortage of blood delivery to the body due to decreased ability of myocardial contraction.

Defibrillation

Applying an electrical shock to the heart in order to stop fibrillation and restore normal heart contractions.

Diastole

The phase of relaxation and dilation of the heart chambers between contractions.

Endocarditis

Inflammation of the endocardium and possibly the heart valves, due to rheumatic fever, bacteria, syphilis, etc.

Fibrillation

Fibrillation is the rapid, irregular or unsynchronized contraction of the muscle fibers of the heart.

Flutter

Abnormal, rapid pulsation of the heart.

Heart murmur

Pathologic heart sound produced when blood flows across one of the heart valves, loud enough to be heard with a stethoscope.

Hypercholesterolemia

The condition of excessively high cholesterol level in the blood.

Hyperlipidemia

The condition of excessively high lipid level in the blood.

Hypertension

The condition of higher than normal blood pressure.

Hypertriglyceridemia

The condition of excessively high triglyceride level in the blood.

Hypotension

The condition of lower than normal blood pressure.

Hypertensive heart disease

This is a disease including a number of complications relating to hypertension. The heart is subject to the burden of pumping blood counter to the increased resistance to arterial flow, and the vessels gradually lose elasticity due to heightened pressure.

Ischemic heart disease

This is coronary artery disease with insufficient blood flow to the myocardium (ischemia), which may cause chest pain and myocardial necrosis.

Mitral insufficiency (mitral regurgitation)

The mitral valve does not close properly when the left ventricle pumps blood so that some blood leaks into the left atrium.

Mitral stenosis

This is a disease of the heart valve in which the mitral valve is thickened or the opening is narrowed, mostly due to complications of rheumatic fever.

Myocardial infarction

Necrosis of the myocardium caused by interruption of blood supply to the heart tissues, often as a result of thrombosis or stricture of the coronary arteries.

Myocarditis

Inflammation of the myocardium due mostly to viral infection. This may result in myocardial necrosis or arrhythmia.

Palpitation

Abnormally strong heart beat that can be felt by the person, may be accompanied by chest pain.

Pericardial effusion

Abnormal accumulation of fluid in the pericardial sac.

Pericarditis

Inflammation of the pericardium, caused by rheumatic fever, viral infection, malignant tumor, etc. Symptoms include chest pain, difficulty of breathing, cyanosis, palpitation, valvular murmurs heard through a stethoscope, etc.

Systole

The contracting phase of the ventricles in the pumping cycle.

Tricuspid atresia

A congenital heart disease with a complete absence of the tricuspid valve, which means no atrioventricular connection.

Vasoconstriction

Contraction of the muscular walls of blood vessels like arteries, arterioles and veins, resulting in smaller diameter.

Vasodilator

A substance (drug) that causes dilation of the blood vessels.

Terms for Surgery and Treatment

Angioplasty

Surgical reconstruction of the blood vessel by widening the narrowed portion using a balloon catheter or a stent.

Atherectomy

Surgical procedure to remove fatty plaque from an artery.

Atrial fibrillation ablation

The process of removing rapid, irregular or unsynchronized contractions of the atrium, typically by radiofrequency ablation.

Bypass surgery

Surgical procedure involving rerouting a tubular body part that covey blood or other body fluid.

Pericardiocentesis

Removing pericardial fluid through a needle inserted into the pericardium, for treatment or diagnosis.

Coronary artery bypass graft

Surgical procedure to graft an arterial piece (internal thoracic artery or saphenous vein) onto the coronary artery and bypass a portion which has been narrowed or blocked.

Embolectomy

Surgical removal of embolus (mass of material carried in the blood stream) or thrombus (blood clot), usually of emergency.

Implantable cardiac defibrillator (ICD)

A device combining a cardioverter and a defibrillator into one implantable unit, inserted in the chest to monitor and correct fibrillation and tachycardia.

Mitral commissurotomy

Surgical incision of a commissure in the mitral valve to open up the blood passage.

Open heart surgery

Surgical incision of a heart chamber to correct the inner structure.

Percutaneous transluminal coronary angioplasty

A procedure to improve coronary blood flow by flattening the plaques built up in the coronary artery using a balloon catheter.

Pericardiectomy

Surgical removal of a part or all of the pericardium.

Shunt surgery

A general term for surgical processes resulting in making anatomical shortcuts away from the normal paths for bodily fluid circulation.

Valve replacement

Open heart surgery in which a damaged heart valve is replaced with an artificial one.

Valvotomy

An incision into a narrowed valve in order to restore proper blood flow.

Valvuloplasty

Plastic surgery to repair a heart (or a venous) valve.

Terms for Test and Intervention

Angiography

A medical imaging technique in which an X-ray image is taken to visualize the heart valves or blood vessels, with the help of contrast media injected in the blood stream.

Aortogram

A medical X-ray image taken to visualize the aorta, with the help of contrast media injected in the blood stream.

Arteriography

A medical imaging technique in which an X-ray image is taken to visualize the artery, with the help of contrast media injected in the blood stream.

Cardiac catheterization

Insertion of a catheter in the heart chamber or blood vessel surrounding the heart for diagnostic and interventional purposes.

Cardiac scan

A heart computed tomography (CT) scan; a test to detect calcium deposits in the myocardium, with the help of contrast media injected in the blood stream.

Cardioversion

A treatment of cardiac arrhythmia with a controlled electrical current, to restore normal heartbeat.

Doppler ultrasound

Using Doppler effect of ultrasound wave to measure blood current in vessels.

Echocardiogram

Visual image of the moving heart produced using ultrasound.

Electrocardiogram

ECG or EKG. Record of electrical activities of the heart

Electrophysiology study

An evaluation of the electrical activities of the heart, to assess and diagnose the type of arrhythmia.

Exercise stress test

Test and measurement of the heart's ability to respond to physical stress (during exercise) in a controlled clinical environment.

Holter monitoring

Monitoring the electrical activities of the cardiovascular system continuously for at least 24 hours, with the patient wearing a portable device and having several noninvasive electrodes attached to the chest.

Single-photon emission computed tomography

Nuclear medicine tomographic imaging technique, scanned from multiple angles to produce 3D images.

Thallium test

Thallium stress test is a nuclear imaging test to diagnose the coronary artery and evaluate flow of blood in response to stress during a controlled exercise, after intravenous administration of a radioisotope.

Transesophageal echocardiogram

An alternative form of echocardiogram. A probe containing an ultrasound transducer is passed into the patient's esophagus which is near the heart, to produce better image than by transthoracic procedure.

Venography

A diagnostic procedure in which an X-ray image of the veins is taken after a special dye is injected in the veins.

Ventriculography

A diagnostic procedure in which an X-ray image of the ventricle is taken after a special dye is injected in the ventricle.

Analysis and Meaning of Key Terms

Roots

Term	Term Analysis	Meaning
angi/o :		vessel
angiography [ӕndʒiágrəfi]	-graphy = process of recording	X-ray imaging of cardiovascular part using contrast media
angioma [ӕndʒióumə]	-oma = mass, tumor	benign tumor of blood or lymph vessels
angiospasm [ӕndʒióspǽzəm]	-spasm = sudden, involuntary contraction	vasospasm; sudden, involuntary contraction of blood vessel that may lead to tissue death
angiostenosis [ӕndʒióstənóusis]	-stenosis = narrowing	condition of narrowed blood vessel
aort/o :		aorta (largest artery)
aortic stenosis [eiɔ́:rtik stinousis]	-stenosis = narrowing	condition of narrowed aortic valve or aorta, causing heightened pressure in the left ventricle
arteri/o :		artery
arteriole [ɑ:rtíəriòul]	-ole = small	smallest of arteries that connect to the capillaries
arteriosclerosis [ɑ:rtíəriòuskləróusis]	-sclerois = hardening	condition in which arteries have lost resiliency and hardened
arteriostenosis [ɑ:rtíərioustinousis]	-stenosis = narrowing	condition in which arteries have been narrowed
ather/o :		fatty plaque
atherosclerosis [ӕθərouskəróusis]	-oma = mass, tumor	narrowed condition of the artery caused by plaques (accumulation of fatty deposits, usually cholesterol, atheroma or fibroma)
atheroma [ӕθəróumə]	-oma = tumor, mass	abnormal fatty deposit which develops within walls of arteries
cardi/o :		heart
cardiomegaly [ká:rdiouméɡeli]	-megaly = enlargement	megalocardia; abnormally enlarged heart

Term	Term Analysis	Meaning
cardi/o :		**heart**
cardiomyopathy [kɑ̀:rdioumaiɑ́pəθi]	-my/o = muscle; -pathy = desease	deterioration of or a disease in the myocardium, due to unknown cause
pancarditis [pæ̀nkɑ́:rdáitis]	pan- = all; -itis = inflammation	inflammation of the entire heart (all layers)
pericarditis [pèrikɑ:rdáitis]	peri- = around; -itis = inflammation	inflammation of the pericardium
pericardium [pèrikɑ́:rdiəm]	peri- = around; -um = structure	membranous sac surrounding the heart
embol/o :		**embolus, clogging**
embolus [émbələs]	-us = condition	mass of material carried in the blood stream obstructing the flow
phleb/o :		**vein**
phlebothrombosis [flébɔ́:θrámbousis]	-thromb/o = clot; -osis = abnormal	formation of blood clot in the superficial vein
thrombophlebitis [θrɑ̀mbəflibáitis]	-thromb/o = clot; -itis = inflammation	inflammation of a superfical vein due to blood clot
thromb/o :		**clot**
thrombus [θrɑ́mbəs]	-us = condition	blood clot in vessels that causes thrombosis
vascul/o :		**blood vessel**
avavascular [eivǽskjulər]	a- = not; -ar = pertaining to	lacking blood vessels
cerebrovascular [sèrəbrəvǽskjələr]	cerebr/o = brain; -ar = pertaining to	pertaining to blood vessels in the brain
arti/o :		**atrium**
interatrial septum [intəréitriəl séptəm]	septum = wall	the wall separating the two atria
brady- :		**slow**
bradycardia [brǽdikɑ́:rdiə]	-ia = condition; cardi/o = heart	condition of slow heartbeat
coron/o :		**crown, heart**
coronary artery [kɔ́:rənèri ɑ́:rtəri]	-ary = pertaining to	artery branched from the aorta that supplies blood to the myocardium

Term	Term Analysis	Meaning
isch/o :		**holding back, restriction**
ischemia [iskí:miə]	-emia = blood condition	the condition of obstructed blood supply to the myocardium
scler/o :		**hardening**
sclerotherapy [sklirouθérəpi]	-therapy = treatment	injection of material that hardens and shrinks veins to treat varicose veins, hemorrhoids, etc.
valv/o, valvul/o :		**valve**
valvuloplasty [vǽlvjuləplǽsti]	-plasty = surgical reconstruction	plastic surgery to repair a heart valve, usually to widen stenotic passage
vas/o :		**blood vessel**
vasoconstriction [væ̀sou*u*kənstríkʃən]	-constrict = to narrow	narrowing of blood vessels by constriction
vasodilation [væ̀sou*u*dailéiʃən]	-dilat/o = expand	widening of blood vessels by dilation
ventricul/o :		**ventricle**
interventricular septum [íntərventrikjulər séptəm]	-septum = wall	the wall separating the two ventricles
tachy- :		**fast**
tachycardia [tæ̀kikɑ́:*r*diə]	-ia = condition	condition of fast heartbeat

Abbreviations

Abbreviation	Full Term	Meaning
AFib	Atrial fibrillation	rapid, irregular or unsynchronized contractions of the atrium - a typical arrhythmia
AV	Atrioventricular	of relationship between the atrium and the ventricle
AS	Aortic stenosis	condition of narrowed aortic valve or aorta
ASD	Atrial septal defect	congenital defect in the wall between the two atria, allowing flow between the chambers

Abbreviation	Full Term	Meaning
ASHD	Arteriosclerotic heart disease	heart disease due to the condition of arteries narrowed by plaque built up along the inner walls
BP	Blood pressure	systolic and diastolic blood pressure readings
CABG	Coronary artery bypass graft	grafting artery piece to bypass the blocked portion of coronary artery
CAD	Coronary artery disease	
CCU	Coronary care unit	cardiac intensive care unit in a hospital ward
CHF	Congestive heart failure	condition of severely limited ability by the heart to pump blood
COA	Coarctation of the aorta	congenital condition of constricted aorta in the area in contact with other large vessels nearby
CPK	Creatine phosphokinase	
CPR	Cardiopulmonary resuscitation	emergency procedure to manually preserve brain function until further measures are taken to restore spontaneous blood circulation and breathing for the patient in cardiac arrest
CV	Cardiovascular	pertaining to the circulatory system, i.e. the heart and blood vessels
CVA	Cerebro vascular accident	stroke; loss of brain function when blood supply to the brain is interrupted
DORV	Double outlet right ventricle	congenital heart disease where both of the great arteries (pulmonary artery and aorta) connect to the right ventricle
ECG, EKG	Electrocardiogram	recorded output of the electrical activities of the heart
Echo	Echocardiogram	Visual image of the moving heart produced using ultrasound
HDL	High density lipoprotein	
HHD	Hypertensive heart disease	disease including a number of complications relating to hypertension
HTN	Hypertension	high blood pressure
ICD	Implantable cardiac defibrillator	device inserted in the chest to monitor and correct arrhythmia
IHD	Ischemic heart disease	coronary artery disease with insufficient blood flow to myocardium
IVC	Inferior vena cava	largest vein that carry blood into right atrium from below
LA	Left atrium	
LAD	Left anterior descending coronary artery	

Abbreviation	Full Term	Meaning
LDL	Low density lipoprotein	
LV	Left ventricle	
LVH	Left ventricular hypertrophy	thickening of the myocardium of the left ventricle
MI	Myocardial infarction	Necrosis of the myocardium caused by interruption of blood supply to the heart tissues
MR	Mitral regurgitation	blood backflow through the mitral valve due to not closing properly
MS	Mitral valve stenosis	condition of mitral valve having been narrowed
MVP	Mitral valve prolapse	condition of mitral valve having been prolapsed, preventing normal flow
NSR	Normal sinus rhythm	condition of normal electrical conduction by the sinoatrial node
PAD	Peripheral artery disease	obstruction of arteries not within the heart, aortic arch and the brain
PAT	Paroxysmal atrial tachycardia	supraventricular tachycardia; rapid heart rhythm originating at or above atrioventricular node
PDA	Patent ductus arteriosus	congenital disorder in the heart wherein a newborn's ductus arteries (a shunt vessel connecting the pulmonary artery to the proximal descending aorta) fails to close after birth
PS	Pulmonic stenosis	obstruction of blood flow from the right ventricle to the pulmonary artery
PTCA	Percutaneous transluminal coronary angioplasty	angioplasty of the stenotic coronary artery
PVC	Premature ventricular contraction	contraction of ventricles being initiated too early by Purkinje fibers rather than the sinoatrial node, causing inefficient pumping
RA	Right atrium	
RV	Right ventricle	
SA	Sinoatrial	relating to the sinoatrial node
SPECT	Single photon emission computed tomography	
SVC	Superior vena cava	largest vein that carries blood into right atrium from above
TEE	Transesophageal echocardiogram	echocardiogram taken from the probe inserted in the esophagus
TOF	Tetralogy of Fallot	congenital heart defect involving 4 anatomical anomalies of the heart
VSD	Ventricular septal defect	septum having a hole and not completely separating the two ventricles

Exercises

1. Write the meaning of the following cardiovascular anatomical terms.

① tricuspid valve

atrioventricular valve between the right atrium and the right ventricle

② right ventricle

chamber at the lower right part of the heart that pumps blood out through the aorta

③ pulmonary vein

large blood vessel through which blood flows from the lung to the left atrium

④ left atrium

chamber at the upper left part of the heart that receives blood from the lung

⑤ mitral valve

atrioventricular valve between the left atrium and the left ventricle

⑥ aortic valve

the valve that prevents backflow between the left atrium and the aorta

⑦ aorta

main trunk of the arterial system that carries blood from the left ventricle to the whole body (except lungs) through arteries

⑧ pericardium

membranous sac containing the heart

⑨ epicardium

the outermost layer of the heart wall, contacting pericardium

⑩ endocardium

the innermost layer of the heart wall

⑪ septum

wall separating the left and right chambers of the heart

⑫ arterioles

the smallest of arteries that connect to the capillaries

⑬ capillary

the most numerous and smallest of the body's blood vessels

⑭ coronary artery
artery that supplies blood to the myocardium and other components of the heart

⑮ pacemaker
impulse-generating device to stimulate heart muscles to contract

⑯ sinoatrial node
impulse-generating (pacemaker) tissue located on the wall of the right atrium

2. Write the meaning of the following surgical terms.

① atherectomy
aurgical procedure to remove fatty plaque from an artery

② atrial fibrillation ablation
removing of fibrillation (arrhythmic contractions) of the atrium

③ bypass surgery
surgical procedure involving rerouting a stenotic vessel.

④ pericardiocentesis
removing pericardial fluid through a needle inserted into the pericardium

⑤ coronary artery bypass graft
surgically grafting an arterial piece onto the coronary artery and to bypass a stenotic portion

⑥ endarterectomy
surgical procedure to remove plaque from an artery

⑦ implantable cardiac defibrillator(ICD)
device inserted in the chest to monitor and correct arrhythmia

⑧ mitral commissurotomy
surgical incision of a commissure in the mitral valve

⑨ open heart surgery
surgical incision of a heart chamber to correct the inner structure

⑩ percutaneous transluminal coronary angioplasty
angioplasty of the stenotic coronary artery

⑪ pericardiectomy
surgical removal of a part or all of the pericardium

⑫ phlebectomy

surgical removal of a portion of a vein

⑬ phlebotomy

making an incision in a vein to draw blood

⑭ shunt surgery

surgical process of making anatomical shortcuts away from the normal paths

⑮ valve replacement

open heart surgery in which a damaged heart valve is replaced with an artificial one

3. Correct the spelling of the following terms.

① angiospazm	angiospasm
② arrythmia	arrhythmia
③ cardiomecgaly	cardiomegaly
④ diastrole	diastole
⑤ febrilation	fibrillation
⑥ flotter	flutter
⑦ hyperipidemia	hyperlipidemia
⑧ hypotention	hypotension
⑨ palpitasiion	palpitation
⑩ pericardiac effusion	pericardial effusion
⑪ phlebologyist	phlebologist
⑫ regergitation	regurgitation
⑬ vasocontricsion	vasoconstriction

4. Write the full name of the following abbreviations.

① ASD	trial septal defect
② B.P.	blood pressure
③ CABG	coronary artery bypass grafting
④ CAD	coronary artery disease
⑤ CHF	congestive heart failure

⑥ COA coarctation of the aorta

⑦ CPR cardiopulmonary resuscitation

⑧ ECG, EKG electrocardiogram

⑨ HTN hypertension

⑩ IHD ischemic heart disease

⑪ LAD left anterior descending coronary artery

⑫ MI myocardial infarction

⑬ MR mitral regurgitation

⑭ NSR normal sinus rhythm

⑮ PDA patent ductus arteriosus

⑯ PS pulmonic stenosis, pulmonary stenosis

⑰ PTCA percutaneous transluminal coronary angioplasty

⑱ PVC premature ventricular contraction

⑲ SVC superior vena cava

⑳ VSD ventricular septal defect

5. Construct medical terms that mean the following.

- Use vas/o to construct terms that mean the following.

1. decrease of diameter of blood vessels vasoconstriction
2. dialation of the blood vessels vasodilation, vasodilatation

- Use arteri/o to construct terms that mean the following.

3. small branch of an artery arteriole
4. hardening and loss of elasticity in arteries arteriosclerosis
5. narrowing of effective cross-section areas in arteries arteriostenosis

- Use cardi/o to construct terms that mean the following.

6. disease of heart muscles cardiomyopathy, myocardiopathy
7. inflammation of all layers of the heart wall pancarditis
8. membranous structure surrounding the heart pericardium

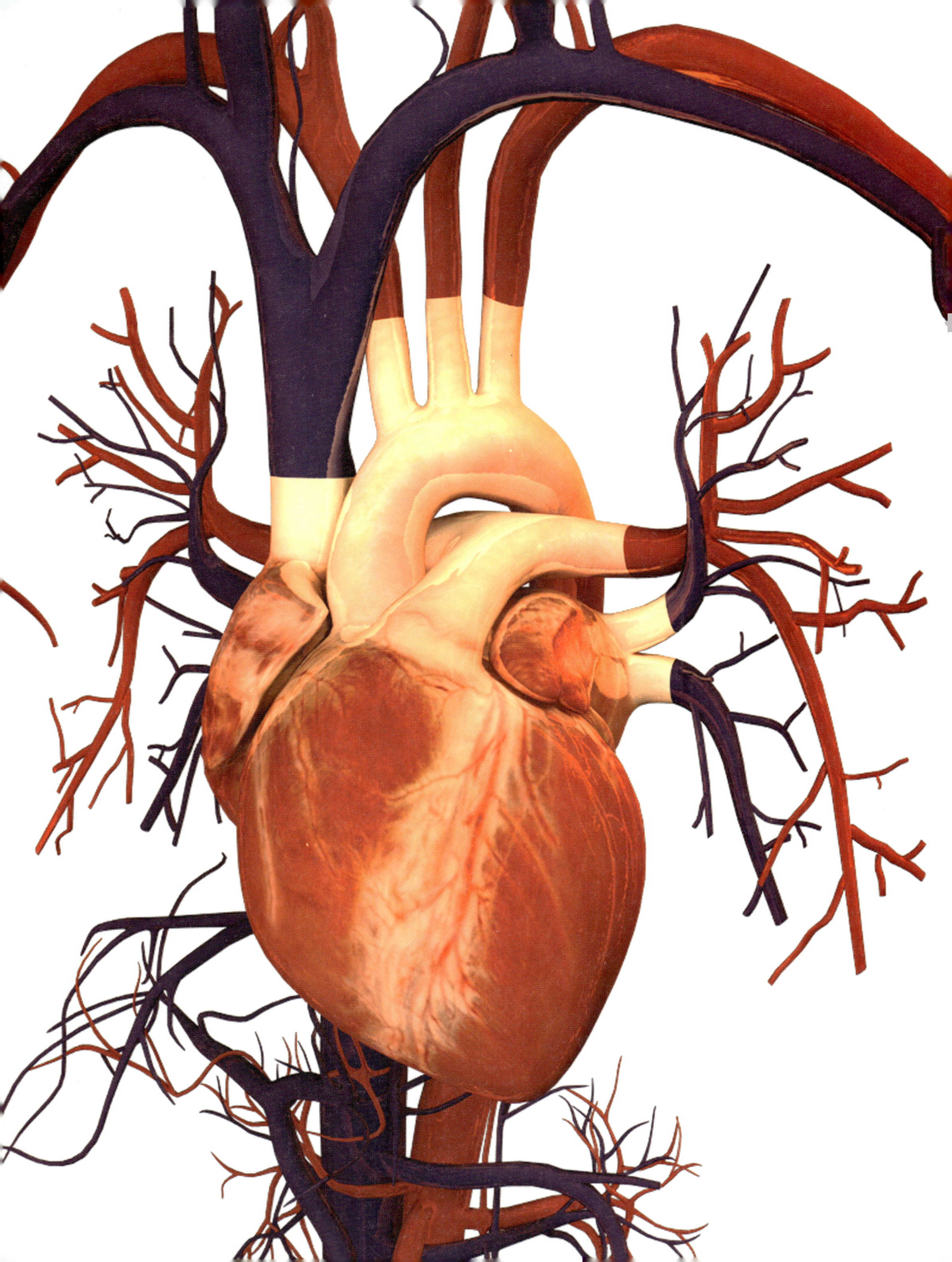

Chapter 13

Blood and Immune/Lymphatic System

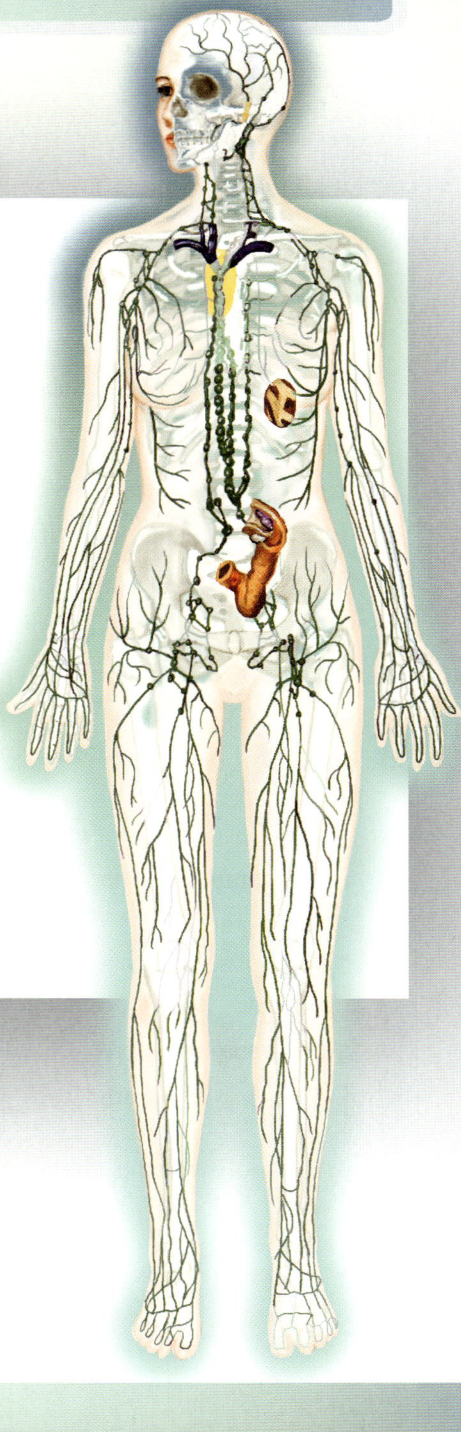

Chapter Contents

- Prolog
- Anatomical Terms
- Terms for Symptoms and Diseases
- Terms for Surgery and Treatment
- Terms for Test and Intervention
- Analysis and Meaning of Key Terms
- Abbreviations
- Exercises

Learning Objectives

- Describe components of the blood.
- Locate parts of the lymphatic system.
- Analyze, define and pronounce terms relating to the blood and lymphatic system.
- Define abbreviations relating to the blood and the lymphatic system.

Prolog

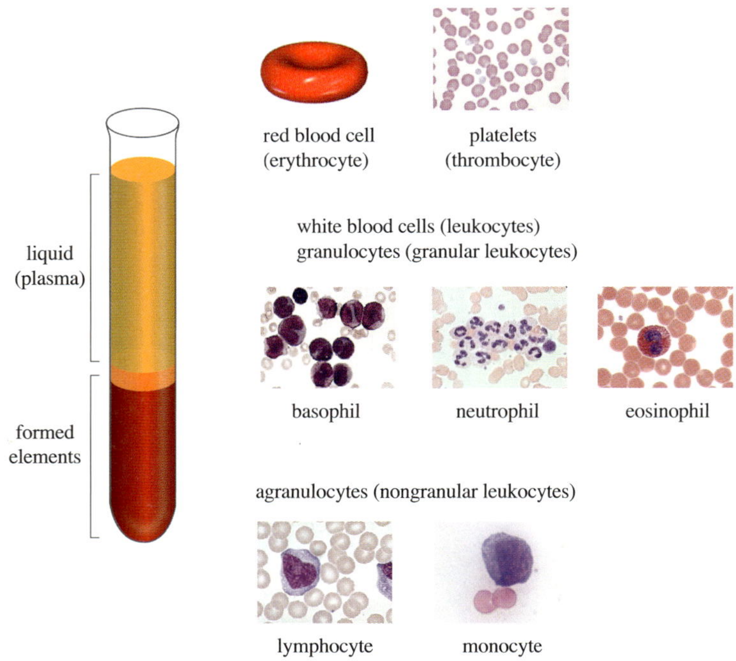

Figure 13-1 Components of the blood

Blood plasma transports fats, proteins, gases, salts and hormones as well as blood cells, and picks up waste materials to and from destination organ cells throughout the body. The fats such as triglycerides, phospholipid and cholesterol are transported to tissues by attaching to proteins. Proteins present in blood plasma are mostly albumins, globulins and fibrinogen.

- Blood plasma transports blood cells, gases, fats (as triglycerides, phospholipid and cholesterol), salts, proteins (albumins, globulins and fibrogens) and hormones.

- Serum is plasma with fibrinogen and and other clotting factors removed.
- Blood cells start out as hemocytoblasts (blood stem cells) in the process called hematopoiesis. Hemocytoblasts develop into three different blood cell types : erythrocytes (red blood cells), leucocytes (white blood cells), thrombocytes (platelets). Each process is called erythropoiesis, leukopoiesis, thrombopoiesis, respectively.

Erythrocytes are shaped like discs with the concave center. They contain hemoglobin that contains iron that binds with oxygen or carbon dioxide. After reticulocytes mature to become erythrocytes, they leave the red bone marrow and enter the bloodstream, where they can be counted in a clinical test. The erythrocyte is destroyed after about 120 days.

Leukocytes fight against infections after they migrate from the bloodstream into the infected tissues. They are classified as either granular or agranular.

The granular leukocytes (granulocytes) are further classified as either eosinophils, basophils or neutrophils. The eosinophils release chemicals that can neutralize toxic substances into the bloodstream. The basophils release histamine, a natural toxin that initiates inflammatory process by dilating the blood vessels. The dilation increases blood flow into the site of the infection, thereby speeding recovery. Neutrophils, also known as polymorphonuclear leukocytes, devour bacteria and other harmful matter.

The agranular leukocytes (agranulocytes) are further classified as either monocytes or lymphocytes. Monocytes act much like neutrophils, ingesting harmful microbes. Lymphocytes' functions are important in the immune system.

Thrombocytes (platelets) initiate blood clotting when hemorrhage occurs. By releasing the clotting agents such as prothrombin and fibrinogen, a platelet lump is formed where a vessel has ruptured to halt hemorrhage.

The type of blood a patient can receive in a transfusion depends on the presence or absence of the A, B, AB or O antigens. If the person receives the wrong type of blood, antibodies will be formed against the specific antigen as they recognize the antigen to be foreign to the body. This is an antigen-antibody reaction. If a person with type A blood receives type B blood or vice versa, the person will generate antibodies. A person with type AB blood doesn't generate antibodies with any type blood, enabling him / her to receive all types of blood.

A person with type O blood need type O blood for transfusion, but he/she can donate to another person with any type blood. The antigen-antibody reaction may cause agglutination of erythrocytes. Therefore, the blood must be cross-matched before it is transfused into a patient. In cross-matching, the donor's blood must be mixed with the recipient's blood and analyzed for agglutination.

Memory key

- Type A blood has type A antigens. Type B blood has type B antigens. Type AB blood has antigens of both types, while type O blood doesn't have either.

There are several other blood antigens. The most important is the Rh antigen, which was discovered while examining the blood of the Rhesus monkeys. Most people are Rh positive, which means they have the Rh antigen. The rest of them who don't have the Rh antigen are Rh negative.

The lymphatic system consists of vascular system, lymph fluid, lymph nodes, the thymus gland, the spleen, the tonsils and the Peyer's patches. The lymphatic system serves several important functions in the body. They move various materials to and from body tissues, and transports lipids from the digestive system. Lymphocytes and monocytes in the system help the body defend against infections.

The vascular system consists of three types of vessels, the smallest of which are lymphatic capillaries present in all body tissues and originate in capillary beds with those of the circulatory system. Plasma constantly seeps out of arterial capillaries and is absorbed in the body tissues. This fluid, which has become the interstitial fluid, picks up bacteria and cellular wastes and seeps back into the circulatory system or into the lymphatic capillaries.

The fluid that has entered lymphatic capillaries and has become lymph, drains into lymphatics (larger lymphatic vessels) and again drains into right and left lymph ducts, the largest lymphatic vessels. The right lymph duct receives lymph from the right side of the head, neck, chest and the right arm. The left lymph duct receives lymph from the rest of the body. The left duct is also known as the thoracic duct. Both lymph ducts drain into the bloodstream.

Some lymphatics drain into lymph nodes. Lymph nodes are distributed at various sites in the body. They fuction as filters for lymph and contain a lot of phagocytes that devour bacteria. This process is called phagocytosis. When there is infection, the lymph node becomes swollen and tender due to abnormal increase in the number of bacteria. This condition is called lymphadenopathy. The sites of lymph node clusters are cervix (neck), under the mandible (lower jaw), axilla (armpit) and groin.

The thymus gland, located near the heart in the thoracic cavity, doubles as a lymphatic organ and an endocrine gland. It secretes thymosin, a hormone that stimulates bone marrows to produce T-cells which mature in the thymus.

Memory key

- The lymphatic system drains fluids, carries nutrients, hormones, oxygen and lipids, and fights against infections.
- The spleen stores blood and contains many phagocytes.

Tonsils are made of lymphatic tissue, and filter out bacteria. There are three pairs of tonsils located in the throat. The palatine tonsils are at the back of the oropharynx. The pharyngeal tonsils (adenoids) are in the nasopharynx. The lingual tonsils are near the base of the tongue. Peyer's patches are in the small intestine and are lymphatic filters.

Anatomical Terms

Erythrocyte

Shaped like small discs, erythrocytes contain hemoglobin that contains iron to carry and deliver oxygen to cells in all parts of the body.

Leukocyte

Leucocytes are relatively large and round but appear white due to lack of hemoglobin. In the process called phagocytosis, they destroy pathogens and remove dead tissues to protect the body.

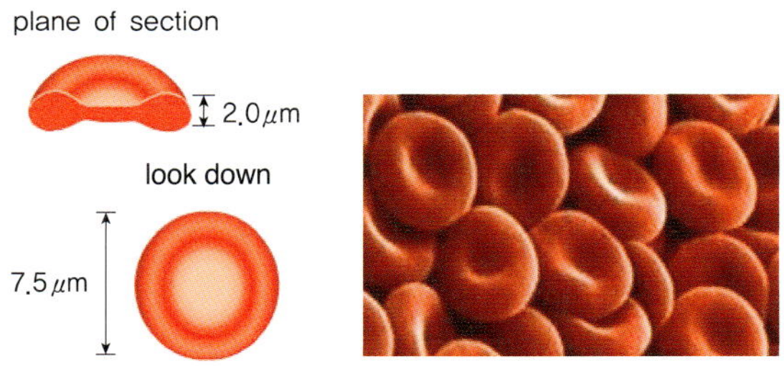

Figure 13-2 Erythrocyte

Platelet

Platelets (thrombocytes) attach to the connective tissue of damaged and open blood vessel site and release materials that help stop hemorrhage by clotting. They are built up with globulin, a type of protein.

Granulocyte

A type of leukocyte that contains granules in the cytoplasm.

Neutrophil

A type of granulocyte that makes up 55~70% of all leukocytes. It is responsible for defense of the body through phagocytosis.

Eosinophil

A type of granulocyte that makes up about 1~3% of all leukocytes. It is known to be involved in inflammatory and allergic responses.

Basophil

A type of granulocyte that makes up only under 1% of all leukocytes. It is involved in inflammatory responses and releases heparin, an anticoagulant.

Agranulocyte

A type of leukocyte that contains no granules in the cytoplasm.

Monocyte

A mobile macrophage, the largest of all leukocytes that moves around in the body for phagocytosis.

Lymph

Lymph is a transparent body fluid like plasma that is transformed from the plasma as the result of the capillary exchange. It drains from all over the body into lymphatic vessels and eventually back to bloodstream.

Lymphatic vessel

A vessel through which lymph flows, distributed in the body much like veins.

Thoracic duct

This is also known as the left lymph duct. Lymph drained from all parts of the body, except from the right side of the body superior to the midriff, flows through the thoracic duct into the vein.

Lymphocyte

A type of leukocyte that is responsible for immune function. It is produced in medulla ossea or lymphatic tissues. T-cells and B-cells are major types of lymphocytes.

Lymph node

Small oval tissues shaped like peas, the lymph nodes are major suppliers of the lymphocytes. They remove harmful bacteria and toxins and produce antibodies.

Lymphatic tissue

Lattice-like network of tissue containing lymphocytes in interstitium, distributed loosely or clustered like those at lymph nodes.

Tonsil

A collection of lymphoid tissues in the oral cavity formed as a mass, responsible for immune function.

Spleen

The largest lymphatic organ in the body that produces lymphocytes and destroys old erythrocytes and thrombocytes.

Thymus

The thymus is a specialized organ involved in immunoresponses and produces mature T-cells.

Terms for Symptoms and Diseases

Hemolytic anemia

A condition in which excessive destruction of erythrocytes causes reduction of their life from the normal 120 days, resulting in anemia.

Pernicious anemia

A condition in which reduction in the concentration of vitamin B_{12} in the blood, required for the development and maturing of erythrocytes, causes formation of megaloblasts (abnormally large erythrocytes) in the blood.

Hemolysis

Hemolysis is the destruction of blood cells and subsequent release of hemoglobin.

Hemophilia

A group of hereditary genetic disorders that impair the body's ability to control blood clotting. It takes the patient much longer time to stop hemorrhage when a blood vessel is broken.

Sickle cell anemia

A hereditary form of hemolytic anemia, mainly affecting people of African origin, in which mutated hemoglobin distorts erythrocytes into a crescent shape, causing them to become stuck in capillaries.

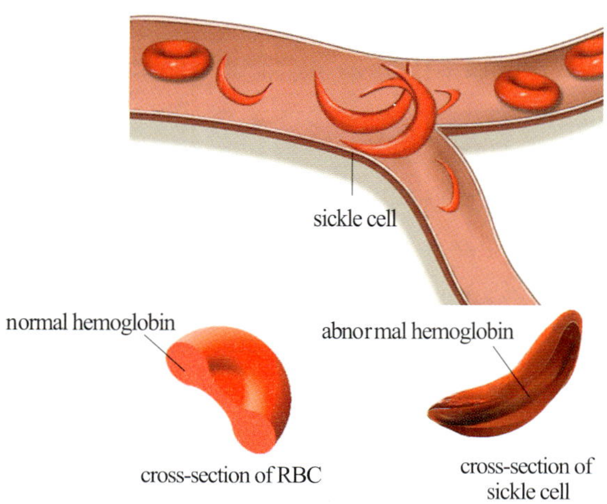

Figure 13-3 Sickle cell anemia

Sepsis

A serious systemic infection and inflammation caused by the presence of pathogenic microbes or their toxins in the bloodstream.

Congestion

The condition in which local overfullness of venous blood occurs in an internal organ or tissue.

Hemostasis

The process of limiting hemorrhage by the natural physiological contraction of the damaged vessel, blood clotting or by external physical means.

Bubo

Inflamed swelling of a lymph node due to infection, frequently occurring in the armpit or the groin.

Edema

Swelling due to unusual amount of buildup of interstitial tissue fluid beneath the skin or in a cavity

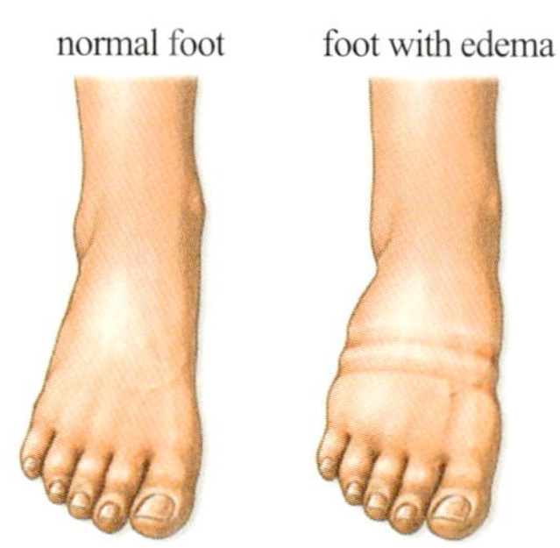

Figure 13-4 An example of edema

Hemorrhage

Escaping of blood components (especially erythrocytes) from the circulatory system.

Hyperemia

An increase in the quantity of blood flow to a body part.

Lymphoma

A malignant tumor in the lymph node, with symptoms including enlarged lymph nodes, large lump on the neck or armpit.

Immunosuppression

Suppression of immune responses detrimental to the body, in cases such as autoimmune disorder or rejective response of an organ transplant, with administration of drugs or radiation therapy.

Lymphocytosis

An increase in the number or proportion of lymphocytes in the blood, that can be observed in pathological condition like infection by pathogen or leukemia.

Lymphocytopenia

Abnormally low number of lymphocytes in the blood, due to inherited or acquired causes.

Terms for Surgery and Treatment

Bone marrow transplantation

This is a method of cancer treatment in which the patient's diseased bone marrow is replaced with healthy counterpart. This is usually performed when the patient's bone marrow is quite deteriorated due to radiation therapy or chemotherapy, especially in cases with leukemia as immunotherapy.

Transfusion

Intravenous infusion of healthy donor's blood or its components into the patient whose own blood or its components are not enough.

Lymph node biopsy

Microscopic examination of a sample lymph node tissue taken from the living body.

Lymphangiography

A medical imaging technique in which contrast media is injected into the patient's lymphatic system and an X-ray picture is taken to visualize the lymph vessels often in the lower parts of the body.

Terms for Test and Intervention

Complete blood count (CBC)

Counting of blood cells (RBC, WBC, platelets, etc.) present in a sample volume of the patient's blood and examining them. For RBC (erythrocyte), concentration of hemoglobin, HCT (hematocrit, packed cell volume ratio), MCV (mean RBC volume), MCH (mean hemoglobin amount in RBC), MCHC (mean concentration of hemoglobin), hemoglobin index, etc. are output, which often help in diagnosis of diseases.

Erythrocyte sedimentation rate (ESR)

The rate at which erythrocytes sediment in a period of one hour. After the venous blood mixed with anticoagulant in a test tube is left standing for a given amount of time, the blood cells in the plasma sediment at the bottom. The speed at which the sedimentation is occurring is measured. This technique can be helpful in diagnosis of various conditions including immune disorders, infections and inflammations, myeloma, wounds, with monitoring the response to therapy.

C-reactive protein (CRP) test

A specific protein that reacts with C-polysaccharide of Pneumococcus is involved in inflammation and breakdown of tissues. CRP is found in the blood serum 14~24 hours after inflammation or tissue breakdown. This test is used for monitoring prognosis.

Arterial blood gas analysis (ABGA)

A sample blood is taken from the artery of a patient, often with artificial breathing suffering from respiratory or circulatory disease, to analyze oxygen concentration, efficiency of carbon dioxide transportation, etc.

Analysis and Meaning of Key Terms

Blood

Term	Term Analysis	Meaning
hemat/o, hem/o :		**blood**
hemolysis [himɑ́ləsis]	-lysis = breakdown, destruction, separation	breakdown of blood cells, esp. RBC
hematologist [hi:məta:lədʒust]	-logist = specialist	scientist or doctor specializing in blood
hematology [hèmətɑ́lədʒi]	-logy = study of	study of blood and related organs and diseases
erythr/o :		**red**
erythrocyte [erə́θrosàit]	-cyte = cell	red blood cell
leuk/o :		**white**
leukocyte [lú:kəsàit]	-cyte = cell	white blood cell
myel/o :		**bone marrow, spinal cord**
myelogenous [màiəlɑ́dʒənəs]	-genous = produced by	produced by the bone marrow
myeloid [máiəlɔ́id]	-oid = resembling, derived from	pertaining to bone marrow or spinal cord
reticul/o :		**net, network**
reticulocyte [ritíkjuləsàit]	-cyte = cell	immature erythrocyte that have RNA of reticular shape before maturing
thromb/o :		**blood clot**
thrombocyte [θrɑ́mbəsàit]	-cyte = cell	platelet
thrombolysis [θrɑmbɑ́ləsis]	-lysis = destruction, breakdown, separation	breakdown of blood clots by pharmacological means
thrombosis [pèrikɑ:rdáitis]	-osis = abnormal condition	abnormal clotting of blood inside a vessel, obstructing circulation

Term	Term Analysis	Meaning
chrom/o :		color
hyperchromia [hàipərkriumiə]	-ia = condition hyper- = excessive, above normal	excessively high level of hemoglobin in the erythrocyte
hypochromia [hàipəkroumiə]	-ia = condition hypo- = deficient, below normal	excessively low level of hemoglobin in the erythrocyte
normochromia [normokroumiə]	-ia = condition norm/o = normal	normal level of hemoglobin in the erythrocyte
immun/o :		immunity, protection
immunodeficiency [ìmjənoudifíʃənsi]	-deficiency = lack of	lacking immune response
immunology [ìmjənάlədʒi]	-logy = study of	study of immune system

Lymph

Term	Term Analysis	Meaning
lymphaden/o :		lymph node
lymphadenitis [limfæ̀dənάitis]	-itis = inflammation	inflammation of the lymph node, causing swelling
lymphadenopathy [limfæ̀dənάpəθi]	-pathy = disease	disease of the lymph node, usually meaning lymphadenitis
lymphangi/o :		lymph vessel
lymphangitis [limfæ̀ndʒiάitis]	-itis = inflammation	infection/inflammation of the lymphatic vessels
lymph/o :		lymph
lymphedema [limfidémə]	-edema = accumulation of fluid, swelling	swelling due to lymphatic vessel blockage and local retention of fluid
lymphoma [limfóumə]	-oma = tumor	tumor of the lymph node, usually malignant
splen/o :		spleen
splenomegaly [splì:nəmégəli]	-megaly = enlargement	enlargement of the spleen
splenorrhagia [splì:nərájah]	-rrhagia = bursting forth	bursting forth (bleeding) of the spleen
splenorrhaphy [splì:nəráhfe]	-rrhaphy = surgical suturing	surgical suturing of the spleen

Term	Term Analysis	Meaning
thym/o :		thymus gland
thymectomy [θaiméktəmi]	-ectomy = excision, surgical removal	surgical removal of the thymus

Suffixes

Term	Term Analysis	Meaning
-blast :		Immature cell
hemocytoblast [henə́sidəblast]	hem/o = blood, cyt/o = cell	immature blood cell
lymphoblast [limfəblast]	lymph/o = lymph	immature lymphocyte
monoblast [mɔ́noblast]	mon/o = one, single	immature mononuclear leukocyte
-crit :		separation
hematocrit (HCT) [himǽtəkrit]	hemat/o = blood	percentage of RBC in the blood
-cytosis :		increase in the number of cells
anisocytosis [anisəsítoseə]	anis/o = unequal	significant size variation of RBCs
leukocytosis [lù:kəsaitóusis]	leuk/o = white	increase in the number of RBCs
poikilocytosis [poilkiləsítosəs]	poikil/o = variation, irregularity	presence of RBCs with abnormal shape
-emia :		blood condition
anemia [əní:miə]	an- = no, not, lacking	too few RBCs or too low hemoglobin content
erythremia [erə́tgremiə]	erythr/o = red	polycythemia vera, the condition in which the bone marrow produces too many blood cells, esp. RBCs
-emia :		blood condition
hyperbilirubinemia [hàipərbilərub-ə́nemiə]	hyper- = excessive, above normal; bilirubin/o = bilirubin	presence of excess bilirubin in the blood
hypercholesterolemia [hàipərkəlèstər-əli:miə]	hyper- = excessive, above normal	presence of excess cholesterol in the blood

Term	Term Analysis	Meaning
-emia :		blood condition
hyperlipidemia [hàipərlìpədí:miə]	hyper- = excessive, above normal	condition of excess lipid in the blood
leukemia [lu:kí:miə]	leuk/o = white	cancer of the blood, having too many WBCs produced in the bone marrow
-penia :		deficiency, decrease
erythrocytopenia [erəthrosàitəpí:niə]	erythr/o = red, cyt/o = cell	erythropenia, deficiency of RBCs in the blood
leukocytopenia [lookosàitəpí:niə]	leuk/o = white, cyt/o = cell	leucopenia, deficiency of WBCs in the blood
pancytopenia [pansitopí:niə]	pan- = all, cyt/o = cell	deficiency of RBCs, WBCs and platelets in the blood
thrombocytopenia [θrɑ̀mbousàitəpí:niə]	thromb/o = clotting, cyt/o = cell	thrombopenia, deficiency of platelets in the blood
-phoresis :		transmission, carrying
electrophoresis [ilèktroufərí:sis]	electr/o = electric	method of separating and analyzing large molecules such as proteins or DNA, using electric field to move the charged molecules dispersed in a gel
-poiesis :		production, formation
erythropoiesis [irìθroupoií:sis]	electr/o = red	production of RBCs in bone marrow
hematopoiesis [hì:mətoupɔi:sis]	hemat/o = blood	production of blood cells
-poietin :		hormone regulating the production of blood cells
erythropoietin [irìθroupɔ́iətən]	erythr/o = red	glycoprotein hormone that controls erythropoiesis
-stasis :		stopping, controlling
hemostasis [hìməstéisis]	hem/o = blood	the process of keeping bleeding in check
-immune :		immunity, protection
autoimmune disease [ɔ̀:touimjú:n dizí:z]	auto- = self	the condition of abnormal immune response against one's own tissues

Abbreviations

Abbreviation	Full Term	Meaning
ABO	A, B, O blood groups	blood grouping system by antigen type
CBC c.b.c	Complete blood count	blood cell count of RBCs, WBCs, platelets; blood panel
Diff	Differential count	measuring percentage of each type of WBCs
Eos	Eosinophil	an acid-loving granular type WBC that fights parasite infections
ESR	Erythrocyte sedimentation rate	the rate at which RBCs precipitate in an hour
Hb, Hgb	Hemoglobin	iron-containing substance in RBCs that transport oxygen
HCT, HcT	Hematocrit	percentage by volume of RBCs in a sample of blood
Lymphs	Lymphocytes	a non-granular type WBC in the lymphatic immune system, including NK cells, T cells and B cells
Mono	Monocyte	a non-granular mononuclear type WBC in the immune system
PMN	Polymorphonuclear	having a nucleus with lobes of diverse shapes
Polys	Polymorphonuclear leukocytes	a granular polymorphonuclear type WBC, usually referring to neutrophil
R.B.C., rbc	Red blood cell	erythrocyte
Segs	Segmented neutrophils	a granular polymorphonuclear type WBC, with segmented nuclei
W.B.C., wbc	White blood cell	leukocyte
Ab	Antibody	a protein produced by B-lymphocytes that binds to a specific antigen
Ag	Antigen	a foreign substance that stimulates the production of an antibody
AIDS	Acquired immune deficiency syndrome	
HIV	Human immunodeficiency virus	the agent attacking the immune system and causing AIDS
Ig	Immunoglobulin	antibody occurring naturally in the body

Exercises

1. Name three proteins in the blood plasma.

albumin, globulin, fibrinogen

2. What is (are) difference(s) in the following terms?

① Plasma and serum

plasma : fluid of blood after blood cells are removed

serum : plasma after blood clotting factor including fibrinogens is removed

② eosinophils, basophils, and neutrophils

eosinophil : leukocyte responsible for combating parasites and releasing chemicals that can neutralize toxic substances into the bloodstream

basophil : leukocyte responsible for releasing histamine, a natural toxin that initiates inflammatory process by dilating the blood vessels

neutrophil : large leukocyte that devours bacteria and other harmful matters

③ A, B, AB, and O type blood

Type A blood contains antigen type A.

Type B blood contains antigen type B.

Type AB blood contains both antigens type A and B.

Type O blood contains neither type A nor type B antigen.

3. Define the following medical terms.

① phagocyte

immune cells, usually large leukocytes in the lymph nodes or other organs, that destroy and ingest harmful foreign particles and pathogens

② thymosin

hormone secreted by thymus that stimulates the development of T-cells (T-lymphocytes) in the bone marrow

③ pharyngeal tonsil

adenoid; a lymphatic tissue covered by ciliated epithelium, found in the posterior wall of the nasopharynx at the back of the throat

④ T lymphocyte

lymphocyte initiated by the thymus that can recognize specific antigens and control other immune cells

⑤ B lymphocyte

lymphocyte developed by the bone marrow that produce antibodies

4. Name four lymph nodes.

cervical lymph node (in the neck)

submandibular lymph node (below the mandible, lower jaw)

axillary lymph node (in the armpit)

inguinal lymph node (in the groin)

Chapter 14

Respiratory System

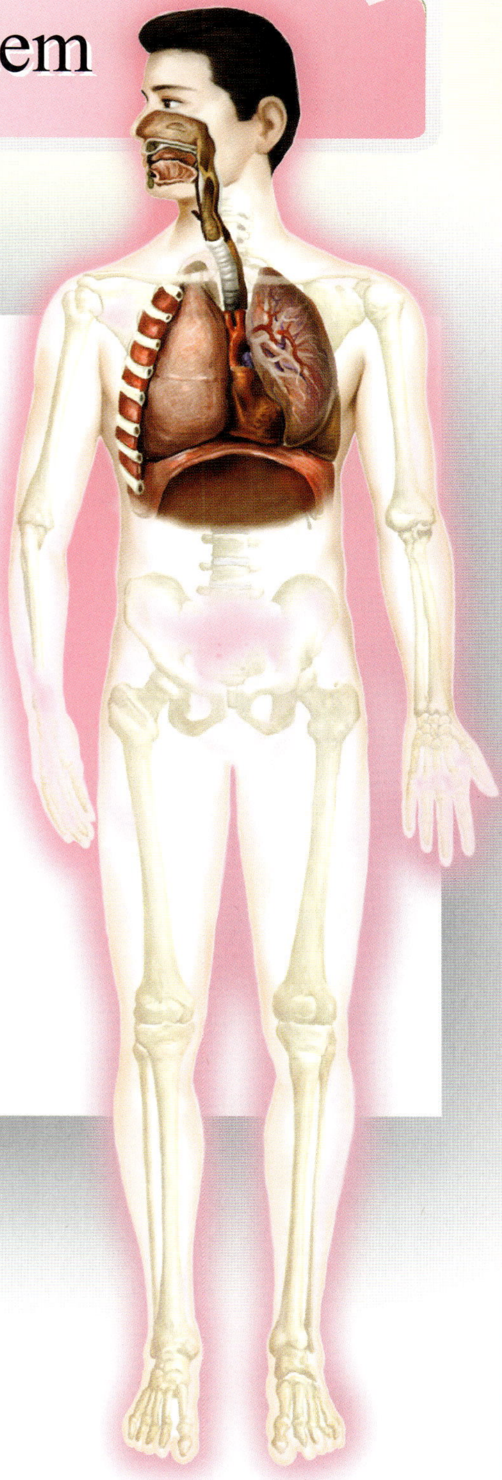

Chapter Contents

- Prolog
- Anatomical Terms
- Terms for Symptoms and Diseases
- Terms for Surgery and Treatment
- Terms for Test and Intervention
- Analysis and Meaning of Key Terms
- Abbreviations
- Exercises

Learning Objectives

- Learn the structure, names of the organs and their locations in the upper and lower respiratory tract.
- Analyze and understand terms relating to the respiratory system.
- Pronounce and define anatomical terms relating to the respiratory system.
- Pronounce and define symptomatic terms relating to the respiratory system.
- Pronounce and define surgical terms relating to the respiratory system.
- Define abbreviations commonly used in the respiratory system.

Prolog

The respiratory system is a collection of organs whose function is to supply blood with oxygen extracted from the air and discharge carbon dioxide by breathing air into and out of the body. The upper respiratory tract consists of the nose, nasal cavity, pharynx and larynx. The lower respiratory tract consists of the trachea, bronchi, and lungs.

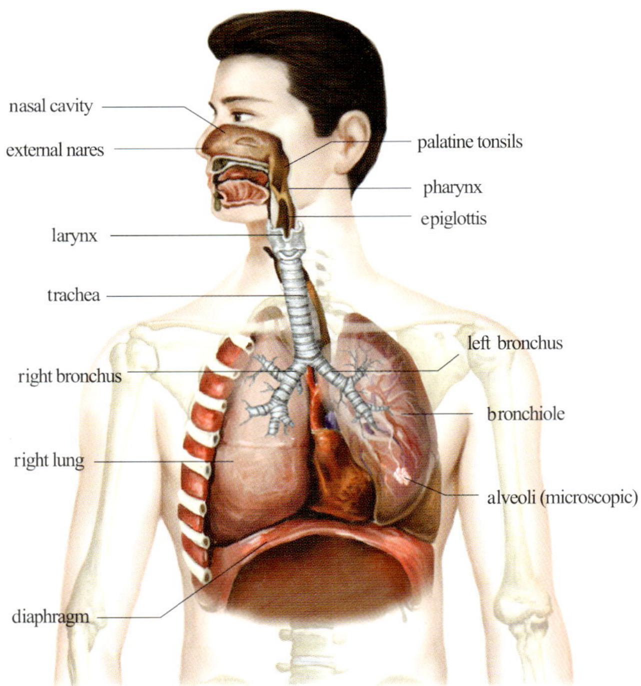

Figure 14-1 Structure of the respiratory system

This chapter is written for the reader to understand the structure and function related to the respiratory system, and to learn the related terms.

Anatomical Terms

Nose, Nasal cavity and Paranasal Sinuses

Nose

The nose is a cartiaginous and bony tissue structure with a mucous membrane and fine hair in the nostrils. The entering air is heated and humidified while it passes through the hairy nasal cavity. The cilia in the nose excrete dust and foreign materials.

Nasal septum

The medial wall separating the left and right nasal cavities.

Nasal cavity

The air space that extends from the nostril to the uvula.

Paranasal sinuses

Empty pairs of air spaces in the skull connected to the nasal cavities and covered with mucous membranes. The cavities heat up the air during inhalation, and help resonate voice from the vocal cord.

Frontal sinus

Superior to the eyes, in the frontal bone which forms the hard part of the forehead.

Ethmoidal sinus

The small air space in the ethmoid bone.

Maxillary sinus

Inferior to the eyes, in the maxillary bones and largest of the paranasal sinuses.

Sphenoidal sinus

In the sphenoid bone of the skull.

Memory key

- The left and right nasal cavities of the nose are separated by the nasal septum. Frontal, ethmoidal, maxillary and sphenoidal sinuses comprise the paranasal sinuses.

Pharynx, Larynx and Trachea

Pharynx

The pharynx is the muscular passage for food and air, consisting of nasopharynx through which air from the nose passes toward the larynx, oropharynx through which food from the mouth passes toward the esophagus, and laryngopharynx where the pharynx and the larynx meet.

Nasopharynx

The region of the passage superior to the soft palate posterior to the nasal cavity.

Oropharynx

The region of the passage posterior to the oral cavity and contains the tongue base, the tonsils and the posterior wall of the pharynx.

Laryngopharynx

The region where the pharynx and larynx are connected.

Adenoid

A lymphatic pharyngeal tonsil tissue posterior to the nasal cavity, which appears degenerated in adults.

Tonsil

Collection of lymphoid tissues on the sides of the throat.

Palatine tonsils

Lymphatic tissues on the palatine, on both sides of the soft palate at the back of the throat.

Pharyngeal tonsil

The adenoid, posterior to the nasal cavity on the back wall of the pharynx.

Lingual tonsil

Small wart-like lymphatic tissue protrusions at the surface of the tongue base.

Larynx

The organ that controls breath and produces voice, between the pharynx and the trachea.

Epiglottis

A flap made of elastic cartilage tissue at the entrance of the larynx, which admits air but automatically blocks foreign matter, including food when swallowing, going into the trachea.

Vocal cords

The organ in the mid-larynx that generates vocal sound.

Glottis

The space between the vocal cords in the larynx, or the structure that surrounds the opening.

Laryngeal cartilage

The supporting skeleton for the larynx, consisting of 9 cartilages including 3 unpaired and 3 paired.

Thyroid cartilage

Also known as Adam's apple, this is the largest of the laryngeal cartilages that protrudes in front of the larynx.

Cricoid cartilage

A ring of hyaline cartilage that forms the inferior and posterior part of the larynx

Trachea

The passageway, anterior to and running in parallel with the esophagus, for the air to enter the bronchi. It is 10~11 cm long and starts at the lower end of the cricoid cartilage toward the lung, consisting of a series of tracheal cartilage rings, stacked up and attached to each other with fundiform ligament, to form a tube.

Memory key

- The pharynx consists of nasopharynx, oropharynx and laryngopharynx. The larynx is enclosed in C-shaped rings of cartilage.

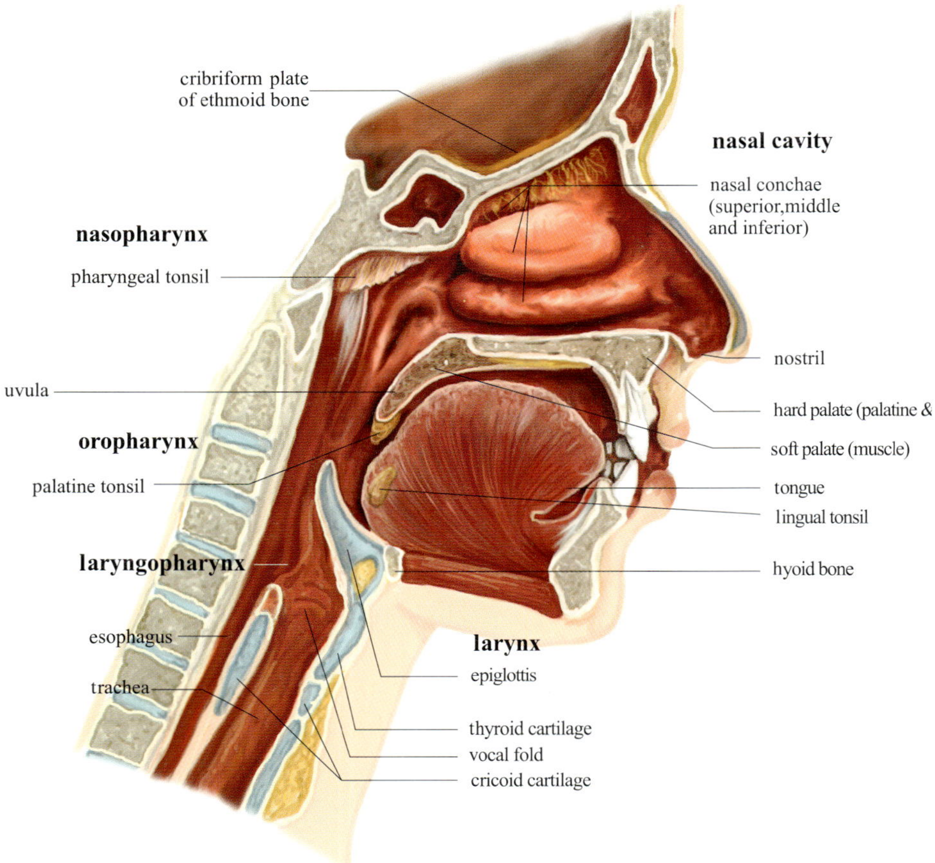

Figure 14-2 Structure of the upper respiratory tract

Bronchus and Lung

Carina

The carina of trachea is a cartilaginous ridge within the trachea where the air path divides into two bronchi.

Bronchus

The trachea divides into left and right bronchi, at the level of the 4th thoracic

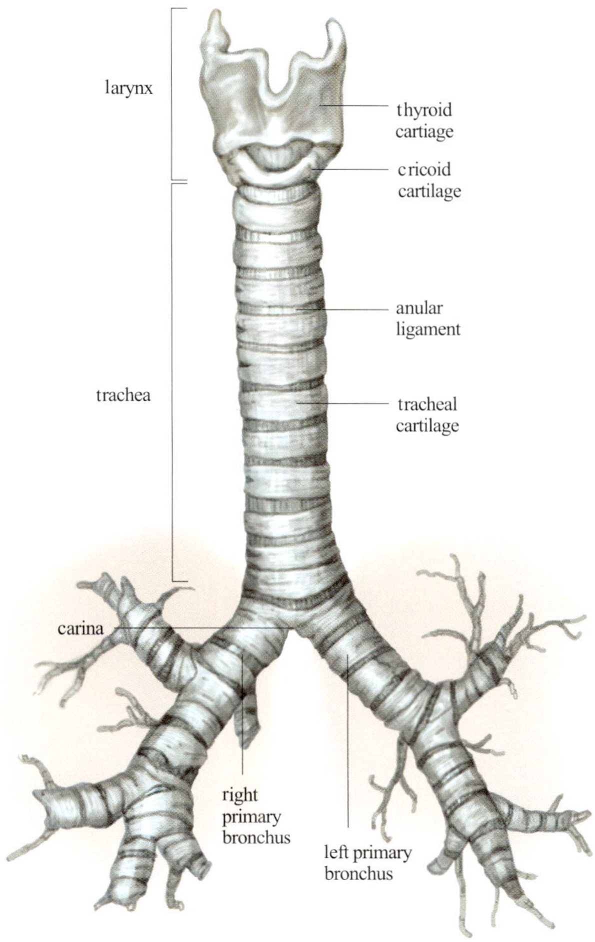

Figure 14-3
Larynx, trachea and bronchi

vertebra. The bronchi are the air passage and deliver air into the left and right lungs. The right bronchus is shorter and wider than its counterpart on the left. The goblet cells that make up the bronchi secrete mucous fluid to catch foreign materials, while the cilia on the lining move foreign materials for absorption or excretion.

Bronchioles

The thin air passages of diameter no larger than 1 *mm* in the bronchial tree which is branched out from the main bronchi.

Alveolar ducts

The tiny ducts at the end of the bronchial tree that connect the bronchioles to alveolar sacs and alveoli.

Alveolar sac

An alveolar sac is a basic gas exchange unit at a terminal end of the bronchial tree, and contains many alveoli. Alveolar sacs surround alveolar ducts and are clustered around them like grapes.

Alveoli

Alveoli located at the ends of the alveolar ducts and contained in the alveolar sac are tiny air cavities where oxygen and carbon dioxides are exchanged.

Lung

Two semi-conical organs in the pleural cavity. The right lung is divided into three lobes, while the left one is divided into two.

Apex of lung

The rounded upper part of each lung.

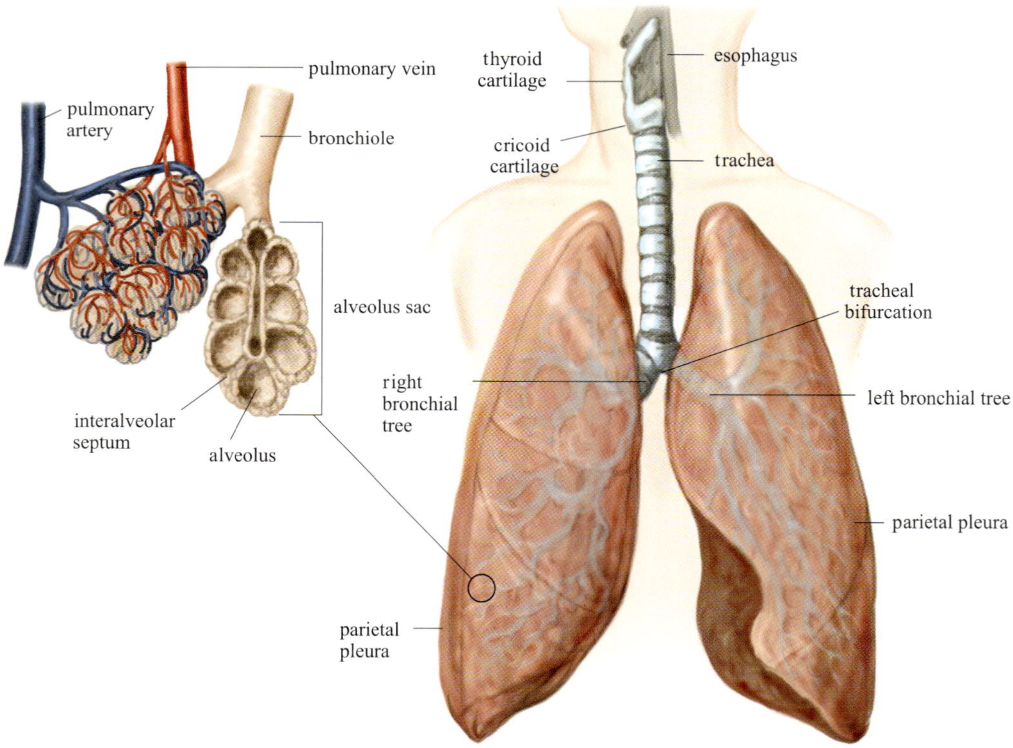

Figure 14-4 Structure of the lower respiratory tract

Base of lung

The broad and concave bottom part of each lung resting upon the convex surface of the diaphragm.

Memory key

- The trachea divides into the left and right bronchi at the level of the 4th thoracic vertebra. The linings of the bronchi secrete mucus fluid. The cilia on the lining move to excrete foreign materials.

Pleural and Mediastinal Cavities

Pleura

The thin and serous double-layer membrane surrounding each lung. Between the inner, visceral pleura and the outer, parietal pleura is the pleural cavity filled with pleural fluid that lubricates relative movement of the layers, however, it takes some effort to separate the two layers.

Parietal pleura

The outer membranous layer inside the chest that covers the lung.

Visceral pleura

The inner membranous layer that directly covers the lung.

Pleural cavity

The space that separates the two pleural layers and contains pleural fluid that serves as lubricant to prevent friction between the two layers while breathing.

Diaphragm

The muscular membrane that separates the thoracic and abdominal cavities.

Mediastinum

Mediastinum is a group of tissues and organs in the thorax that separate the left and right pleural cavities. It lies between the lungs, behind the sternum, in front of the thoracic vertebrae, below the pharynx, and above the diaphragm. It includes the heart, aorta, trachea, esophagus and the thymus.

Memory key

- The mediastinal cavity is at the center of the thoracic cavity, and contains the heart, aorta, trachea and esophagus.
  The pleural cavity contains a small quantity of pleural fluid as lubricant.

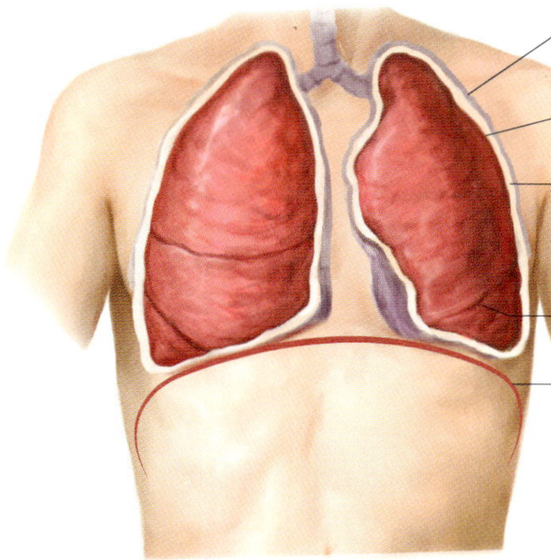

Figure 14-5 Structure of the pleura

Terms for Symptoms and Diseases

Adenoiditis

Acute or chronic inflammation of the adenoid, the pharyngeal tonsil.

Anoxia

The condition in which a tissue is severely deprived of oxygen.

Aphonia

Loss of voice due to dysfunction of a vocal organ.

Apnea

A sleep disorder in which breathing is temporarily suspended.

Asbestosis

Chronic fibrosis of the lungs due to inhalation of asbestos particles.

Aspiration

The entry of food or foreign material into the lower respiratory tract or the lungs.

Asthma

A chronic inflammatory respiratory disease caused by hypersensitivity reactions associated with reversible airflow obstruction and bronchospasm. Symptoms include coughing, wheezing, shortness of breath and stricture of air passage.

Atelectasis

Collapse or closure of the lung as the alveoli are deflated.

Bradypnea

Abnormally slow breathing rate.

Bronchiectasis

Permanent enlargement of parts of the bronchi and bronchioles associated with destruction of their muscles and elastic tissues.

Bronchitis

Inflammation of the mucous membrane of the bronchus.

Bronchiolitis

Inflammation of the bronchioles and alveoli.

Bronchospasm

Sudden spasm of the smooth muscle in the walls of the bronchi, related to asthma or bronchitis.

Cheyne-Stokes respiration

Abnormal pattern of breathing characterized by progressively deeper breathing, followed by a gradual decrease that results in a temporary stop in breathing called apnea.

Chronic obstructive pulmonary disease

Chronic obstruction of the air flow through the bronchi related to the pulmonary emphysema and chronic bronchitis.

Cough

Sudden explosive discharge of air from the pulmonary alveoli upon trigger by the nervous system in a defensive response.

Crackles

Abnormal sound of inhalation with short high rustling noise.

Cyanosis

Blue discoloration of the skin due to lack of oxygen in the blood.

Cystic fibrosis

A genetic disorder, in which the exocrine glands produce large amount of viscous mucus, causing respiratory and digestive problems.

Dyspnea

The condition of impaired breathing, or shortness of breath.

Dysphonia

Difficulty in producing vocal sounds due to the dysfunctional larynx.

Emphysema

An abnormal accumulation of air in tissues or organs, especially in the lungs.

Empyema

A condition in which pus from infected tissue collects in a cavity.

Epistaxis

Bleeding from inside the nose.

Eupnea

Normal, healthy breathing.

Hemoptysis

Coughing up (discharge through the mouth) of blood from the respiratory tract.

Hemothorax

The condition of blood accumulation in the pleural cavity.

Hiccup

Repeated involuntary contraction of the diaphragm and the corresponding closure of the glottis, resulting in temporary blockage or air inhalation and the "hic" sound.

Hydrothorax

The condition of serous fluid accumulation in the pleural cavity.

Hypercapnia

The condition of abnormally high concentration of carbon dioxide in the blood.

Hyperpnea

Deep and rapid respiration, normally during or following exercise or at high altitude, or abnormally due to anemia or other respiratory condition.

Hypocapnia

The condition of abnormally low concentration of carbon dioxide in the blood.

Hypopnea

Overly shallow breathing or low respiratory rate.

Hyperventilation

A condition of excessive amount of air ventilation in the alveoli.

Hyperresonance

An exaggerated chest resonance heard in various abnormal pulmonary conditions.

Hypoventilation

A condition of decreased amount of air ventilation needed for gas exchange in the alveoli.

Hypoxemia

Deficiency in the concentration of oxygen in the blood.

Hypoxia

Deficiency in the concentration of oxygen in the body tissues.

Laryngitis

Inflammation of the larynx typically caused by viral infection.

Lung abscess

Collection of pus in the lung tissue with an infection.

Lung cancer

Carcinoma in the lung(s).

Metabolic acidosis

The condition of low pH level when the body produces too much nonvolatile acid or loses bicarbonates.

Metabolic alkalosis

The condition of high pH level when the body produces too little nonvolatile acid or gains bicarbonates.

Obstructive sleep apnea

Repeated cessation of breath while sleeping due to pharyngeal airway obstruction.

Orthopnea

Having shortness of breath when lying flat, inducing the patient to sit up while sleeping.

Pansinusitis

Inflammation of all paranasal sinuses.

Paradoxical respiration

An abnormal condition in which the chest deflates during inhalation and inflates during exhalation.

Paroxysmal nocturnal dyspnea

Spasmodic shortness of breath at night, even when sitting up.

Pharyngitis

Inflammation of the pharyngeal mucous membrane and/or lymphatic tissue caused by bacteria or viral infection.

Pleural effusion

Inflammation of the pleura with sharp breathing pain causes excess serous fluid accumulation leaking out of the cavity.

Pleural friction rub

The noise generated when the two layers of the pleura move and rub against each other.

Pleurisy

Inflammation of the pleura accompanied by pleural effusion.

Pneumoconiosis

Chronic lung disease leading to proliferation of fibrous tissues and lung damage, caused by inhalation of dust such as silica and asbestos.

Pneumonia

Inflammation of the lungs caused by pneumococcal or viral infection.

Pneumothorax

Accumulation of air or other gas in the pleural cavity.

Pulmonary abscess

Collection of pus in the lung tissue with an infection.

Pulmonary edema

The condition in which alveoli are filled with leaked serous fluid in lung congestion.

Pulmonary embolism

The condition in which the pulmonary artery is blocked by thrombus, air, fatty lump in circulation.

Pyothorax

Empyema (accumulation of pus) in the pleural cavity.

Pursed lip breathing

The method of slow exhaling for carbon dioxide discharge through tightly pressed, pursed lips.

Rales

Abnormal sound of breath heard with a stethoscope, with crackling noise made by air passing through bronchioles or alveoli filled with fluid.

Respiratory acidosis

Higher than normal concentration of carbon dioxide and lower than normal pH level in the blood, due to inadequate amount of carbon dioxide exhausted by breathing.

Respiratory alkalosis

Lower than normal concentration of carbon dioxide and higher than normal pH level in the blood, due to excessive amount of carbon dioxide exhausted by breathing.

Rhinorrhea

Mucus exudate from the nose.

Rhonchi

Dry rattling noise heard during breathing, due to fluid lined in the bronchial tubes.

Silicosis

Chronic nodular fibrosis in the lungs due to inhalation of sand, silica, rock dust, etc.

Sinusitis

Inflammation of the paranasal sinus caused by viral, bacterial, fungal infection or allergic rhinitis.

Sneezing

Nervous irritation in the respiratory tract triggering a sudden convulsive expulsion of air.

Sputum

Mucous coughed up from the lining between the lung and the larynx.

Stridor

High pitch noise generated by air passing a narrow obstruction in the upper respiratory tract.

Tactile fremitus

Vibration felt on the wall of the chest while examining the thorax.

Tachypnea

The state of breathing faster than normal.

Tonsillitis

Inflammation of the tonsil.

Upper Respiratory Infection

Infection in the nasal cavities, pharynx and larynx.

Wheeze

The sound of breathing through the stricture of air passage.

Terms for Surgery and Treatment

Adenoidectomy

Surgical removal of the adenoid.

Bronchoplasty

Surgical repair or reconstruction of the bronchus.

Cricothyreotomy

An emergency surgical procedure in which a hole is cut through the patient's neck into the trachea in order to relieve blockage in the upper respiratory tract.

Decortication

Surgical removal (peeling) of the surface layer, the fibrous membrane (that has become inelastic thus obstructing lung expansion) of the pleural cavity.

Laryngectomy

Surgical removal of a part of the larynx.

Laryngoplasty

Surgical reconstruction of the larynx (usually for voice).

Laryngostomy

Surgical creation of an artificial air path in the larynx.

Lobectomy

Surgical excision of a lung lobe.

Pleurectomy

Surgical excision of the parietal pleura.

Pleurodesis

A treatment to form adhesion between the visceral and the parietal pleurae.

Pneumonectomy

Surgical excision of a whole lung.

Pulmonary Embolectomy

Surgical removal of emboli (blood clot) out of the pulmonary artery.

Rhinoplasty

Reconstructive surgery of the nose.

Segmental resection, Segmentectomy

Surgical removal of a part of an organ.

Septoplasty

Surgical reconstruction of the nasal septum.

Septotomy

Surgical incision of the nasal septum.

Thoracotomy

Surgical incision into the pleural space of the chest.

Thoracoplasty

Surgical procedure of the chest, involving resection of some ribs and realignment of the diseased lung.

Tonsillectomy

Surgical removal of a tonsil.

Tracheoplasty

Surgical reconstruction of the trachea.

Tracheostomy

Surgical process of cutting into the trachea through the neck and inserting a tube, in order to make an artificial air passage for breathing.

Tracheotomy

Surgical process of cutting into the trachea.

Uvulectomy

Surgical removal of the uvula.

Uvulopalatopharyngoplasty

Making incision of the uvula, soft palate, tonsils or pharynx for patients with sleep apnea or severe snoring in order to ease air passage and help breathing.

Video-assisted Thoracic Surgery (VATS)

Surgical procedure with minimal incision of the chest using a thoracoscope (tiny endoscopic video camera) and remotely controlled surgical equipment.

Wedge resection

Surgical removal of a local part of the lung.

Terms for Test and Intervention

Acid-Fast Bacilli (AFB) smear

Examination of the patient's sputum for verification of presence of acid-fast bacilli, the pathogen for tuberculosis.

Arterial Blood Gas Analysis

Analysis of the arterial blood for levels of oxygen, carbon dioxide and other gases.

Bronchography

Radiography of the bronchus, with administration of contrast agent in the bronchial tube through a catheter.

Bronchoscopy

Visual examination of the bronchus with an endoscope.

Continuous Positive Airway Pressure

Application of continuous positive pressure to maintain a continuous level of positive airway pressure in a spontaneously breathing patient.

Chest computed tomography

X-ray computed tomography of the thorax.

Laryngoscopy

Visual examination of the larynx with an endoscope.

Lung biopsy

Microscopic examination of a sample tissue from the lung by the pathologist.

Mediastinoscopy

Visual examination of the mediastinum with a mediastinoscope inserted through incision superior to the sternum.

Polysomnography

A multiparameter technique to record and evaluate the patient's sleep pattern.

Positron Emission Tomography (PET)

A medical imaging technique using detection of gamma rays produced by positrons emitted from radionuclides injected in the vein.

PPD (Purified Protein Derivative test)

A screening test for tuberculosis, where a small dose of tuberculin is injected in the skin in order to evaluate the response.

Pulmonary angiography

X-ray imaging technique for pulmonary blood vessels with injection of contrast agent in the pulmonary artery.

Pulmonary function test

A general evaluation of the respiratory system for pulmonary function or disease.

Thoracoscopy

Examination of the pleura using a thoracoscope (a type of endoscope).

Thoracentesis

Medical procedure to drain fluid from the pleural cavity, using a needle.

Ventilation/Perfusion scan

Nuclear medical imaging technique for diagnosis of pulmonary embolism or other diseases.

Analysis and Meaning of Key Terms

Diseases

Term	Term Analysis	Meaning
adenoid/o :		adenoids
adenoiditis [æ̀dənɔidáitis]	-itis = inflammation	acute or chronic inflammation of the adenoid
alveol/o :		alveolus, air sac
alveolitis [æ̀lviəláitis]	-itis = inflammation	inflammation of the alveoli in the lung
bronchi/o, bronch/o :		bronchus
bronchiectasis [brὰŋkiéktəsi]	-ectasis = dilation, expansion	permanent enlargement of the bronchus, accompanied by cough and sputum
bronchitis [brɑ:ŋkaitis]	-itis = inflammation	inflammation of the mucous membrane of the bronchus
bronchiol/o :		bronchioles
bronchiolitis [brὰŋkiouláitis]	-itis = inflammation	inflammation of the bronchioles, common in young children due to viral infection, causing shortness of breath
laryng/o :		larynx, voice box
laryngitis [lærindʒaitis]	-itis = inflammation	Inflammation of the larynx usually caused by viral infection, often resulting in fever and hoarseness
pneumat/o, pneum/o :		air, lung
pneumoconiosis [nju̇:mo*u*kò*u*nióu-sis]	coni/o = dust; -osis = abnormal condition	abnormal condition of the lungs caused by inhalation of dust
pneumon/o, pulmo/o :		lungs
pneumonia [nju:móunjə]	-ia = state, condition	pathological condition (inflammation) of the lungs, caused by viral or bacterial infection
rhin/o :		nose
rhinitis [rainάitis]	-itis = inflammation	inflammation of the mucous membrane of the nose

Term	Term Analysis	Meaning
sinus/o :		sinuses
pansinusitis [pænsainəsáitis]	pan- = all -itis = inflammation	inflammation of all the sinuses
tonsill/o :		tonsils
tonsillitis [tɑ̀nsəláitis]	-itis = inflammation	inflammation of the tonsils

Roots

Term	Term Analysis	Meaning
adenoid/o :		adenoids
adenotome [ǽdinətoum]	-tome = cutting instrument	instrument for surgical excision of the adenoids
bronchi/o, bronch/o :		bronchus
bronchodilator [brɑ̀ŋkədiléitər]	-or = person or thing dilat/o = dilation, widening	a drug used to dilate the bronchus to relieve bronchoconstriction
bronchoscopy [brɑ̀ŋkəskəpi]	-scopy = visual examination	visual examination of the bronchus using a bronchoscope
muc/o :		mucus
mucolytic [mjù:koulítik]	-lytic = destruction, breakdown	serving to dissolve mucus
nas/o, rhino: nose		
nasolacrimal [néizouléækrimәl]	lacrim/o = tear gland -al = pertaining to	pertaining to the nose and tear gland
nasopharyngeal [nèizoufəríndʒiəl]	pharyng/o = pharynx -al = pertaining to	pertaining to the nasopharynx
ox/o :		oxygen
anoxia [ænáksiə]	an- = not; -ia = state of	condition of severe or total lack of oxygen
hypoxia [haipɑ:ksiə]	hypo- = deficient, abnormally low -ia = state of	condition of abnormally low oxygen
pector/o :		chest, breast
pectoral [péktərəl]	-al = pertaining to	pertaining to the chest

Term	Term Analysis	Meaning
pharyng/o :		pharynx, throat
pharyngoglossal [færinggouglɔ́:səl]	gloss/o = tongue -al = pertaining to	pertaining to the pharynx and tongue
pleur/a, pleur/o :		pleura, pleural cavity
pleuralgia [pluræ̀ldʒiə]	-algia = pain	pain of the pleural cavity or muscle ribs
rhin/o :		nose
rhinorrhea [ràinərí:ə]	-rrhea = discharge	
rhinoplasty [ráinəplæ̀sti]	-plasty = surgical reconstruction	reconstructive surgery of the nose
spir/o :		respiration, breathing
spirometer [spàiərɑ́mitər]	-meter = measuring device	a device used to measure the flow pattern and volume of air inspired and expired by the lungs
steth/o :		chest
stethoscope [stéθəskòup]	-scope = instrument used to examine	medical device for listening to internal sounds of the body
thorac/o :		chest
thoracentesis [θɔ́:rəsentí:sis]	-centesis = surgical puncture to aspirate fluid	needle drainage of fluid from the pleural space; thoracocentesis
thoracoplasty [θɔ́:rəkouplæ̀sti]	-plasty = surgical reconstruction	surgical reconstruction of the thorax, usually involving resection of ribs

Suffixes

Term	Term Analysis	Meaning
-capnia :		carbon dioxide condition
hypercapnia [haipərkǽpniə]	hyper- = too high, excessive	abnormally high concentration of carbon dioxide in the blood
hypocapnia [haipɔ́kǽpniə]	hypo- = too low, deficient	abnormally low concentration of carbon dioxide in the blood

Term	Term Analysis	Meaning
-ectomy :		surgical excision
pneumonectomy [njù:mounéktəmi]	pneumon/o = lungs	surgical excision of a lung
adenoidectomy [æ̀dənɔ̀idéktəmi]	adenoid/o = adenoids	surgical excision of the adenoid
lobectomy [loubéktəmiə]	lob/o = lobe	surgical excision of a lobe of the lung
tonsillectomy [tɑ̀nsəléktəmi]	tonsili/o = tonsils	surgical excision of a tonsil
-metry :		measurement
spirometry [spairɑmtíri]	spir/o = breathing	measurement of the flow pattern and volume of air inspired and expired by the lungs
-phonia :		voice
aphonia [eifóuniə]	a- = not	loss of voice due to dysfunction of the vocal organ
dysphonia [disfóuniə]	dys- = bad, difficult, abnormal	the condition of having difficulty to produce voice
-pnea :		breathing
apnea [æpní:ə]	a- = not	temporary suspension of breathing
bradypnea [brǽdipní:ə]	brady- = slow	abnormally slow breathing
dyspnea [dispní:ə]	dys- = difficult	condition of impaired breathing
orthopnea [ɔ́:rθəpní:ə]	ortho- = straight	having shortness of breath when lying flat, inducing the patient to sit up while sleeping
tachypnea [tǽkipní:ə]	tachy- = fast	unusually fast breathing
-ptysis :		spitting
hemoptysis [himɑ́təsis]	hem/o = blood	coughing up of blood from the respiratory tract
-rrhea :		discharge
rhinorrhea [ràinərí:ə]	rhin/o = nose	fluid discharge from the nose

Term	Term Analysis	Meaning
-spasm :		sudden, involuntary contraction
bronchospasm [brάŋkəspæ̀zəm]	bronchi/o, bronch/o = bronchus	sudden involuntary contraction of the bronchus
laryngospasm [læriŋgouspæ̀zəm]	laryng/o = larynx, voice box	sudden involuntary closure of the larynx
-stomy :		forming a new opening
laryngostomy [læriŋgástəmi]	laryng/o = larynx, voice box	surgical creation of an artificial air path into the larynx through the neck
tracheostomy [trèikiάstəmi]	trache/o = trachea, windpipe	surgical process of cutting into the trachea through the neck for an artificial air passage
-thorax :		chest
hemothorax [hi:məθɔ́:ræks]	hem/o = blood	state of blood collection in the pleural cavity
pneumothorax [n*j*ù:mo*u*θɔ́:ræks]	pneum/o = air	state of air collection in the pleural cavity
pyothorax [pὰiəθɔ́:ræks]	py/o = pus	state of pus collection in the pleural cavity
-tomy :		process of cutting
thoracotomy [θɔ̀:rəkάtəmi]	thorac/o = chest	surgical incision into the pleural space of the chest
sinusotomy [sainəsátəmi]	sinus/o = sinuses	surgical incision of the sinus

Abbreviations

Abbreviation	Full Term	Meaning
ABGA	Arterial Blood Gas Analysis	analysis of the arterial blood for levels of oxygen, carbon dioxide, etc.
AFB	Acid Fast Bacillus	sputum test for presence of acid-fast bacilli
ARDS	Acute Respiratory Distress Syndrome	serious medical condition with widespread inflammation of the lung
COPD	Chronic Obstructive Pulmonary Disease	chronic obstruction of the air flow through the bronchi related to the pulmonary emphysema and chronic bronchitis
CPAP	Continuous Positive Airway Pressure	application of continuous positive pressure to maintain a continuous level of positive airway pressure in a spontaneously breathing patient
DPI	Dry Powder Inhaler	a device to deliver dry powdered medication to the lung
DVT	Deep Vein Thrombosis	thrombi formed in deep veins (usually in the leg) that may break free to cause pulmonary embolism
ERV	Expiratory Reserve Volume	maximal volume of air that can be exhaled from normal exhalation end
FEV	Forced Expiratory Volume	volume of air exhaled under forced condition
FRC	Functional Residual Capacity	volume of air remaining in the lungs at normal exhalation end
FVC	Forced Vital Capacity	volume of air moved from deepest inhalation to the maximal exhalation
IC	Inspiratory Capacity	maximal volume of air that can be inhaled from normal exhalation end
IPPB	Intermittent Positive Pressure Breathing	respiratory therapy to mechanically help breathing with positive pressure at intervals
IPPV	Intermittent Positive Pressure Ventilation	respiratory therapy to mechanically force ventilation with positive pressure at intervals
IRV	Inspiratory Reserve Volume	maximal volume of air that can be inhaled from normal inhalation end
LLL	Left Lower Lobe	the inferior lobe of the left lung
LUL	Left Upper Lobe	the superior lobe of the left lung
MDI	Metered Dose Inhaler	device that delivers s specific amount of aerosolized medication to the lungs through inhalation

Abbreviation	Full Term	Meaning
MDR	Multi Drug Resistant	a condition in which pathogens are resistant to multiple antimicrobials
MEFR	Maximal Expiratory Flow Rate	maximal air flow rate during exhalation
NPPV	Noninvasive Positive Pressure Ventilation	positive pressure ventilation where an air tube does not penetrate into the respiratory tract
NSCLC	Non Small Cell Lung carcinoma	any epithelial lung cancer other than small cell lung cancer, relatively insensitive to chemotherapy
OSA	Obstructive Sleep Apnea	repeated cessation of breath while sleeping due to pharyngeal airway obstruction
PCP	Pneumocystis (Carinii) Pneumonia	pneumonia due to fungal infection in people with weak immunity, involving alveolar sacs
PEEP	Positive End Expiratory Pressure	the air pressure in the lungs at the end of exhalation
PEFR	Peak Expiratory Flow Rate	peak air flow rate during exhalation
PFT	Pulmonary Function Test	general evaluation of the respiratory system for pulmonary function
PIP	Peak Inspiratory Pressure	highest level of pressure applied to the lungs during inhalation
PPD	Purified Protein Derivative	Mantoux test - screening test for tuberculosis using intradermal injection
RLL	Right Lower Lobe	the inferior lobe of the right lung
RML	Right Middle Lobe	the middle lobe of the right lung
RUL	Right Upper Lobe	the superior lobe of the right lung
RV	Residual Volume	volume of air remaining in the lungs after maximal exhalation
SCLC	Small Cell Lung Cancer	lung cancer involving smaller than normal cells with little cytoplasm
SOB	Shortness of Breath	difficulty in breathing, dyspnea
TB	Tuberculosis	disease by bacterial infection causing tubercles mainly in the lungs
TLC	Total Lung Capacity	total volume of air in the lungs at maximal inhalation
TV	Tidal Volume	volume of air moved during normal breathing
URI	Upper Respiratory Infection	acute infection in the upper respiratory tract (nose, sinuses, pharynx, larynx)
VC	Vital Capacity	volume of air that can be exhaled after deepest inhalation

Exercises

1. Write the terms for the following respiratory anatomical parts.

① medial wall separating the left and right nasal cavities
nasal septum

② the small air space in the ethmoid bone ethmoidal sinuses

③ the region where the pharynx and larynx are connected
laryngopharynx

④ collection of lymphoid tissue on the sides of the throat
tonsils

⑤ the organ that controls breath and houses vocal cords, between the pharynx and the trachea larynx

⑥ the flap at the laryngeal entrance that controls air and food passage
epiglottis

⑦ the organ in the larynx that generates voice vocal cord

⑧ Adam's apple, the cartilage that protrudes in front of the larynx
thyroid cartilage

⑨ thin air passages in the bronchial tree branched out of the main bronchus
bronchioles

⑩ the sacs at the terminal end of the bronchial tree that contain many alveoli
alveolar sacs

⑪ the outer membranous layer inside the chest that covers the lung
parietal pleura

⑫ the space that separates the two pleural layers and contains pleural fluid
pleural cavity

⑬ the muscular membrane that separates the thoracic and abdominal cavities
diaphragm

2. Write the meaning of the following surgical terms.

① surgical reconstruction of the bronchus — bronchoplasty

② emergency surgical procedure in which a hole is cut through the patient's neck into the trachea in order to relieve blockage in the upper respiratory tract — cricothyroidotomy

③ surgical removal of a part of the larynx — laryngectomy

④ surgical reconstruction of the larynx — laryngoplasty

⑤ surgical excision of a lobe of the lung — lobectomy

⑥ surgical excision of the parietal pleura — pleurectomy

⑦ treatment to form adhesion between the visceral and the parietal pleurae — pleurodesis

⑧ surgical excision of a whole lung — pneumonectomy

⑨ surgical incision into the pleural space of the chest — thoracotomy

⑩ surgical removal of the whole larynx — total laryngectomy

⑪ surgical reconstruction of the trachea — tracheoplasty

⑫ surgical removal of the uvula — uvulectomy

⑬ surgical removal of a local part of the lung — wedge resection

3. Spell the following words correctly.

① Trachia — trachea

② Preula — pleura

③ Dyspnia — dyspnea

④ Pneumosorax — pneumothorax

⑤ Ashma — asthma

⑥ Bronchoscophy — bronchoscopy

⑦ Trachostomy — tracheostomy

⑧ Thorasentecis — thoracentesis, thoracocentesis

⑨ Neumonia — pneumonia

⑩ Spirometeor spirometer

⑪ Bronchiecktasis bronchiectasis

⑫ Pansinucitis pansinusitis

4. Write the full term for the following abbreviations.

① ABGA Arterial Blood Gas Analysis

② ARDS Acute Respiratory Distress Syndrome

③ COPD Chronic Obstructive Pulmonary Disease

④ CPAP Continuous Positive Airway Pressure

⑤ DVT Deep Vein Thrombosis

⑥ PIP Peak Inspiratory Pressure

⑦ TV Tidal Volume

⑧ TLC Total Lung Capacity

⑨ URI Upper Respiratory Infection

⑩ VC Vital Capacity

5. Construct medical terms that mean the following.

- Use **-pnea** to construct terms that mean the following.

1. temporary suspension of breathing apnea
2. condition of impaired breathing dyspnea
3. having shortness of breath when lying flat, inducing the patient to sit up while sleeping orthopnea
4. unusually fast breathing tachypnea

- Use **-ectomy** to construct terms that mean the following.

5. surgical excision of the adenoid adenoidectomy
6. Surgical excision of a whole lung pneumonectomy
7. surgical excision of the larynx laryngectomy
8. surgical removal of emboli (blood clot) from the pulmonary artery embolectomy

- Use **bronchi/o** to construct terms that mean the following.

9. permanent enlargement of the bronchi and bronchioles
   bronchiectasis
10. inflammation of the bronchus bronchitis
11. visual examination of the bronchus with a bronchoscope
   bronchoscopy

- Use **pneumon/o** to construct terms that mean the following.

12. accumulation of air or other gas in the pleural cavity
   pneumothorax
13. inflammation of the lungs caused by pneumococcal or viral infection
   pneumonia
14. lung condition with proliferation of fibrous tissues and lung damage caused by inhalation of dust such as silica and asbestos
   pneumoconiosis

Chapter 15

Digestive System

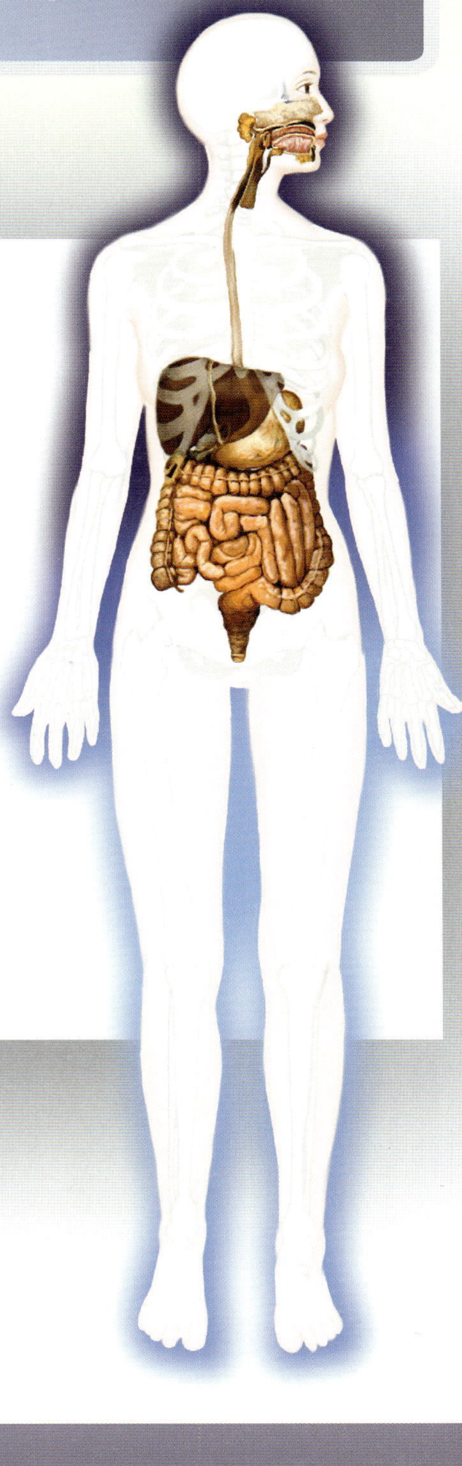

Chapter Contents

- Prolog
- Anatomical Terms
- Terms for Symptoms and Diseases
- Terms for Surgery and Treatment
- Terms for Test and Intervention
- Analysis and Meaning of Key Terms
- Abbreviations
- Exercises

Learning Objectives

- Define alimentary canal and describe its functions.
- Define accessory digestive system and its functions.
- Be familiar with the digestive process and related terms.
- Explain functions of each organ in the digestive system.
- Define terms for tests relating to the digestive system.
- Define terms for diseases and treatments relating to the digestive system.
- Define abbreviations used in the digestive system.

Prolog

Digestive organs can be divided into the alimentary canal (digestive tract, or gastrointestinal tract) and the accessory digestive system. Food is broken down into small pieces in the alimentary canal and the nutrients are absorbed into the blood in the surrounding organs.

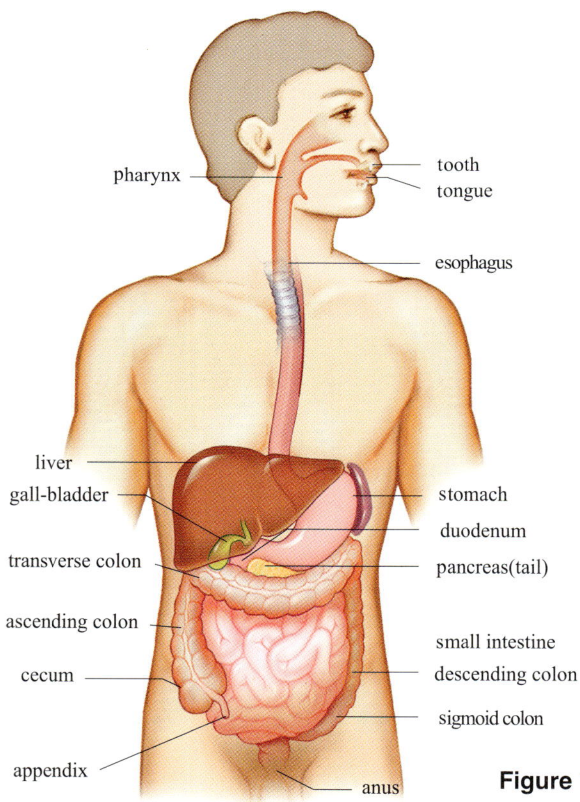

Figure 15-1 The digestive system

The alimentary canal includes the mouth, pharynx, esophagus, stomach, small intestine, colon connected to the anus.

The accessory digestive system includes the teeth, tongue, gallbladder and several digestive glands (salivary glands, liver, pancreas). Secretions from these glands break down the food to molecular level.

Oral Cavity

The oral cavity is where the digestive system begins, and consists of lips, palate, gingiva, salivary glands, teeth and tongue.

There are three main functions of the oral cavity :

First, it ingests food as the first stop in the alimentary canal. Chewing action is performed in concert by the lower jaw, teeth, tongue and lips. Decomposition of carbohydrates in the food is helped by digestive enzymes in the saliva. The resulting food is sent to the esophagus.

Second, the oral cavity characterizes and resonates the sound generated in the larynx, the result of which is voice. Consonants are made through cooperative movements and shaping of the tongue, soft palate, lips, cheeks, etc.

Third, it tastes the food. The tongue specializes in tasting, however, it is known that other parts of the oral mucous membranes can identify the taste of food.

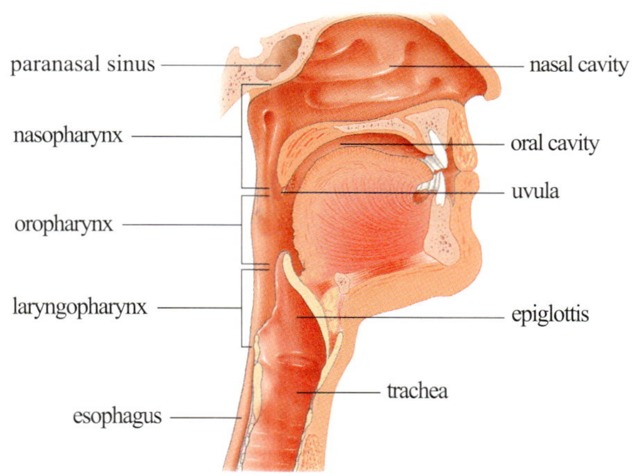

Figure 15-2 Location of the oral cavity

Memory key

- Functions of the oral cavity include chewing food while mixing it with saliva, tasting, producing voice and controlling breath.

Gastrointestinal Tract Activities

Activities of the gastrointestinal tract include ingestion of food, propulsion (movement), mechanical digestion, chemical digestion, absorption and defecation. The organ where chemical digestion occurs is either the direct producer of or near the glands that produce digestive enzymes. The mucous membranes of the stomach and the intestines secrete mucus for protection and lubrication of their inner surface.

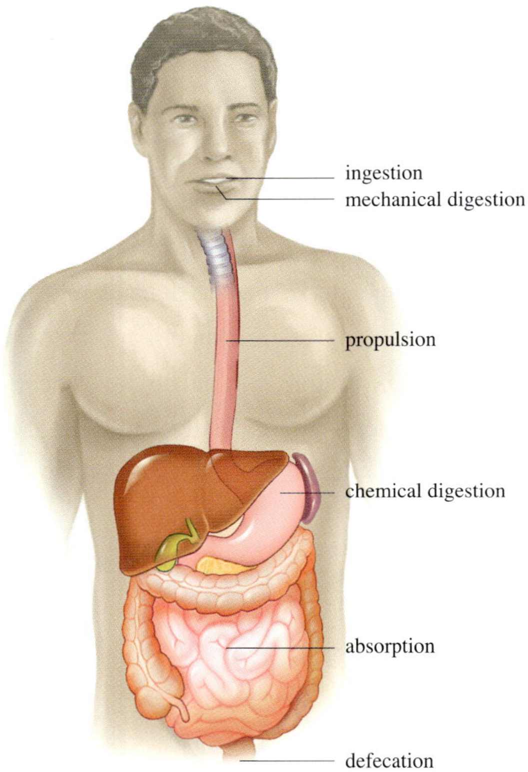

Figure 15-3 Activities of the gastrointestinal tract

Anatomical Terms

Oral Cavity

Lips

The outer muscular protruded folds at the opening of the mouth, sensitive to touch and temperature of food as the entry of the digestive tract.

Cheek

The thick, soft skin on each side of the face between the temple and the chin. The cheeks are the walls on the left and right sides of the oral cavity. They hold food along with the tongue in the process of mastication (chewing). They also help control the breathing process.

Buccal cavity

The part of the oral cavity bound by the cheeks, teeth, gums and the palate.

Frenulum lingua

A fold of mucous membrane attaching the underside midline of the tongue to the floor of the oral cavity. If this is unusually short, limiting the mobility of the tongue, the condition is called ankyloglossia.

Palate

The ceiling part of the oral cavity, composed of the anterior bony hard palate and the posterior fleshy soft palate.

Hard palate

The hard anterior part of the oral ceiling that occupies about 2/3 of the palate.

Soft palate

The soft posterior part of the oral ceiling that occupies about 1/3 of the palate.

Uvula

The fleshy protrusion hanging in the rear from the soft palate. It is at the border between the oral cavity and the pharynx. When food is swallowed, it folds back to prevent the food from entering the nasopharynx.

Gingiva

The gum consisting of mucosal tissue, covering the alveolar processes (tooth pockets in the maxilla and the mandible).

Salivary glands

The oral glands, including parotid, sublingual and submandibular and other minor glands that secrete digestive fluids such as amylase and maltase.

Parotid gland

The largest of salivary glands, a pair of inverted triangular shaped, inferior and anterior to the ears, 4-5 cm long, 3 cm wide and 2 cm thick. These glands secrete saliva through the Stensen's duct.

Sublingual gland

The pair of salivary glands, smallest of the three major pairs of salivary glands, under the tongue.

Submandibular gland

The second largest pair of salivary glands beneath the lower jaws. These glands secrete saliva through the Wharton's duct.

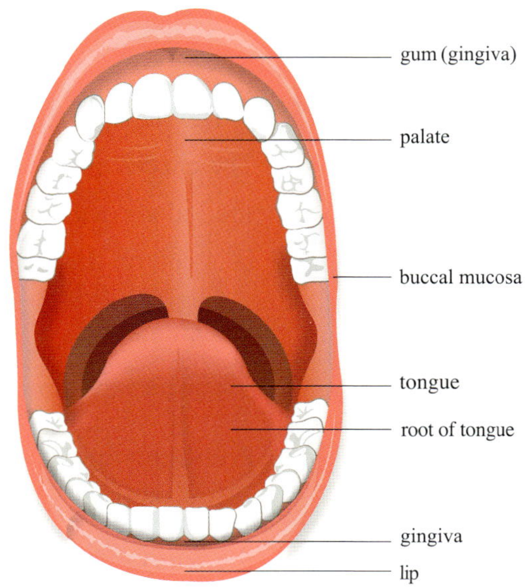

Figure 15-4 Front view of the oral cavity

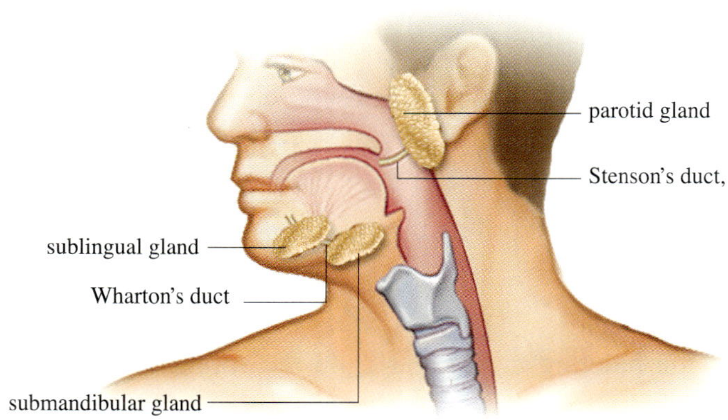

Figure 15-5 Salivary glands and ducts

Memory key

- Major salivary glands are parotid, submandibular and sublingual glands. The saliva contains amylase, which help start digestive process of carbohydrates.

Teeth, tooth

Teeth are calcified hard tissue structure embedded in the alveolar processes of the maxilla and mandible. A tooth can be divided into the crown, neck and root, and consists of 3 layers of calcified tissues : enamel, dentin, cementum. Teeth are classified by function and shape as incisors, canine cuspids, premolars (bicuspids), molars (multicuspids).

Enamel

Enamel is the hardest but brittle, white superficial layer of the tooth, covering the neck and crown.

Dentin

Dentin, the layer under the enamel, is yellowish and softer than the enamel, and occupies most of the tooth volume.

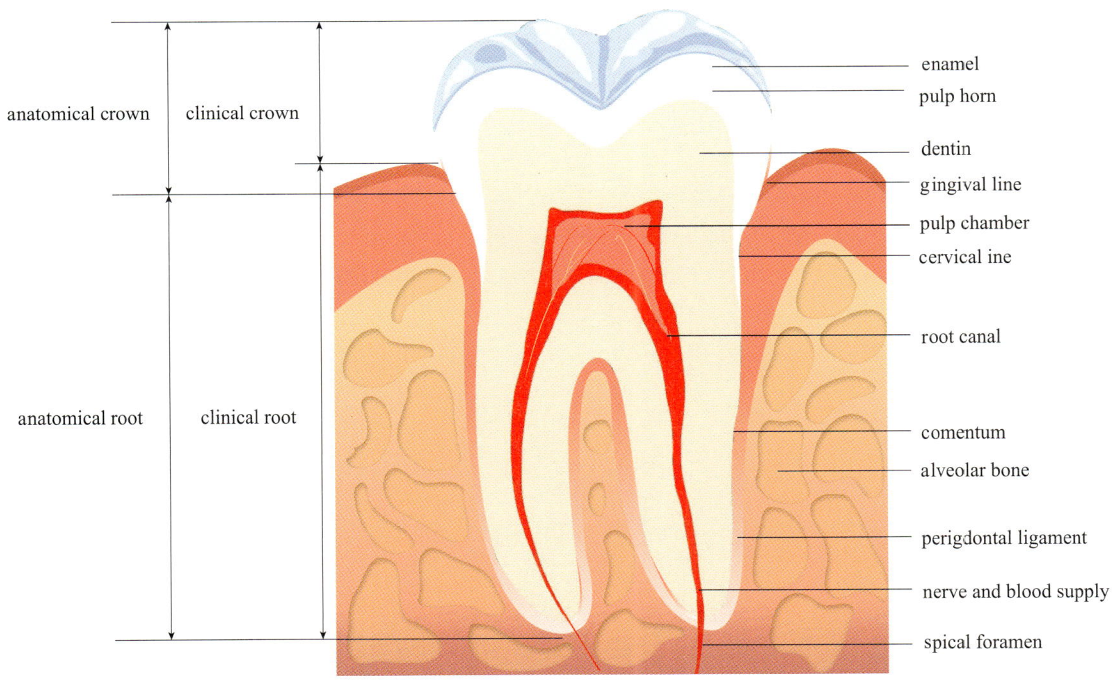

Figure 15-6 Structure of tooth

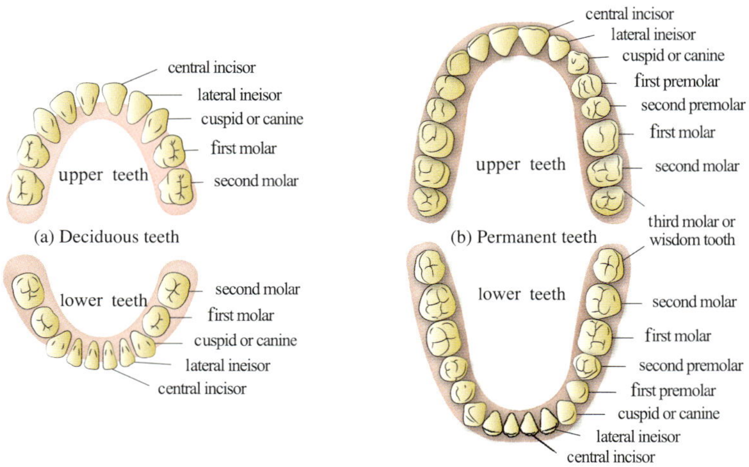

Figure 15-7 Deciduous and permanent teeth

Cementum

Cementum is a specialized bone covering the root of the tooth and lacking in blood vessel.

Dental pulp

Dental pulp, filling the cavity in the dentin, is a soft connective tissue containing nerve and blood vessel.

Memory key

- Teeth are named by shape as incisors, canine cuspids, premolars (bicuspids), molars (multicuspids). The structure of the tooth includes dental pulp, enamel, dentin and cementum. The crown extends out of the gingiva, while the root is buried under the gingiva.

Deciduous teeth

Typically 20 primary teeth are formed during the period 6 months through about 3 years after birth.

Permanent teeth

Typically 32 teeth are grown from alveolar processes in children about 6 years and up, designed to function for life.

Tongue

As the flexible muscular tissue at the bottom of the oral cavity, the tongue is the most versatile in shape. Its functions include positioning the food for chewing, mixing food with digestive fluid, characterizing the voice by reshaping the oral cavity, tasting and sensing touch.

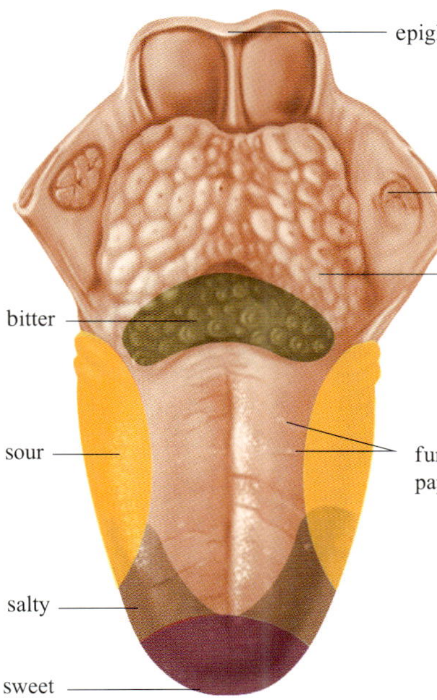

Figure 15-8 Taste map of the tongue

Memory key

- The rough part of the tongue is populated with papillae that can sense bitter, sour, salty and sweet tastes.

Pharynx, Esophagus and Stomach

Pharynx

The food from the mouth moves back and passes through oropharynx and laryngopharynx. These are the passageway for solid and liquid food plus the air. However, the nasopharynx doesn't function as a digestive organ

Oropharynx

The tube between the oral cavity and the esophagus, through which the food and air pass.

Laryngopharynx

The part between the palate and the esophagus.

Nasopharynx

The part between the end of the nasal cavity and where it meets the rear end of the oral cavity.

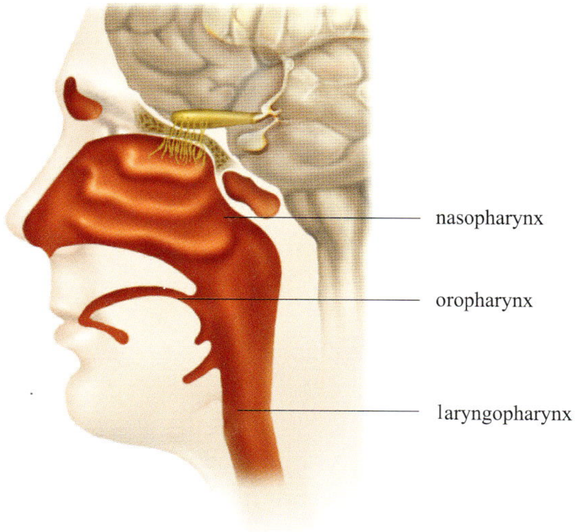

Figure 15-9 Pharynx

Esophagus

The esophagus is a muscular tube of about 25 cm in length. The normally contracted esophagus expands and help food move, and the epiglottis closes the entrance to the larynx when it passes laryngopharynx. While the food moves down the long tube of the esophagus, it passes through the thoracic mediastinum and the esophageal hiatus of the diaphragm to the abdominal cavity. The esophagus meets the stomach at the cardiac orifice. The food moves down the esophagus by peristalsis, and enters the stomach through the lower esophageal sphincter.

Stomach

The stomach is the enlarged part of the gastrointestinal tract just inferior to the esophagus. It is a temporary container for food where proteolysis starts, and the food is partly digested to become chyme. It is located at the upper left quadrant of the peritoneal cavity, and much of it is covered by the liver and the diaphragm. The size of an adult's stomach varies between 15 and 25 cm, while the diameter and volume depend on how much food is contained in it.

Rugae (plural of ruga)

When the stomach is empty, the mucous wall of the stomach shrinks to form longitudinal folds, or wrinkles, known as the rugae.

Cardiac region, cardia

Being close to the heart, cardia is the region close to the cardiac orifice where the food transfers from the esophagus to the stomach.

Fundus

The dome-shaped top part of the stomach, located under the diaphragm level and superolaterally to the cardia.

Body

The middle part of the stomach connected to the funnel-shaped pyloric region. The diameter of the pyloric antrum gradually decreases to become pyloric canal, which ends at the pylorus.

Pylorus

The pylorus continues until the pyloric sphincter which meets the duodenum (the first part of the small intestine). It controls emptying the stomach.

Greater curvature

The convex curvature, at the lateral part of the stomach.

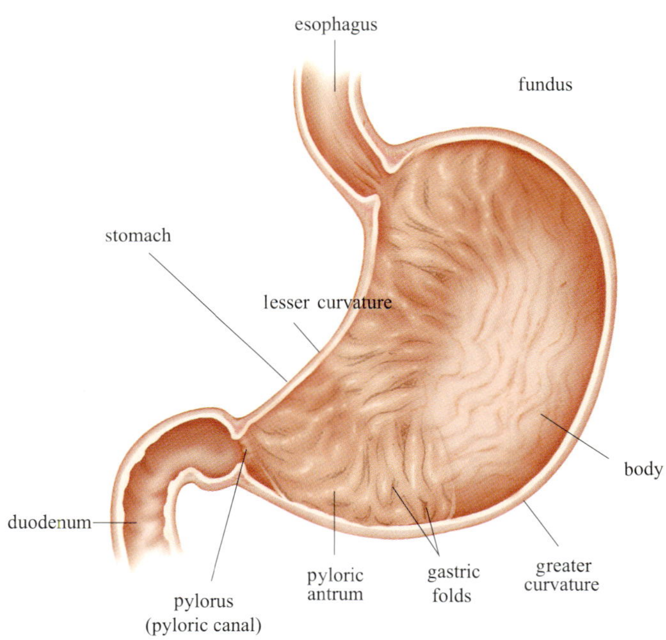

Figure 15-10 Stomach

Lesser curvature

The concave curvature, at the medial part of the stomach.

Memory key

- Food enters the stomach through the lower esophageal sphincter, and it moves to the small intestine through the pyloric sphincter and the duodenum.
- Food in the stomach mixes with gastric digestive fluid to become chyme.

Small and Large Intestines, Peritoneum

Small intestine

The small intestine is a very important digestive organ. It is the longest organ (about 6 m) of the alimentary canal, extending between the stomach and the large intestine. This organ digests food and absorbs nutrients.

Duodenum

Duodenum is of a relatively stable, horseshoe-shaped part between the pylorus and the jejunum, and surrounds the head part of the pancreas. The name origin means length of 12 fingers.

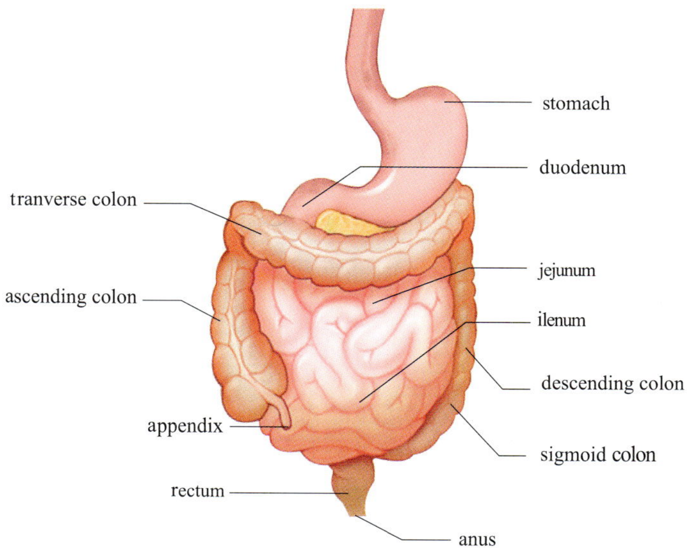

Figure 15-11 Small and large intestines

Jejunum

The jejunum is about 2.5 m long, between the duodenum and the ileum.

Ileum

The ileum is about 3.5 m long, and meets the large intestine at the ileocecal valve.

Memory key

- The small intestine's 3 sections are duodenum, jejunum and ileum.
- Waste material (chyme to become feces) is passed to the large intestine through the ileocecal valve.

Large intestine

The large intestine, about 1.5 m long and about 6 cm in diameter, starts at the ileocecal valve and terminates at the anus, and surrounds the small intestine on three sides. It absorbs water from the waste chime, and sends the solid waste to the rectum for discharge.

Cecum

The cecum is at the beginning part of the large intestine and the appendix is attached to it.

Vermiform appendix

The thin blind-ended tube connected to the cecum. The local place of pain when acute appendicitis occurs is called McBurney's point.

Colon

Often synonymous with the large intestine, the colon is the portion that connects the cecum and the rectum, and consists of the ascending colon, transverse colon, descending colon and sigmoid colon.

Rectum

The tube that is about 20 cm long, between the sigmoid colon and the anus.

Anus

Anus is at the end of the rectum, also being the terminating part of the gastrointestinal tract, and purges the waste.

Peritoneum

The serous membrane that encloses the abdominal viscera. It can be divided into parietal peritoneum and visceral peritoneum. The potential space between the two layers is the peritoneal cavity. As variations of the serous membrane, there are mesentery, mesocolon, omentum, etc.

Mesentery

The membrane that attaches the small intestines to the rear wall of the abdomen.

Mesocolon

The membrane that attaches the colon to the rear wall of the abdomen.

Omentum (greater, lesser)

The layer of the peritoneum that surrounds and supports the abdominal organs and the stomach.

Memory key

- The large intestine is about 6 cm in diameter, about 1.5 m long, absorbs water and vitamin K and B, and removes waste material.

Liver, Biliary system and Pancreas

Liver

The liver is the largest internal organ in the body located at the upper right quadrant of the abdominal cavity, just below the diaphragm. Arterial blood is supplied through the hepatic artery, and venous blood rich in nutrients from the digestive tract is carried to the liver through the hepatic portal vein. Functions of the liver are : production of bile; carbohydrate metabolism - synthesis, analysis and storage of glycogen; lipid metabolism - processing of fatty acids; protein metabolism - generation of ammonia, urea and synthesis of plasma proteins such as blood clotting factor; blood cell formation; storage of vitamins and minerals such as iron; and detoxification of harmful substances. The bile from the liver flows through a pair of hepatic ducts and the common bile duct, to the gallbladder where it is stored, or drains to the duodenum.

Memory key

- The liver helps digestion of food by delivering bile; detoxifies harmful materials; metabolizes carbohydrates, fats and proteins; stores glycogen, vitamins A, D, E, K and minerals such as iron and copper.

Hepatic duct

The duct through which bile produced by the liver flows to the gallbladder.

Gallbladder

The pear-shaped sac that sits beneath the right lobe of the liver and stores bile.

Common bile duct

Common bile duct is where the common hepatic duct and the cystic duct join. Thence it joins the pancreatic duct. The united duct eventually enters the duodenum.

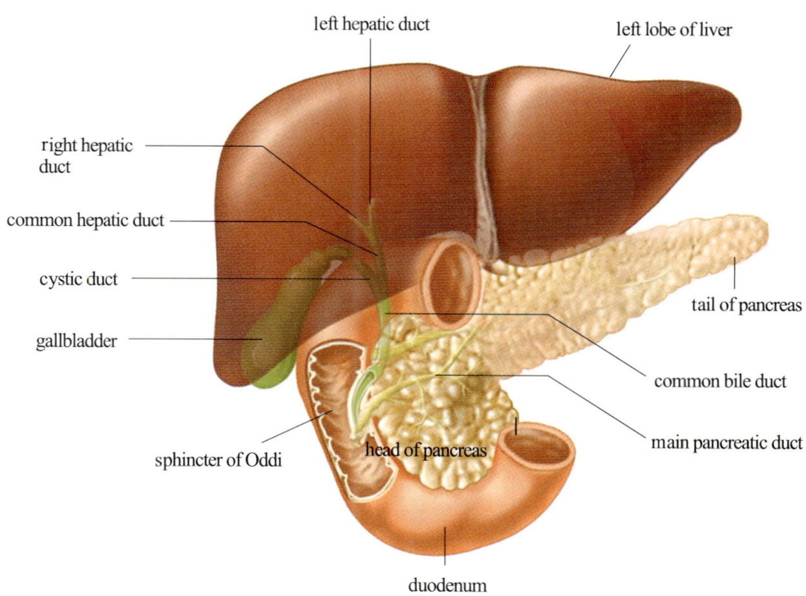

Figure 15-12 Liver, biliary system and pancreas

Pancreas

The pancreas is a soft, fish-shaped glandular organ, partially surrounded by the duodenum. The pancreas performs both endocrine and exocrine functions. The exocrine function is to release pancreatic juice as the digestive enzymes into the duodenum. In the endocrine part of the pancreas, beta cells secrete insulin, and the alpha cells secrete glucagon, released into the bloodstream.

Sphincter of Oddi

The sphincter at the opening end of the common bile duct is a muscular valve that controls release of bile and pancreatic juice into the duodenum.

Ampulla of Vater

This is the united part of the common bile duct and the pancreatic duct of about 1.5 cm long, connected to the duodenum.

Memory key

- The pancreas secretes insulin and glucagon that control blood sugar level, and releases pancreatic juice into the duodenum.

Terms for Symptoms and Diseases

Oral Cavity

Symptoms

- **Aphagia**
  Symptom of inability or refusal to swallow.
- **Dysphagia**
  Symptom of difficulty in swallowing due to pain or other cause.
- **Glossodynia**
  Lasting sensation of burning or stinging on the tongue.

- **Xerostomia**

Dryness of the mouth usually due to reduced salivary flow. Possible causes include dysfunctional salivary gland, systemic disease, dried oral mucous membrane, psychogenic tension, etc.

- **Halitosis**

A symptom of notably unpleasant odor from or through the mouth, due to dental plaque, oral disorder or gastrointestinal disease.

- **Leukoplakia**

White patches of keratosis on the mucous membranes of the oral cavity or the tongue, which is often a precursor of squamous cell carcinoma.

- **Ptyalism, hypersalivation, sialorrhea**

Flow of excess saliva from the mouth.

- **Dental plaque**

Bacterial adhesion on the surface of the teeth or dental prosthesis.

- **Dental calculus**

Calcified and hardened dental plaque from continual accumulation.

Inflammations and infections

- **Cheilitis, chilitis**

Inflammatory disease of the lips.

- **Stomatitis**

Inflammation of the mucous membranes in the oral cavity due to bacterial, viral or fungal infection.

- **Aphthous stomatitis**

Recurrent appearance of mouth ulcers on the oral mucous membrane, a.k.a. canker sore.

- **Glossitis**

Inflammation of the tongue, with vesicles, fissure or loss of papillae on the surface as the symptoms. White or gray spots appear on the tip or side edges.

- **Periodontal disease**

Disease of the periodontal tissue initiated by bacteria in the dental plaque.

- **Pulpitis**

Inflammatory disease of the pulp in the tooth.

- **Uvulitis**

  Inflammatory disease of the uvula.

- **Parotitis, parotiditis**

  Inflammatory disease of the parotid gland.

- **Epidemic parotitis, mumps**

  A acute inflammation of the parotid gland caused by paramyxo virus, prevalent in children. Often propagated by droplets, it is highly contagious and frequently occurs in late winter and spring. Routine vaccinations have dropped the incidence to a low level.

- **Sialadenitis**

  Inflammatory disease of the salivary gland.

Congenital anomalies

- **Cleft palate**

  A congenital condition in which the two plates of the palate are not completely joined.

- **Cleft lip, harelip**

  A congenital condition in which the upper lip has a fissure and is not continuous but has a gap, leaving an opening when the mouth is closed. In some cases the condition is extended to the nose. Cheiloplasty can be performed to correct the condition.

- **Dental caries**

  Tooth decay, the condition in which the tooth enamel is eroded by the acid produced from bacterial fermentation of sugar, starch, etc.

Tumors

- **Epulis**

  Any benign tumor that occurs in the gingiva.

- **Tongue cancer**

  An oral cancer occurring in the tongue.

Pharynx, Esophagus and Stomach

Symptoms

- **Anorexia**

  Symptom of poor or no appetite resulting in excessive weight loss.

- **Dyspepsia**

  A disorder of digestion, characterized by indigestion felt in the upper middle abdomen. It usually accompanies heartburn, feeling full too early, upper abdominal bloating, discomfort, and nausea during and after meal.

- **Regurgitation**

  Reflux of swallowed food back to the oral cavity. It can also mean reflux of blood due to a defect in a heart valve.

- **Emesis**

  Vomiting of food from the stomach through the esophagus and the mouth.

- **Nausea**

  Feeling sick with the desire to vomit.

- **Eructation, belching**

  The act of expelling gas from the stomach through the mouth with accompanying noise.

- **Bulimia**

  Ingesting abnormal amount of food due to excessive appetite.

- **Hematemesis**

  Vomiting of blood due to hemorrhage in the upper digestive tract.

- **Polyphagia**

  An abnormal condition of eating large amount of food due to excessive hunger, caused by dysfunctional central nervous system.

Inflammations and infections

- **Adenotonsilitis**

  Bacterial or viral infection of the oropharynx or nasopharynx.

- **Pharyngitis**

  Inflammation of the pharynx, causing sore throat.

- **Tonsillitis**
  Inflammation of the tonsils.

- **Esophagitis**
  Inflammation of the esophagus.

- **Gastritis**
  Inflammation of the inner lining of the stomach, acute or chronic. Symptoms include upper central abdominal pain and burning sensation at night or between meals, blood in stool, stomach ache, etc.

- **Gastroduodenitis**
  Inflammation of the stomach and the duodenum.

- **Gastroenteritis**
  Inflammation of the mucous membranes of the stomach and intestine. Symptoms include loss of appetite, nausea, vomiting, stomach ache, diarrhea, etc.

Disorder and disease due to metabolisms, growth, nutrition or unknown causes

- **Esophageal ring**
  A ring of mucosal tissue at the lower part of the esophagus can cause difficulty in swallowing. The patient may feel as if something is hanging in the throat.

- **Esophageal spasm**
  A condition in which abnormal contraction of the esophageal muscle makes it difficult to swallow food and can cause regurgitation. Pain can be felt below the breastbone and may propagate to the jaw and arms.

- **Esophageal varices**
  Dilation of the veins in the lower part of the esophagus. Causes are cirrhosis, parenchymal liver disease, duodenal ulcer, pancreatitis or hepatic portal hypertension.

- **Esophagotracheal fistula**
  An abnormal connection between the esophagus and the trachea.

- **Gastroesophageal reflux disease (acid reflux)(GERD)**
  Chronic symptom of mucosal damage by stomach acid flowing up the esophagus with accompanying heartburn and chest pain.

• **Gastric ulcer**

Painful ulcer on the mucosal linings of the stomach or the small intestine. Symptoms include pain or burning sensation in the stomach between meals and in the evening.

• **Duodenal ulcer**

Ulcer occurring at the duodenum is the most common ulcer of the gastrointestinal type. Damage in the lesion goes deeper than the mucous membrane layer, where the underlying muscle is exposed.

• **Peptic ulcer**

Damage of the mucous membrane that exposes the underlying muscle layer of the digestive organ.

• **Gastroptosis**

Abnormal condition in which the stomach droops down excessively. It is considered abnormal when the low point of the stomach at rest is below the horizontal level of the navel viewed with an X-ray image.

• **Pylorospasm**

Disorder due to spasmodic contraction of the pyloric sphincter.

• **Pyloric stenosis**

Constriction of the pyloric region causing obstruction of chyme movement.

Tumor

• **Zollinger-Ellison syndrome**

An endocrine tumor grown from non-beta islet cells in the pancreas. The non-beta cells secrete hormone gastrin which stimulates production of gastric acid. In Zollinger-Ellison syndrome, the tumor causes excessive secretion of gastrin which in turn induces excessive production of gastric acid, with consequent severe digestive ulceration.

• **Stomach cancer**

Abnormal growth of the malignant tumor from the lining of the stomach. Early symptoms include pain when eating food, blood in stool, dark colored stool, loss of appetite, chronic indigestion, vomiting, unpleasant breath, fatigue, loss of weight, etc.

Small and Large Intestines, Peritoneum

Symptoms

- **Borborygmus**

  Rumbling noise in the stomach and intestines made by movement of gas accompanying the peristaltic motion.

- **Flatus, flatulence**

  The expulsion of gas from the large intestine through the rectum out of the anus.

- **Constipation**

  Defecation (bowel movement) that is infrequent and hard to make.

- **Diarrhea**

  The condition in which the feces contains excessive watery material.

- **Steatorrhea**

  The presence of excessive amount of fat in the feces.

- **Tympanites**

  The condition of bulged abdomen as a result of excessive accumulation of gas in the stomach and the intestines. It is more common in patients with peritonitis or typhoid.

- **Ascites**

  An accumulation of fluid containing significant amount of protein and other cells in the peritoneal cavity.

- **Tenesmus**

  Continuously feeling the need to excrete feces or urine after being unable to discharge satisfactorily.

- **Melena**

  Dark, tarry feces containing digested blood as the result of gastrointestinal bleeding.

- **Colic**

  Severe and abrupt pain on the waist, caused by the blockage by stones in the urinary tract and the rise in renal pelvis pressure, and the resultant exasperation or spasm of the uretral smooth muscle.

- **Hemoperitoneum**

  Presence of blood in the peritoneal cavity.

- **Pruritus ani**

  Itchiness of the skin at the anus.

- **Hematochezia**

  Bright red blood in the feces, usually related to bleeding in the colon or rectum.

Inflammations and infections

- **Appendicitis**

  Inflammation of the appendix.

- **Enteritis**

  Inflammation of the intestines, usually the small intestine.

- **Duodenitis**

  Inflammation of the duodenum.

- **Ileitis**

  Inflammation of the ileum.

- **Colitis**

  Inflammation of the colon.

- **Ulcerative colitis**

  Inflammation of the colon with accompanying ulcer. Symptoms include feces with blood, purulence and mucus. Treatment involves colectomy or ileostomy depending on the lesion.

- **Enterogastritis**

  Inflammation of the stomach and the intestine.

- **Enterocolitis**

  Inflammation of the small and large intestines.

- **Ileocolitis**

  Inflammation of the ileum and the colon.

- **Diverticulum**

  Local growth (outpouching) of an inner muscular lining of an organ. It can occur at any place of the esophagus, stomach and intestines, with the duodenum and the colon as the most likely organs.

- **Diverticulitis**

  Inflammation of the diverticulum when the waste material fills and stays in the hollow space.

- **Proctitis, rectitis**

  Proctitis is inflammation of the anus and rectum.

- **Peritonitis**

  Inflammation and swelling of the abdominal cavity and the peritoneum that covers the visceral organs.

Disorder and disease due to metabolism, growth, nutrition or unknown causes

- **Volvulus**

  Twisting of the intestine that causes bowel obstruction.

- **Intussusception**

  Telescoping (invagination) of a portion of the intestine in itself.

- **Intestinal obstruction, Ileus**

  Intestinal obstructions include mechanical obstructions caused by hernia, intestinal adhesion, intussusceptions, volvulus, etc. and paralytic obstruction caused by inability to start peristaltic motion. Symptoms are abdominal distention, severe constipation, vomiting, abdominal pain, severe sweating, etc.

- **Enterolith**

  Mineral concretion (stone-like object) in the intestine.

- **Polyp**

  Mushroom-shaped tumor in the mucous membrane of the intestine.

- **Lactose intolerance**

  Disease related to inability to digest lactose, usually due to lack of lactase.

- **Irritable bowel syndrome**

  A chronic disorder with the nerves and muscles of the intestines being oversensitive. Symptoms are repeated digestive discomfort such as stomachache or abdominal bloating after meal or mild stress, diarrhea and constipation.

• **Rectocele, proctocele**

The condition in which a part of the rectum penetrates through a torn lesion in the vaginal wall.

• **Hernia**

An abnormal condition in which a part of an organ penetrates and protrudes through a torn lesion of another organ.

• **Hiatal hernia, hiatus hernia**

The protrusion of the upper part of the stomach into the thorax through a gap of the weak diaphragm.

• **Inguinal hernia**

Protrusion of an object in the abdominal cavity through the inguinal canal. It can be divided into indirect and direct inguinal hernias.

• **Umbilical hernia**

Hernia of the intestine at the site of the umbilicus (navel).

• **Anal fissure**

A lineal tear or ulcer in the skin of the anal canal, accompanied by sharp pain.

• **Anal fistula**

An abnormal connection between the surface of the anal canal and the perianal skin, through which excretions occur.

• **Hemorrhoid**

A condition of dilated perianal vascular structure (varicosity). Internal hemorrhoid is the condition existing inside the anal sphincter, while external hemorrhoid is that of the outside.

• **Peritoneal abscess**

Collection of pus from inflamed tissue in the peritoneum.

Tumors

• **Colorectal cancer.**

Cancer of the colon or the rectum.

Liver, Biliary system and Pancreas

Symptoms

- **Fatty liver**
  The condition of the liver with abnormal accumulation of lipids.
- **Hepatomegaly**
  The state of abnormal enlargement of the liver due to a disease.
- **Hepatomalacia**
  The state of abnormal softening of the liver tissue.
- **Hyperbilirubinemia**
  Unusually high concentration of bilirubin in the blood.
- **Jaundice, Icterus**
  Yellowish pigmentation of the skin, mucous membranes, sclera of the eye, etc., caused by excessive amount of bilirubin in the blood, accompanied by nausea, vomiting, stomachache, dark colored feces, etc.
- **Acholia**
  A condition of little or no bile secretion into the digestive tract.
- **Glycosuria**
  Abnormal condition in which glucose is discharged in the urine.
- **Cholelithiasis, gallstones**
  Pebble-like crystalline concretion formed in the gallbladder or bile duct.
- **Choledocholithiasis**
  Gallstone-like concretion, composed with bile pigments and calcium salt, in the common bile duct.
- **Cholestasis**
  The obstruction of bile flow from the liver to the duodenum.
- **Hypoglycemia**
  Abnormally low blood glucose level.
- **Hyperglycemia**
  Abnormally high blood glucose level.
- **Hypocholesterolemia**
  Lower than normal concentration of cholesterol in the blood.

- **Hypercholesterolemia**

  Higher than normal concentration of cholesterol in the blood.

Inflammations and infections

- **Hepatitis**

  Inflammation of the liver. It can be classified per various causes as viral hepatitis, alcoholic hepatitis, toxipathic hepatitis, etc. General symptoms are fatigue, arthralgia, nausea, loss of appetite, jaundice, etc.

- **Viral hepatitis**

  Hepatitis caused by viral infection. Types of hepatitis are classified by type A, B, C hepatitis viruses.

- **Cholangitis**

  Inflammation of the bile duct caused by bacterial infection or obstruction of the duct by cholelith (gallstone) or tumor.

- **Cholecystitis**

  Acute or chronic inflammation of the gallbladder.

- **Pancreatitis**

  Inflammation of the pancreas.

Disorder and disease due to metabolisms, growth, nutrition or unknown causes

- **Hydrops of gallbladder**

  Abnormal state of serous fluid accumulation in the gallbladder.

- **Biliary stricture**

  Stricture of the bile duct or the common bile duct, typically caused by gallstones. However, cholangitis, cancer of the pancreas or duodenum, ileitis, pancreatitis, roundworms can cause the condition as well.

- **Diabetes mellitus**

  A metabolic disorder caused by lack of insulin or pancreatic dysfunction. Symptoms include polyphagia, polydipsia, polyuria, hyperglycemia, glycouria, etc.

- **Empyema of gallbladder**

  Collection of pus in the gallbladder.

Tumors

- **Hepatoma**
  A malignant tumor of the liver causing hepatomegaly.
- **Cholangioma**
  Cancer of the bile duct.
- **Carcinoma of pancreases**
  Cancer of the pancreas is accompanied by loss of appetite, unusual intestinal gas, systemic physical weakness, loss of weight, stomachache, epilepsy, jaundice, itchiness, diabetic symptoms, etc.

Terms for Surgery and Treatment

Oral Cavity

Cheiloplasty

Surgical procedure to correct cleft lip, including deficiency caused by external injury, noma or tumor.

Stomatoplasty

Plastic surgery on the oral cavity.

Palatoplasty

Plastic procedure to correct the cleft palate. Among many methods, most often the mucous membrane on the nasal side and the muscle of the palate are separated and reconstructed, between 12~18 months after birth.

Glossoplasty

Plastic surgery on the tongue.

Pharynx, Esophagus and Stomach

Adenotonsillectomy

Surgical removal of the adenoids and tonsils.

Esophagectomy

Surgical removal of a part or all of the esophagus.

Esophagostomy

Surgical operation of making an incision into the esophagus to create an opening.

Esophagoplasty

Surgical reconstruction of the esophagus to correct a defect.

Anastomosis

Interconnection between two channels, passages, tubes or vessels. A connection can be end-to-end, or end-to-side or side-to-side, etc. Esophagogastrostomy, gastrogastrostomy, gastroduodenostomy, gastroenterostomy, gastrojejunostomy, gastrocolostomy, etc. can be performed.

Gastrostomy

Surgical procedure to make an opening in the stomach for external connection for feeding nutrients.

Gastrotomy

Surgical incision into the stomach, to remove foreign matter or to stop bleeding from the stomach.

Gastrectomy

Surgical removal of a part or all of the stomach. Total gastrectomy, subtotal gastrectomy or antrectomy, etc. can be performed.

Gastropexy

Surgical fixation of the stomach to the abdominal wall or other part such as diaphragm.

Gastroplasty

Surgical operation, usually done on the stomach and the lower end of the esophagus, to reduce the size of the stomach. This is a method to treat patients with extreme obesity or a problem with the esophagogastric region. A small pouch with a silicone band around the new passage is created at the upper part of the stomach.

Pyloroplasty

Surgical reconstruction in cases of pyloric stenosis, to relieve obstruction of the chyme movement.

Vagotomy

Surgical resection of the vagus nerve, in order to limit stimulation to the stomach, reducing the secretion of acid in the stomach and the gastric motion.

Gastric gavage

Medical device used to supply the stomach with nutrients through the feeding tube inserted into the nose.

Gastric lavage

Washing of the stomach, with sterilized distilled water or saline solution supplied through a tube inserted into the mouth. The fluid is then drained out of the mouth. This procedure is used before and after stomach surgery or to remove toxic substance.

Small and Large Intestines, Peritoneum

Appendectomy

Surgical removal of the vermiform appendix.

Cecectomy

Surgical removal of the cecum.

Colectomy

Surgical removal of all or a part the colon.

Hemorrhoidectomy

Surgical removal of the hemorrhoids.

Diverticulectomy

Surgical removal of a diverticulum.

Celiotomy, laparotomy

Surgical procedure to make an incision to open the abdominal cavity to gain access into the cavity to diagnose and assess the condition.

Colostomy

Surgical operation to make an opening in the abdominal wall and connect it to the colon to make discharge of feces possible.

Ileostomy

Surgical operation to make an opening in the abdominal wall and connect it to the ileum to make discharge of feces possible, after colectomy for ulcerative colitis, ileitis or colon cancer.

Enterostomy

Surgical operation to make an opening in the abdominal wall and connect it to the intestine to make discharge of waste possible. Other similar operations include ileocolostomy, enterocolostomy, colocolostomy, etc.

Cecopexy

Surgical fixation of the cecum.

Enterorrhaphy

Surgical operation to suture the intestines.

Enterolysis

Surgical operation to separate the intestinal self-adhesion or to the abdominal wall.

Herniorrhaphy

Surgical operation to suture and repair hernia.

Polypectomy

Surgical removal of the polyp.

Proctoplasty

Surgical reconstruction to repair the rectum or the anus.

Proctectomy

Surgical excision of the rectum.

Liver, Biliary system and Pancreas

Liver biopsy

Microscopic examination of a sample tissue from the liver.

Hepatotomy

Surgical incision into the liver.

Hepatectomy

Surgical removal of a part of or the whole liver.

Hepatorrhaphy

Surgical operation to suture the liver.

Cholecystotomy

Surgical incision into the gallbladder to remove cholelith or serous fluid.

Cholecystectomy

Surgical removal of the gallbladder. After the operation, the bile from the liver flows directly to the duodenum.

Cholecystostomy

Surgical operation to create an opening in the gallbladder to insert a tube for bile drainage.

Cholecystogastrostomy

Surgical operation to make a connection (anastomosis) between the gallbladder and the stomach.

Choledochoduodenostomy

Surgical operation to make a connection (anastomosis) between the common bile duct and the duodenum.

Choledochotomy

Surgical incision into the common bile duct to verify existence of cholelith and removal.

Choledocholithotomy

Surgical incision into the common bile duct to remove the cholelith.

Choledocholithotripsy

Medical procedure to physically pulverize the cholelith for passing.

Sphincteroplasty (Oddi)

Surgical operation to relieve constriction and reconstruct the sphincter of Oddi.

Radical pancreatoduodenectomy

Surgical operation for pancreatic cancer. The head part of the pancreas, duodenum, pyloric region of the stomach and inferior part of the common bile duct are removed, then anastomosis of the remaining parts is performed.

Sphincteroplasty (Vater)

Surgical operation to relieve constriction and reconstruct the sphincter of Vater.

Pancreatectomy

Surgical removal of all or part of the pancreas.

Pancreaticoduodenectomy

Surgical procedure to remove the head part of the pancreas and the enclosing part of the duodenum, after which anastomosis is performed.

Whipple's operation

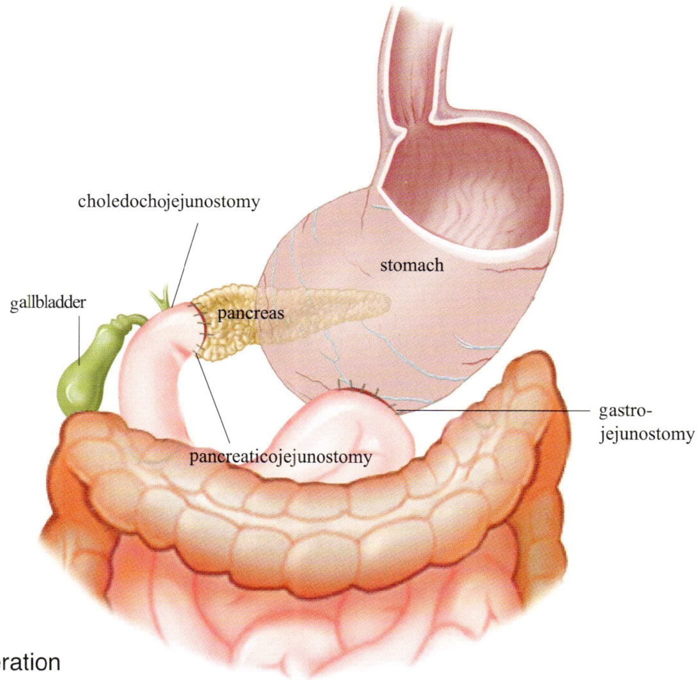

Figure 15-13 Whipple's operation

Terms for Test and Intervention

Endoscopy

An endoscope is a long fiberoptic instrument with a light source and a lens attached at the tip. Endoscopy is visual examination with the instrument inserted into the cavity of the organ. A suspected part of the cavity is further examined with biopsy.

Esophagoscopy

Visual examination of the esophageal tube with an endoscope.

Gastroscopy

Visual examination of the stomach with an endoscope.

Duodenoscopy

Visual examination of the duodenum with an endoscope.

Endoscopic ultrasonography

A medical procedure to examine the digestive tract and the internal organs around the probe of an endoscope, where an ultrasonic activator and a sensor are attached. The method is similar to the regular endoscopy, however, the internal structure beyond the esophageal lining can be examined.

Abdominocentesis, paracentesis

A medical procedure in which the abdominal wall is punctured by a needle to draw abdominal fluid.

Peritoneocentesis

A medical procedure in which the peritoneal cavity is punctured by a needle to draw peritoneal fluid, for the purpose of treatment.

Laparoscopy

Examination of the abdominal cavity using a laparoscope.

Colonoscopy

Visual examination of the colon through the anus, using a colonoscope.

Sigmoidoscopy

Visual examination of the anus, rectum and sigmoid and possible sample extraction using a sigmoidoscope.

Gastrointestinal series

Radiololgic examination of the gastrointestinal tract for tumor, ulcer or other anomalies. Fluoroscopic or X-ray images are taken after the patient swallows barium sulfate solution.

Liver function test

Test of the liver for damage or disease using biochemical blood assays, including SGOT (serum glutamic oxalacetic transaminase or AST), SGPT (serum glutamic pyruvic transaminase or ALT), ALP (alkaline phosphatase), serum bilirubin, etc.

Analysis and Meaning of Key Terms

Term	Term Analysis	Meaning
an/o :		anus
perianal [pèrinal]	peri- = around, -al = pertaining to	pertaining to near the anus
append/o, appendic/o :		appendix
appendectomy [æ̀pəndéktəmi]	-ectomy = excision	excision of the appendix
bil/i :		bile
biliary [bíliéri]	-ary = pertaining to	pertaining to bile
bucc/o :		cheek
buccal mucosa [bʌ́kəl mju:kóusə]	-al = pertaining to, mucosa = mucous membrane	mucous membrane of the cheek
cec/o :		cecum
cecopexy [sí:kəpéksi]	-pexy = surgical fixation	surgical fixation of the cecum

Term	Term Analysis	Meaning
cheil/o :		**lips**
cheilorrhaphy [káiləplæ̀sti]	-rrhaphy = suture	suture of the (cleft) lip
cholangi/o :		**bile duct**
cholangiography [kəlæ̀ndʒiάgrəfi]	-graphy = process of recording	X-ray imaging of the bile duct
cholecyst/o :		**gallbladder**
cholecystitis [kóuləsìstitis]	-itis = inflammation	inflammation of the gallbladder
choledoch/o :		**common bile duct (CBD)**
choledochotomy [kalidəkóutəmi]	-tomy = incision	incision into the common bile duct
col/o, colon/o :		**colon**
colostomy [kəlάstəmi]	-stomy = new opening	surgically making an artificial anus through the abdominal wall connected from the colon
dent/o, odont/o :		**tooth**
edentulous [iːdéntjulas]	e- = without, -ous = pertaining to	without teeth, toothless
duoden/o :		**duodenum**
duodenal [djùːədíːnəl]	-al = pertaining to	pertaining to the duodenum
enter/o :		**small intestine, intestine**
gastroenterology [gæ̀strouèntərάlədʒi]	gastr/o = stomach, -logy = study of study of	the digestive system and its diseases and treatments
esophago/o :		**esophagus**
gastroesophageal [gæ̀strouisafədʒíəl] reflux (GER)	gastr/o = stomach, re- = back, -flux = flow	stomach acid flowing up the esophagus to cause damage on the esophageal lining
gastr/o :		**stomach**
nasogastric [nèizougǽstrik] tube	nas/o = nose, -ic = pertaining to	tube inserted through the nose into the stomach for siphoning out or administrating material

Term	Term Analysis	Meaning
gingiv/o :		gum
gingivitis [dʒìndʒəváitis]	-itis = inflammation	inflammation of the gingiva
gloss/o :		tongue
glossectomy [glɑséktəmi]	-ectomy = excision	surgical removal of the tongue or a part thereof
hepat/o :		liver
hepatocellular [hèpetouséljuːlər]	cellul/o = cell, -ar = pertaining to	pertaining to the cells of the liver
herni/o :		hernia
herniorrhaphy [hə́ːrniɔ́ːrəfi]	-rrhaphy = suture	repair of hernia by means of suture
ile/o :		ileum
ileostomy	-stomy = new opening	surgically making an artificial opening through the abdominal wall connected from the ileum
jejun/o :		jejunum
jejunal [dʒiːdʒúːnəl]	-al = pertaining to	pertaining to the jejunum
labi/o :		lips
labioglossophar-yngeal	gloss/o = tongue, pharyng/o = pharynx	pertaining to the lips, tongue and pharynx
lapar/o :		abdomen
laparoscope [lǽpərəskòup]	-scope = instrument used to visually examine	visual instrument to examine the abdominal cavity
lingu/o :		tongue
sublingual [sʌblíŋgwəl]	sub- = under, -al = pertaining to	pertaining to under the tongue
lith/o :		stone
lithotripsy [liθoutripsi]	-tripsy = crushing	pulverizing gallstone or bilestone for easier pass through the duct

Term	Term Analysis	Meaning
orex/l :		appetite
anorexia [ænəréksiə]	an- = not, lack of; -ia = condition	symptom of poor or no appetite resulting in severe weight loss
or/o :		mouth
oral [ɔ́:rəl]	-al = pertainging to	pertaining to the mouth or speech
pancreat/o :		pancreas
pancreatitis [pǽŋkriətáitis]	-itis = inflammation	inflammation of the pancreas
peritone/o :		peritoneum
ventriculoperitoneal shunt	ventricul/o = ventricles (of the brain); shunt = device used to divert the flow of fluid	artificial passage created for drainage of cerebrospinal fluid from the ventricles to the peritoneal cavity
pharyng/o :		throat,pharynx
pharyngeal [fəríndʒiəl]	-eal = pertaining to	pertaining to the pharynx
proct/o :		rectum
proctoclysis [praktə́kaisis]	-clysis = washing, irrigation	injection of fluid into the rectum for discharge of feces or cleaning
pylor/o :		pylorus
pylorospasm [pailóurəspæzəm]	-spasm = sudden, involuntary contraction	spasmodic contraction of the pyloric sphincter
rect/o :		rectum
rectostenosis	-stenosis = narrowing, stricture	condition of constricted rectum
sialaden/o :		salivary gland
sialadenitis [sàiəlæ̀dináitis]	-itis = inflammation	inflammation of the salivary gland
sigmoid/o :		sigmoid colon
sigmoidoscopy [sigmɔ́idəskòupi]	-scopy = visual examination	visual examination of the sigmoid and the rectum using a sigmoidoscope
steat/o :		fat
steatorrhea [stì:ətəríə]	-rrhea = discharge, flow	presence of excessive amount of fat in the feces

Term	Term Analysis	Meaning
stomat/o :		mouth
stomatitis [stòumətáitis]	-itis = inflammation	inflammation of a part of mucous lining in the mouth
viscer/o :		internal organs
visceroptosis [vìsərəptlsis]	-ptosis = drooping	excessive drooping of internal organs

Abbreviations

Abbreviation	Full Term	Meaning
UPPP	uvulopalatopharyngoplasty	A surgical resection of tissues in the throat (uvula, palate and pharynge) in order to widen the airway of the patient
LAUP	laser assisted uvuloplasty	surgical resection of the unnecessary uvular tissue using laser
LRPP	laser resection palato pharyngoplasty	surgical resection of the unnecessary palatal and pharyngeal tissue using laser
a.c.	ante cibum	(medicine to be taken) before meals
BM	bowel movement	discharge of feces with rectal and anal effort, defecation
b.i.d.	bis in die	(medicine to be taken) twice a day
EGD	esophagogastroduodeno-scopy	upper gastrointestinal endoscopy, including esophagus, stomach and duodenum
GERD	gastroesophageal reflux disease	stomach acid flowing up the esophagus with esophageal damage
GI	gastrointestinal	pertaining to the stomach and intestines
GTT	glucose tolerance test	blood test to evaluate how quickly glucose is cleared form the blood
HAV	hepatitis A virus	
HBV	hepatitis B virus	
HCV	hepatitis C virus	
BE	barium enema	X-ray imaging technique using barium solution as contrast medium filling the colon via the rectum

Abbreviation	Full Term	Meaning
CBD	common bile duct	the duct formed where the hepatic duct and the cholecystic duct join
LFT	liver function tests	Test of the liver for damage or disease using biochemical blood assays
BS	bowel sound	rumbling noise made by contents of the intestine in peristaltic motion
PUD	peptic ulcer disease	damage of the mucous membrane of the gastrointestinal tract
GB	gall bladder	
N&V	nausea and vomiting	
NPO	nil per os	nothing by mouth (not to take any food, drink or medicine by mouth)
p.o.	per os	by mouth (medicine to be taken orally)
p.c.	post cibum	(medicine to be taken) after meals
TPN	total parenteral nutrition	feeding a patient intravenously with nutritional formula, and NPO
UGI	upper gastrointestinal series	examination of the upper gastrointestinal tract with contrast agent and radiologic imaging

Exercises

1. Write medical terms that mean the following.

① discharge of waste material from the body defecation

② oral exocrine gland that secrete digestive fluid salivary gland

③ food tube between the mouth and the stomach esophagus

④ temporarily storage for food where protein digestion starts stomach

⑤ inflammation of the stomach gastritis

⑥ condition of restricted path in the intestine bowel obstruction, intestinal obstruction

⑦ surgical removal of a part or all of the colon colectomy

⑧ surgical removal of the vermiform appendix appendectomy

⑨ surgical removal of a part or all of the liver hepatectomy

⑩ surgical excision of the pancreas and the duodenum pancreaticoduodenectomy

2. Write medical terms that mean the following symptoms or diseases.

① the condition of little or no appetite anorexia

② endoscopic examination of the esophagus, stomach and duodenum esophagogastroduodenoscopy

③ malignant tumor of the liver originating from the liver cells hepatoma

④ symptom of difficulty in swallowing dysphagia

⑤ inflammation of the mucous membrane of the stomach gastritis

3. Write full terms for the following abbreviations.

① ERCP	endoscopic retrograde cholangiopancreatography
② EGD	esophagogastroduodenoscopy
③ GERD	gastroesophageal reflux disease
④ HCV	hepatitis C virus
⑤ CBD	common bile duct
⑥ PUD	peptic ulcer disease
⑦ GB	gallbladder
⑧ TPN	total parenteral nutrition
⑨ UGI	upper gastrointestinal
⑩ NPO	nil per os (nothing by mouth)

4. Write medical terms that mean the following.

① Surgical creation of a passage between the sigmoid colon and the rectum sigmoidoproctostomy

② Surgical creation of a passage between the duodenum and the ileum duodenoileostomy

③ Surgical creation of a passage between the stomach and the jejunum gastrojejunostomy

④ Endoscopic examination of the colon colonoscopy

⑤ Inflammation of the colon colitis

⑥ Surgical creation of an opening into the ileum ileostomy

⑦ Plastic repair of the pylorus pyloroplasty

⑧ Radiographic study of the bile ductss cholangiography

⑨ Radiographic study of the gallbladder cholecystography

⑩ Condition of having a stone in the common bile duct choledocholithiasis

Chapter 16

Urinary System

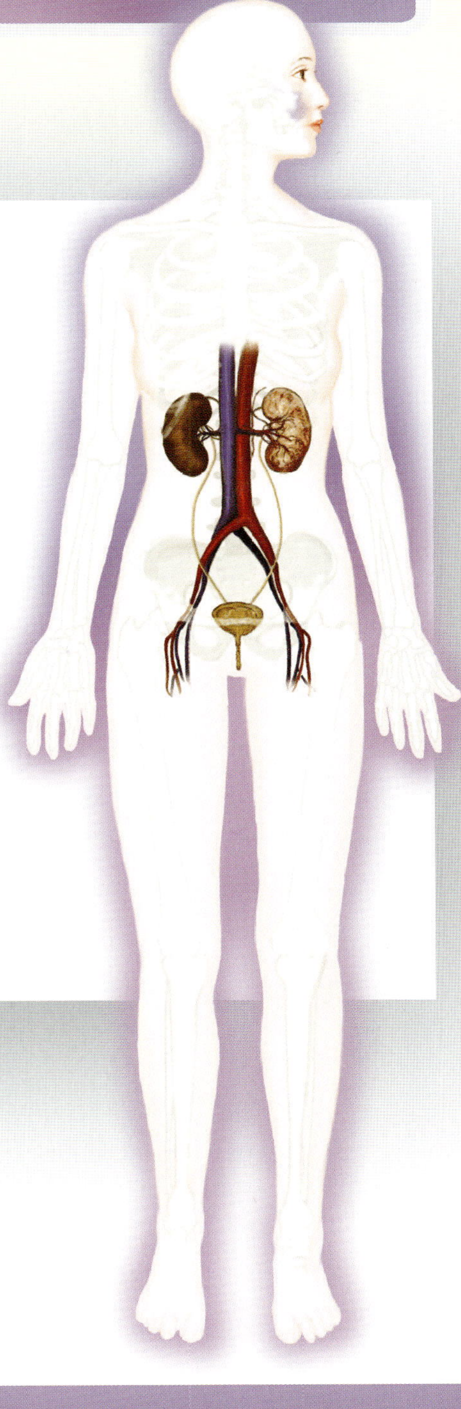

Chapter Contents

- Prolog
- Anatomical Terms
- Terms for Symptoms and Diseases
- Terms for Surgery and Treatment
- Terms for Test and Intervention
- Analysis and Meaning of Key Terms
- Abbreviations
- Exercises

Learning Objectives

- Understand the anatomical structure and functions of the urinary system.
- Learn diseases in the urinary system.
- Learn medical terms for treatment and surgery in the urinary system.
- Pronounce and define medical terms for the urinary system.
- Learn abbreviations used in the urinary system.

Prolog

The urinary system is an excretory system that discharges unnecessary waste material left from the metabolic activities. The most important function is to remove wastes like urea and uric acid from the blood and discharge them through urine. It is also involved in maintaining electrolytic balance by controlling the amount of water, salts and acids, etc. The urinary system consists of a pair of kidneys that form urine, a pair of ureters that transport urine, a urinary bladder that stores urine, and the urethra.

Anatomical Terms

Kidney

The kidney is a bean shaped organ between the peritoneum and the rear abdominal wall in the lumbar region, largely consisting of the renal cortex and the renal medulla. The functional unit of the kidney is called nephron, which consists of the glomerulus and renal tubule. It helps remove waste material from the blood and maintain electrolytic balance with water.

[Composition of the kidney]

- **Cortex**

The superficial part of the kidney that covers the medulla (inner part). It consists of the renal corpuscle and renal tubule.

• **Medulla**

The inner region of the kidney containing the renal pyramids and the collecting tubules.

• **Calyx**

The triangular renal pyramids in the medulla collectively form the calyx.

• **Pelvis**

The calyxes collectively form a (renal) pelvis that funnels urine into the ureter.

• **Hilum**

The gate of the kidney through which renal vein, renal artery, nerves and lymph vessels enter and leave.

Nephron

The functional base unit of the kidney in the renal cortex comprising 3 parts. Each kidney contain 1 ~ 1.25 million nephrons. It filters blood to remove waste material and reabsorb useful material.

[Composition of the nephron]

• **Glomerulus**

A lump of intertwined capillaries enclosed by the Bowman's capsule located in the renal cortex. It is where blood filtration and urine formation starts.

• **Bowman's capsule**

A sac enclosing the glomerulus that collects fluid released from the blood in the glomerular capillaries. It is the beginning part of the renal tubule.

• **Tubule**

The tubular duct that carries the renal fluid filtered at the glomerulus, consisting of the proximal convoluted tubule, Henle's loop and distal convoluted tubule. The fluid in the tubule is drained at the collecting tubule.

Memory key

- The urinary system consists of a pair of kidneys that produce urine, a pair of ureters that carry the urine, the urinary bladder that stores urine, and the urethra that discharge urine out of the body.

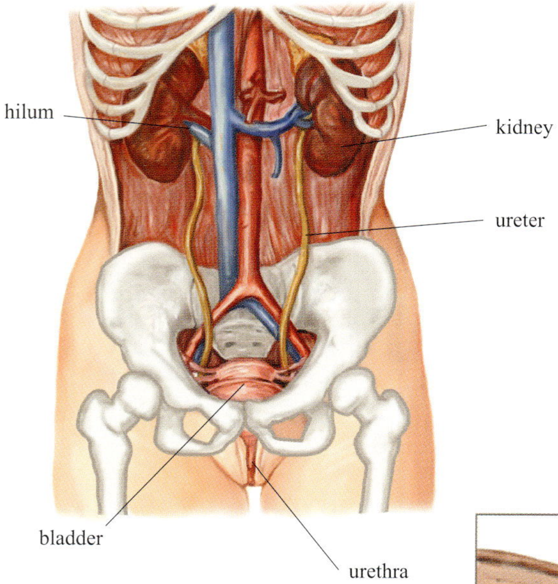

Figure 16-1 Urinary organs

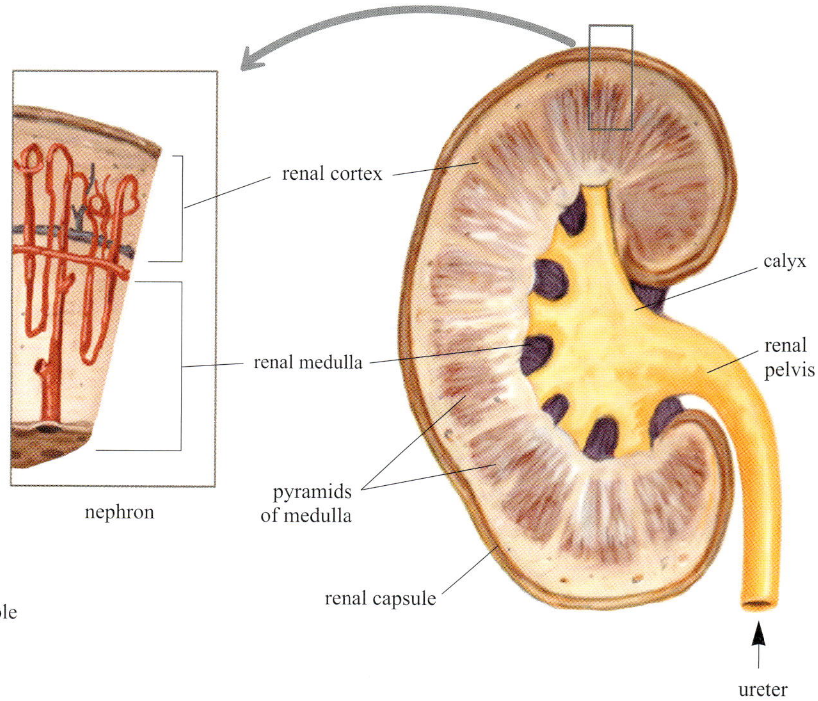

Figure 16-2
Structure of the kidney and the nephron

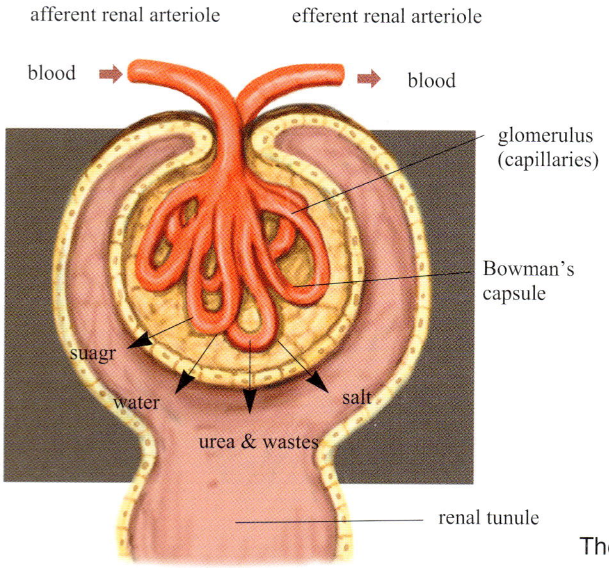

Figure 16-3
The glomerulus & Bowman's capsule

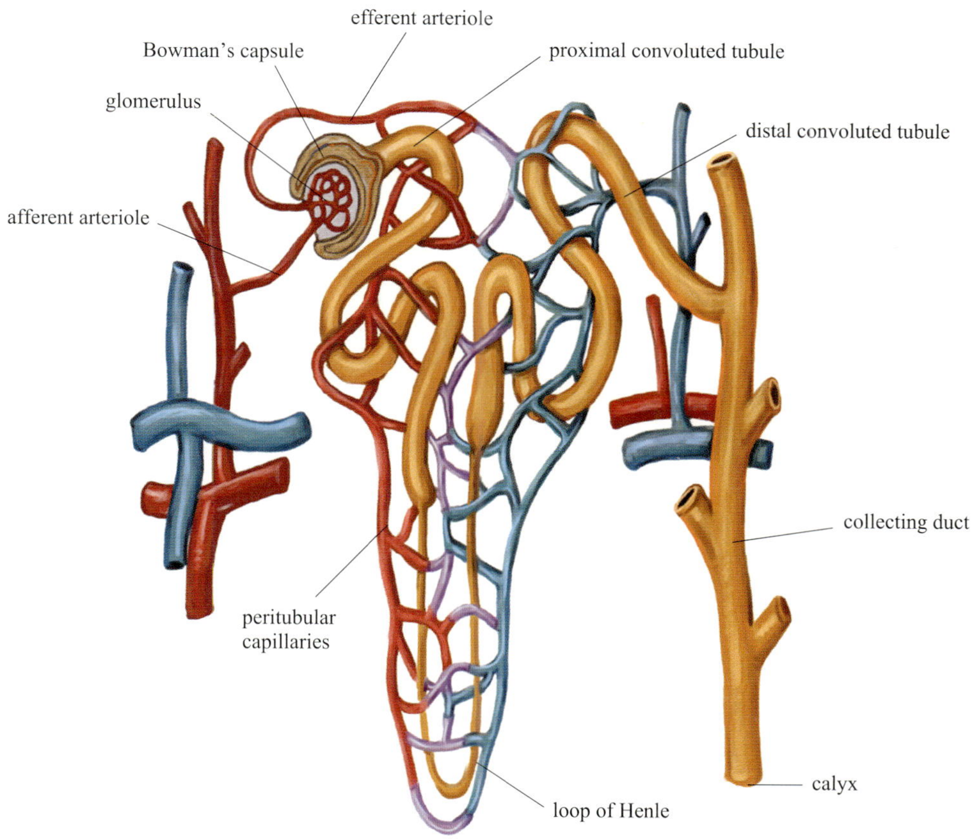

Figure 16-4 The nephron and blood supply

Ureter

A pair of ureters, each 26~33 cm long, carry urine produced in the kidney to the urinary bladder.

Urinary bladder

A temporary storage of urine which will be discharged out of the body. While it collects urine, its size increases while the thickness of the muscular wall decreases.

Trigone

The triangular area on the inner surface of the bladder bound by the orifices of the two ureters and the urethra. The surface of the area is smooth without wrinkles.

Urethra

Urethra is the tube through which urine exits the body, and it is the end part of the urinary tract. It is about 20 cm long for males and 3~5 cm long for females. Females are more susceptible to urethritis. For males, semen is also ejaculated through the urethra.

Urinary meatus

The external orifice of the urethra from which urine is ejected.

Urine

The yellow or amber colored liquid of specific gravity between 1.002 and 1.035, with pH at around 6.5. On average, 1,500~1,800 mL per day of urine is discharged.

Urine Formation & Pathway

The blood that enters the kidney through the renal artery passes the glomerulus where urea, creatinine, water, salt, sugar, etc. are filtered as renal fluid in the Bowman's capsule. Proteins like albumin and blood cells normally should not be included in the fluid.While the renal fluid is carried through the tubule, proper quantity of useful materials like water, electrolytes and nutrients are reabsorbed into the bloodstream. The rest of the fluid is carried as waste (the urine) through the calyx, renal pelvis, ureter, urinary bladder and is discharged out of the body through the urethra.

Memory key

- Urine formation starts as the blood from the renal artery, passes and is filtered at the glomerulus. The filtered renal fluid in the Bowman's capsule is carried through the renal tubule, calyx, pelvis, ureter, urinary bladder and is discharged out of the body through the urethra.

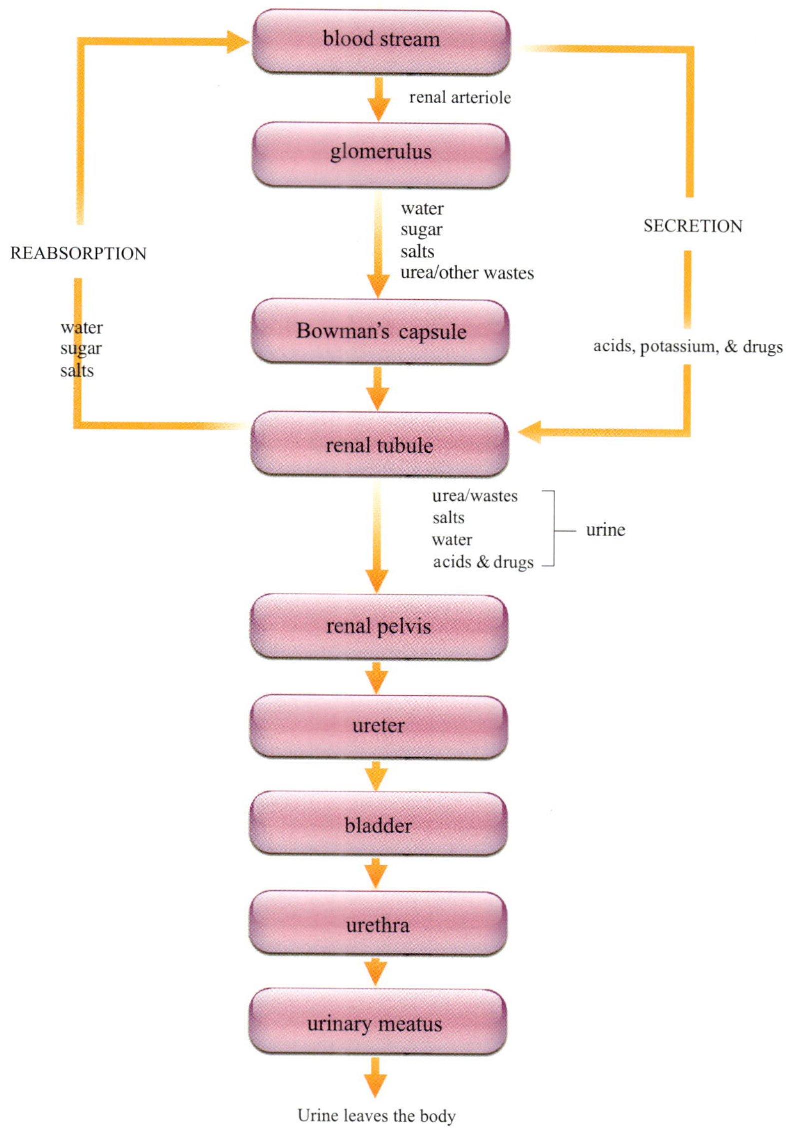

Figure 16-4 Urine formation and pathway

Terms for Symptoms and Diseases

Symptoms

Micturition

The act of urination.

Diuresis

Increase of urine formation and urination, which may be a symptom of diabetes mellitus or diabetes insipidus.

Dysuria

Difficult or painful discharge of urine.

Anuresis

Inability to urinate.

Enuresis

Involuntary urination, especially nocturnal enuresis (night time urinary incontinence, or bedwetting).

Urinary stasis

Stoppage or delay of urinary flow.

Urinary incontinence

Involuntary urination due to inability of the bladder to store urine, possibly caused by neurological disorder, spinal cord injury, weakened pelvic muscles, urinary stasis, bladder dysfunction, etc.

Frequent urination

The need to urinate more often than usual, while the total urinary volume is within normal range.

Urinary urgency

Sudden urge to urinate which is hard to resist.

Urinary retention

Retention of urine in the bladder due to lack of ability to urinate.

Vesical tenesmus

The condition in which continued straining of the bladder to urinate does not result in additional amount of urination, when the patient still has desire to urinate.

Anuria

The condition of lack of urine formation resulting in 100~250 mL of urine discharge per day.

Hematuria

The presence of blood in the urine.

Glycosuria

The presence of glucose in the urine, as a result of excessive carbohydrate intake or diabetes mellitus.

Polyuria

Abnormally large amount of urine, as a symptom of diabetes insipidus, diabetes mellitus or the result of diuretics medication.

Oliguria

The condition of low urine discharge, being under 500 mL per day.

Albuminuria

The presence of albumin in the urine.

Pyuria

The presence of pus in the urine, a symptom of urinary tract infection.

Nocturia

The condition in which the patient needs to wake up to urinate during sleep.

Ketonuria

The presence of ketone in the urine.

Bacteriuria

The presence of bacteria in the urine.

Uremia

Blood poisoning resulting from kidney malfunction and retention of waste products including protein metabolism products that should be excreted as urine. Symptoms include nausea, vomiting, headache, dizziness, poor eyesight, unconsciousness, seizure, azotemia, etc.

Azotemia

The accumulation in the blood of nitrogen-bearing waste products that are usually excreted in the urine.

Acidosis

Abnormally high acidity in the blood and other tissues.

Hyperkalemia

Abnormally high concentration of potassium ions in the blood.

Pitting edema

Abnormal accumulation of serum in a body part that results in swelling, in which case the area does not bounce back after pressing and releasing the area with a finger.

Diseases

Infection & Inflammation

- **Cystitis :** inflammation of the urinary bladder
- **Nephritis :** inflammation of the kidney
- **Pyelitis :** inflammation of the pelvis of the kidney; pyelonephritis
- **Ureteritis :** inflammation of the ureter
- **Urethritis :** inflammation of the urethra
- **Glomerulonephritis**
  Inflammation of the glomeruli, a form of nephritis. Acute glomerulonephritis sometimes occurs with an acute systemic infection. Initial-stage symptoms

are rare; however, in later stages edema, fever, vomiting, oliguria, hematuria, rise of blood pressure, etc. can appear.

- **Pyelonephritis**

  Inflammation of the kidney involving the renal pelvis, caused by bacterial infection. Symptoms include pelvic abscess, pyuria, fever, chill, flank pain, etc.

- **Urinary tract infection (UTI)**

  A collective term for infections in one or more organs of the urinary tract.

Degenerative Vascular Disease

- **Nephrotic syndrome, nephrosis**

  This is a condition caused by degenerative renal tubules leading to damage of the glomeruli and leakage of blood protein into urine. Symptoms include proteinuria, edema and hypoalbuminemia. The lesion is susceptible to infection.

- **Renal failure**

  Renal failure is loss of renal functions, either acute or chronic. Chronic renal failures are caused by chronic glomerulonephritis, chronic pyelonephritis, hypertension, etc. Usual treatment for this condition is dialysis to remove waste products like creatinine, urea, nitrogen, etc. and subsequent kidney transplant if possible. Renal failure is an end-stage renal disease, and it is fatal if not treated properly.

Other Abnormal Conditions

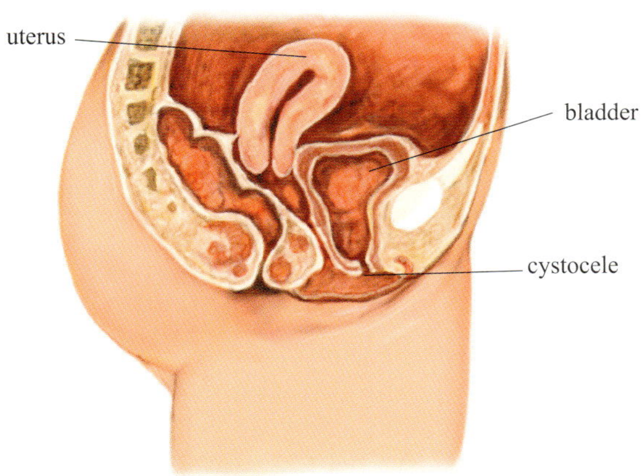

Figure 16-5 Cystocele

- **Cystocele**

  Hernial intrusion of the bladder through the wall between the bladder and the vagina.

- **Nephroptosis**

  Abnormal condition in which the kidney floats and drops down from its original position. The treatment is by nephropexy.

- **Ureterectasis :** Distension or dilation of the ureter.

- **Renal hypertension :** Hypertension caused by kidney disease

- **Polycystic kidney disease**
  A genetic disorder of the kidneys characterized by the presence of multiple fluid-filled cysts and abnormal kidney enlargement.

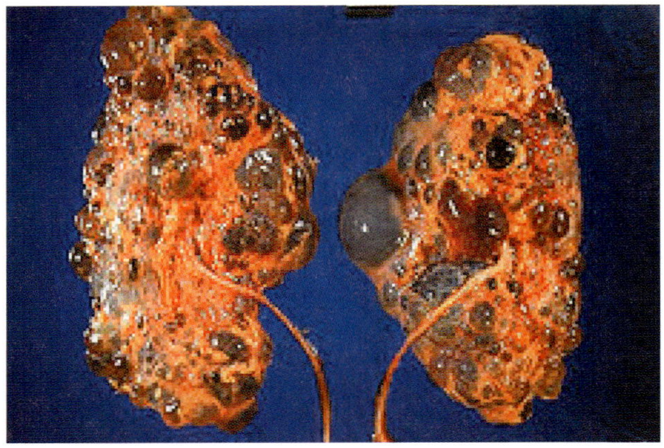

Figure 16-6 Polycystic kidney disease
source : http://en.wikipedia.org/wiki/Polycystic_kidney_disease

Urinary Obstruction

- **Hydronephrosis**
  A condition in which the urine generated in the kidney can't flow freely due to renal calculi, stricture, tumor, hypertrophy of prostate gland, etc., causing kidney distension and malfunction.
- **Nephrolithiasis, renal calculus**
  Commonly known as "kidney stone", nephrolithiasis is a solid concretion formed in the kidney, causing hematuria, pain in the flank, etc.
- **Ureterolithiasis**
  The presence of calculus (kidney stone) in the ureter.

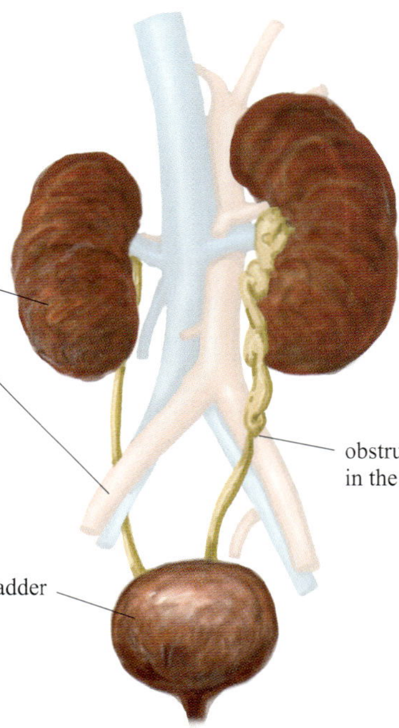

Figure 16-7 Hydronephrosis

- **Ureterostenosis**

  Stricture of the ureter.

Tumors

- **Hypernephroma**

  Malignant tumor typically in the adult's renal tissue. The usual initial symptom is hematuria.

- **Wilms' tumor**

  Malignant tumor that typically occurs in children under 5. Symptoms include pain in the flank, hematuria, weight loss, anemia, anorexia, etc.

Terms for Surgery and Treatment

Nephrectomy

Surgical removal of a kidney.

Nephrolithotomy

Surgical removal of the calculus by incision into the kidney in the case of nephrolithiasis.

Nephropexy

Surgical fixation of the kidney in the case of nephroptosis.

Pyelolithotomy

Surgical removal of the calculus from the renal pelvis.

Pyelotomy

Surgical incision into the renal pelvis of a kidney.

Ureterectomy

Surgical excision of all or a part of the ureter.

Kidney transplantation

Transplanting a healthy kidney of another person into the patient with renal failure.

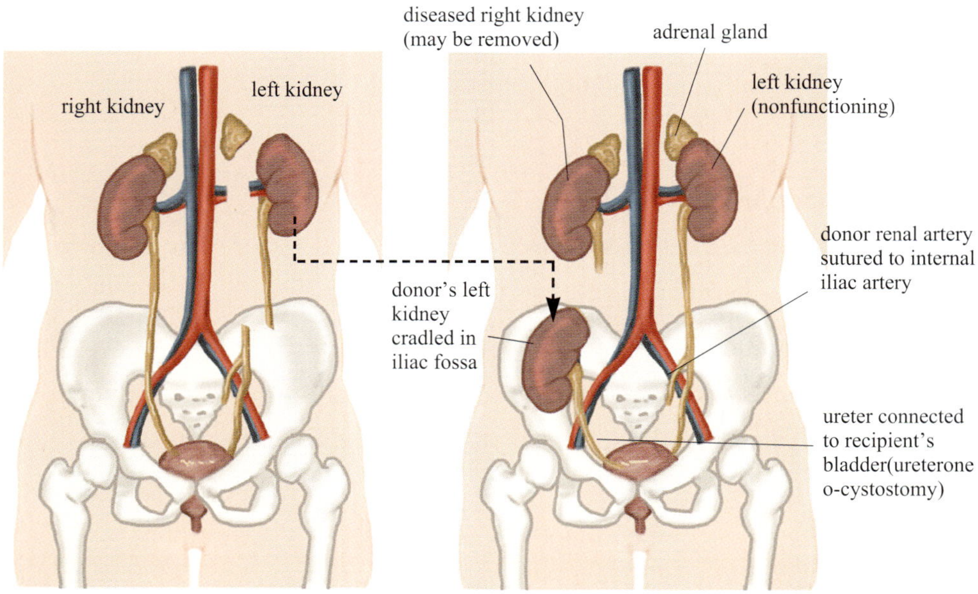

Figure 16-8 Donor's kidney and transplantation into the recipient's right side

Dialysis

A process of removing wastes from blood for patients with renal failure. There are two main types of dialyses :

- **Hemodialysis (HD)**

  In hemodialysis, the blood is pumped into an artificial kidney machine to filter out waste material and returned to the patient's body.

- **Peritoneal dialysis (PD)**

  A dialysate (special solution for dialysis) is run through a tube into the peritoneal cavity, where, given enough time, waste material in the blood is exchanged, after which the dialysate is removed. This method is used when hemodialysis is unsuitable or for patients with cardiovascular disease or prone to hemorrhage.

Memory key

- A patient with renal failure is given hemodialysis or peritoneal dialysis to remove waste material from the blood.

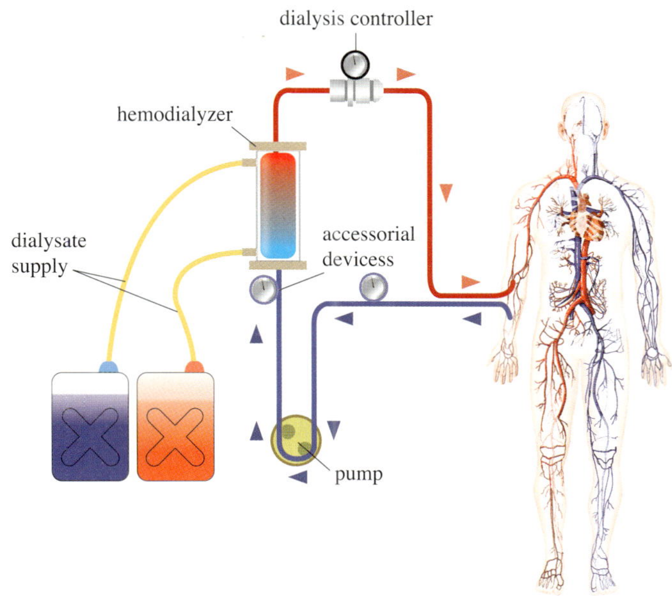

Figure 16-9 Schematic diagram of hemodialysis

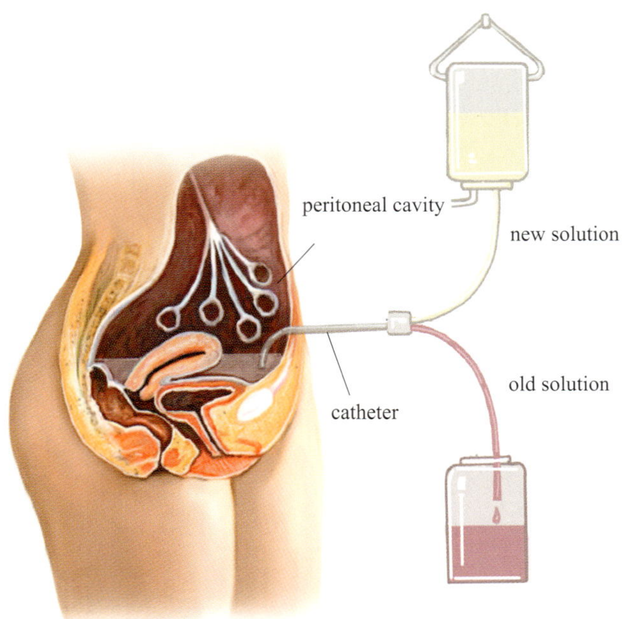

Figure 16-10 Peritoneal dialysis

Terms for Test and Intervention

Cystoscopy

Visual examination of the interior lining of the urinary bladder using a cystoscope.

Urethroscopy

Visual examination of the interior of the urethra using a urethroscope.

KUB (kidney, ureter, bladder)

An X-ray imaging technique without contrast medium to evaluate the urinary organs for location, size and outline.

Intravenous pyelography

An X-ray imaging technique with intravenous injection of contrast medium to visualize activities in the urinary tract. The flow of the contrast medium through the kidney, ureter, bladder and urethra can be seen during the process of excretion from the body. Renal functions, cystic tumor, infection, hydronephrosis, nephrolithiasis, etc. can be diagnosed.

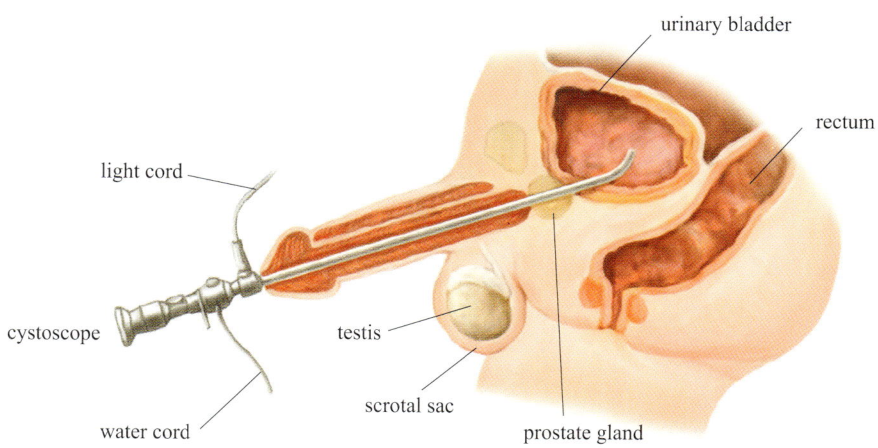

Figure 16-11 cystoscope insertion into the urinary bladder of a male

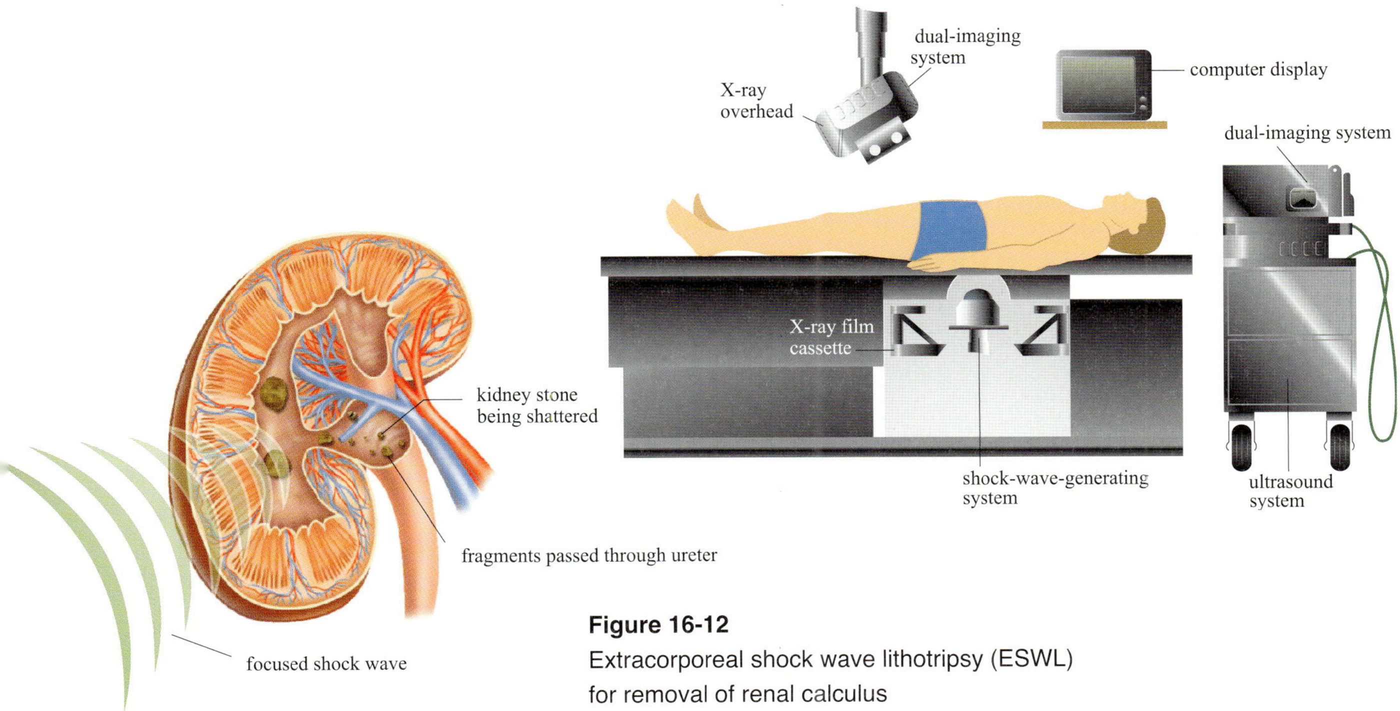

Figure 16-12
Extracorporeal shock wave lithotripsy (ESWL) for removal of renal calculus

Retrograde pyelography

An X-ray imaging technique for the kidney, ureter and bladder, with injection of contrast medium through a catheter inserted into the urethra.

Renal biopsy

A sample tissue of the kidney is taken for diagnostic purposes. The procedure can be performed with either open or closed technique.

Voiding cystourethrogram

An X-ray imaging technique, with injection of contrast medium through a catheter inserted into the urethra. Images of the bladder, ureter and urethra are taken before, during and after urination.

Renal angiography

An X-ray imaging technique for blood vessels in the kidney, for diagnosis of renal cell carcinoma or the condition of the vessels in a patient with hypertension.

Extracorporeal shock wave lithotripsy

A noninvasive surgical procedure involving ultrasonic shock wave, in order to break up urinary calculus for easy passing through the urinary tract, usually when the calculus is located upstream of the urinary bladder.

Blood urea nitrogen

A test to measure the amount of blood urea, a nitrogenous waste product. Excessive levels of BUN can cause unconsciousness or death.

Creatinine clearance test

A test to evaluate the ability to remove blood creatinine. The amount of creatinine discharged in the urine in a 24 hour period is measured.

Urinalysis

The comprehensive analysis of urine, used widely in the diagnosis of the urinary system. Color, pH, sugar, ketone, hemoglobin, etc. are included in the urine chemical analysis.

Urinary catheterization

Insertion of a soft tube into the patient's bladder through the urethra, that allows free urine drainage for the purpose of treatment or diagnosis. This is performed in the case of urethral damage or after surgery on the bladder or the urethra.

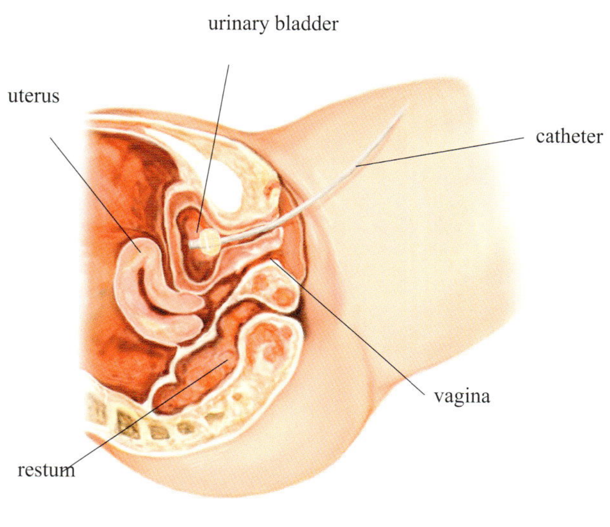

Figure 16-13 Foley cathter inserted into female's bladder

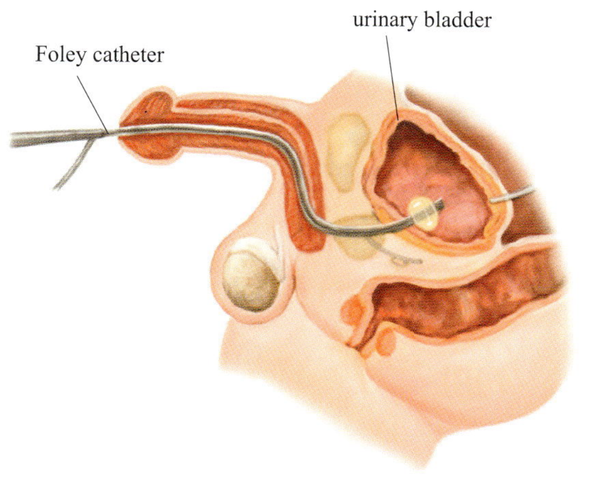

Figure 16-14 Foley cathter inserted into male's bladder

Analysis and Meaning of Key Terms

Term	Term Analysis	Meaning
nephr/o :		kidney
nephrolithiasis [nefraliθáiəsis]	-iasis = abnormal condition; lith/o = stone	kidney stone
nephropathy [nəfrápəθi]	-pathy = disease	kidney disease
nephrolithotomy [nefraliθátəmi]	-lith = stone; -tomy = process of cutting	surgical removal of the kidney stone
ren/o :		kidney
renal hypoplasia [rí:nəl háipoupléiʒə]	-al = pertaining to; -plasia = development; hypo- = under, below normal	underdevelopment of the kidney
pyel/o :		renal pelvis
pyelonephritis [pàiəlounifráitis]	-itis = inflammation	inflammation of the renal pelvis
pyelogram [pàiəlougræm]	-gram = record	X-ray image of the kidney, ureter and bladder
cyst/o :		bladder
cystitis [sistaitis]	-itis = inflammation	inflammation of the urinary bladder
cystoscope [sístəskòup]	-scope = instrument for visual, examination	instrument for visual examination of the urinary bladder
glomerul/o :		glomerulus
glomerulonephritis [gloumèrjulounə-fráitis, glə-]	-itis = inflammation; nephr/o = kidney	inflammation of the glomeruli, a form of nephritis
urethr/o :		urethra
urethrocystitis [jurə̀θrousístaitis]	cyst/o = bladder; -itis = inflammation	inflammation of the urethra and the bladder
ureter/o :		ureter
ureteral [juərí:təral]	-al = pertaining to	pertaining to the ureter
ureterolith [ju:təroulíθ]	-lith = stone	stone stuck in the ureter

Term	Term Analysis	Meaning
ur/o :		**urine, urinary tract**
uremia [juərí:miə]	-emia = blood condition	blood poisoning due to the kidney not being able to filter out waste materials
urologist [juərálədʒist]	-logist = specialist	physician specializing in urology
cortic/o :		**cortex, outer layer**
cortical [kɔ́:rtikəl]	-al = pertaining to	pertaining to the outer layer (of the kidney)
medull/o :		**medulla**
medullary [médəlèri]	-al = pertaining to	pertaining to the inner part (of the kidney)
vesic/o :		**urinary bladder**
vesicotomy [vèsəkátəmi]	-tomy = incision	surgical incision into the urinary bladder
lith/o :		**stone, calculus**
lithotripsy [líθətrìpsi]	-tripsy = crushing	surgical procedure to break up kidney stone by ultrasonic shock wave

Abbreviations

Abbreviation	Full Term	Meaning
ADH	antidiuretic hormone, vasopressin	antidiuretic hormone secreted by the pituitary gland
ARF	acute renal failure	abrupt loss of kidney function
ATN	acute tubular necrosis	death of tubular epithelial cells that form the renal tubules of the kidney
BUN	blood urea nitrogen	test for concentration of blood urea, a nitrogenous waste product from digestion of protein
CAPD	continuous ambulatory peritoneal dialysis	peritoneal dialysis performed continuously all day

Abbreviation	Full Term	Meaning
Cath	catheter, catheterization	soft tube inserted in the body to allow drainage or administration of fluid
CCPD	continuous cycling peritoneal dialysis	peritoneal dialysis performed automatically by machine all night
CKD	chronic kidney disease	progressive loss of renal function over a long period
CRF	chronic renal failure	end stage renal disease that requires kidney replacement therapy
Cysto	cystoscopic examination	visual examination of the urinary bladder with cystoscope
ESRD	end-stage renal disease	end stage renal disease that requires kidney replacement therapy
ESRF	end-stage renal failure	end stage renal disease that requires kidney replacement therapy
ESWL	extracorporeal shock wave lithotripsy	noninvasive surgical procedure to break up kidney stone by ultrasonic shock wave
GU	genitourinary	relating to the genital and urinary systems of the body
HD	hemodialysis	dialysis using artificial dialysis machine to remove waste materials from the blood
IVP	intravenous pyelogram	X-ray image taken of the urinary tract with intravenous contrast medium
K^+	potassium electrolyte	potassium ion concentration in the blood
KUB	kidney, ureter and bladder	X-ray imaging of the urinary tract without contrast medium
Na^+	sodium electrolyte	sodium ion concentration in the blood
PD	peritoneal dialysis	dialysis of the blood involving dialysate in the peritoneal cavity
PKU	phenylketonuria	metabolic disorder due to lack of liver enzyme PAH needed to metabolize amino acid phenylananine
RP	retrograde pyelogram	X-ray image taken with contrast medium injected through urethral catheter
UTI	urinary tract infection	infection that affects part of the urinary tract
U/A	urine analysis	array of tests performed on the urine
VCUG	voiding cystourethrogram	X-ray image taken before, during and after urination, with injection of contrast medium through a catheter inserted into the urethra

Exercises

1. Write the medical term for the following organs.

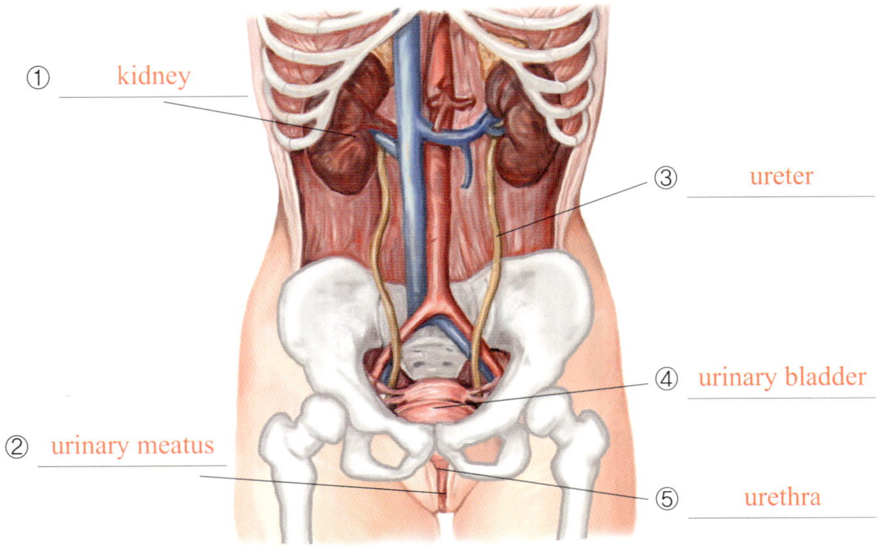

2. Write the medical terms for the following organ parts.

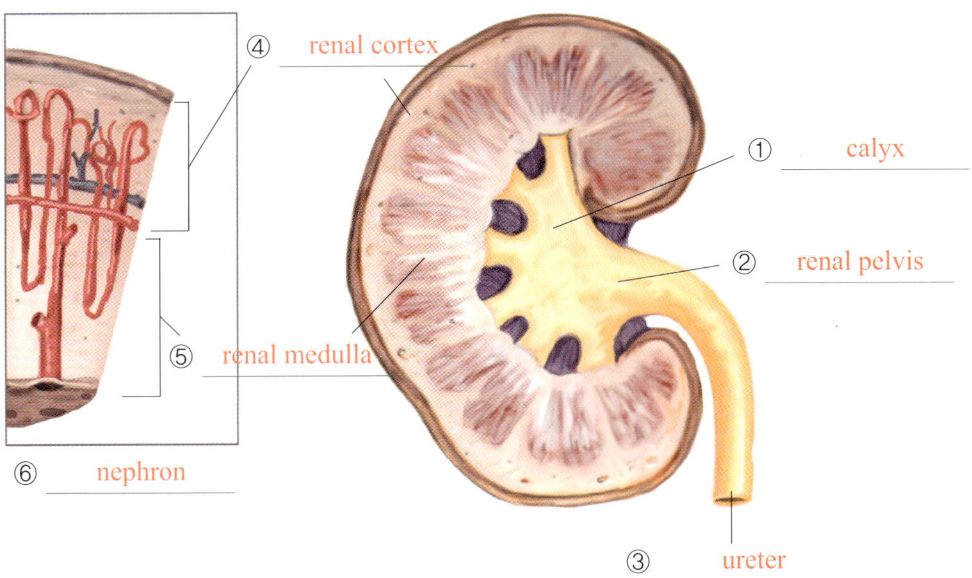

3. Write the meaning of the following medical terms.

- kidney
  a pair of kidney bean-shaped organs that filter out waste products from blood, producing urine
- ureter
  the tube that carries urine from each kidney down to the urinary bladder
- nephron
  the basic structural and functional unit of the kidney that filters the blood
- renal pelvis
  the funnel-like part that collect urine from the calyxes and connected to the ureter
- urinary bladder
  the balloon-like storage sac for urine flowing from the kidneys through the ureters
- urethra
  the tube through which urine from the bladder exits the body
- cystitis
  inflammation of the urinary bladder
- glomerulonephritis
  a form of renal inflammation involving the glomeruli
- hydronephrosis
  overfilling of the kidney due to obstruction in the flow of urine
- nephrolithiasis
  the condition of mineral concretion to form kidney stone
- pyelitis
  inflammation of the renal pelvis
- renal failure
  loss of renal functions, acute or chronic
- uremia
  blood poisoning due to the inability of the kidney to filter out waste materials
- urethritis
  inflammation of the urethra

- anuria

  condition of the kidney producing very little urine

- chronic renal failure

  end stage renal disease that requires kidney replacement therapy

- dysuria

  difficult or painful discharge or urine

- nephrotic syndrome

  renal disease caused by damaged renal tubules and glomeruli resulting in blood protein leakage, swelling, edema, etc.

- oliguria

  lower than normal urine production and discharge

- polycystic kidney

  genetic disorder in which multiple fluid-filled cysts form in the kidneys

- glycosuria

  presence of glucose in the urine often a sign of diabetes mellitus

- lithotripsy

  breaking-up of kidney stone by means of ultrasonic shock wave

- intravenous pyelogram

  X-ray image taken of the urinary tract with intravenous contrast medium

- pyelogram

  X-ray image of the kidney, ureter and bladder

- cystoscopy

  visual examination of the bladder using a cystoscope

- nephrolithotomy

  surgical removal of the calculus by incision into the kidney

- hemodialysis

  dialysis of the blood using artificial dialysis machine to remove waste matrial

4. Write full terms and the meaning for the following abbreviations.

① ARF — acute renal failure / abrupt loss of kidney function

② BUN — blood urea nitrogen / test for the amount of blood urea, a nitrogenous waste product digestion of protein

③ CKD — chronic kidney disease / progressive loss of renal function over a long period

④ CRF — chronic renal failure / end stage renal disease that requires kidney replacement therapy

⑤ ESRF — end-stage renal failure / end stage renal disease that requires kidney replacement therapy

⑥ ESWL — extracorporeal shock wave lithotripsy / noninvasive surgical procedure to break up kidney stone by ultrasonic shock wave

⑦ HD — hemodialysis / dialysis of the blood using artificial dialysis machine to remove waste matrial

⑧ KUB — kidney, ureter and bladder / X-ray imaging of the urinary tract without contrast medium

⑨ PD — peritoneal dialysis / dialysis of the blood involving dialysate in the peritoneal cavity

⑩ UTI — urinary tract infection / infection that affects part of the urinary tract

5. Write medical terms that mean the following.

① a tube through which urine in the bladder is discharged : urethra

② the smallest structural and functional unit in the kidney : nephron

③ involuntary urination, especially that occurs during sleep : enuresis

④ urine test used widely in the diagnosis of the urinary system : urinalysis

⑤ inflammation of the glomeruli, a form of nephritis : glomerulonephritis

Chapter 17

Male Reproductive System

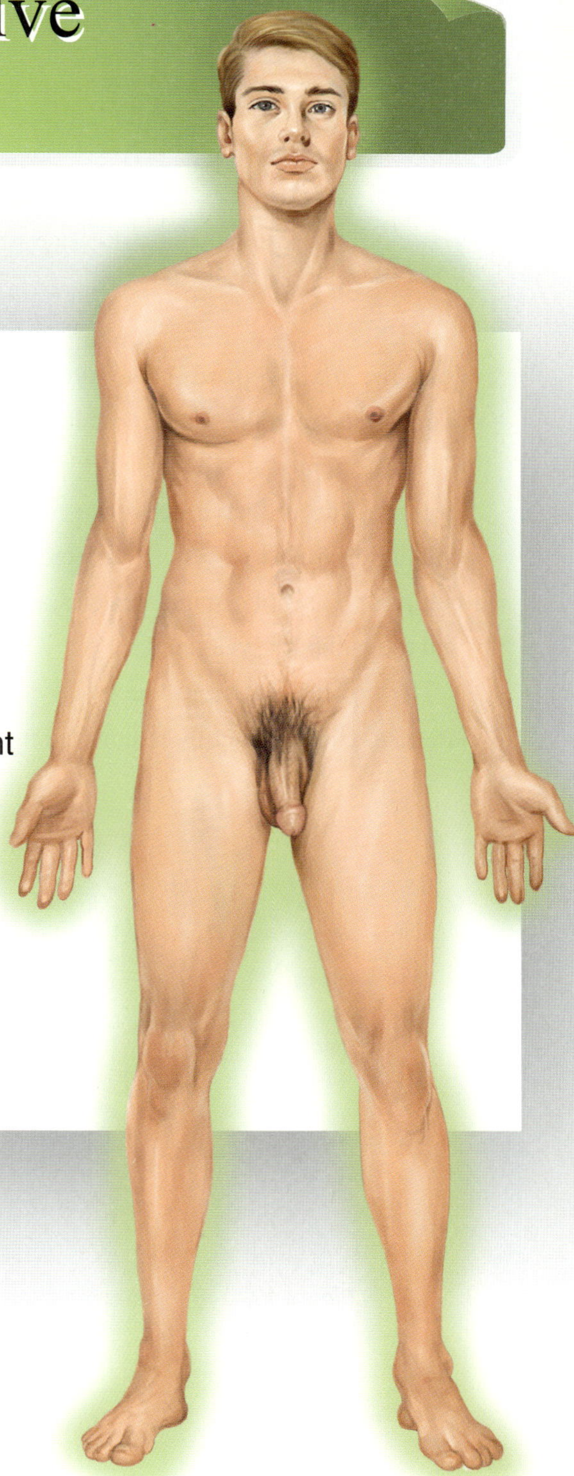

Chapter Contents

- Prolog
- Anatomical Terms
- Terms for Symptoms and Diseases
- Terms for Surgery and Treatment
- Terms for Test and Intervention
- Analysis and Meaning of Key Terms
- Abbreviations
- Exercises

Learning Objectives

- Understand anatomical structure and functions of the male reproductive system.
- Understand diseases of the male reproductive system.
- Understand types of sexually transmitted diseases.
- Learn medical terms for treatment and surgery in the male reproductive system.
- Pronounce and define medical terms for the male reproductive system.
- Learn abbreviations related to the male reproductive system.

Prolog

In the male reproductive system, sperm is produced in the testes and transferred from the male reproductive organ to the female reproductive organ. The male reproductive system is divided into internal and external reproductive organs. The external reproductive organs are the penis and the scrotum containing a pair of testes and epididymides. The internal reproductive organs comprise a pair of seminal vesicles, a pair of ejaculatory ducts, the prostate gland and the bulbourethral gland.

The typical male reproductive system produces billions of sperm cells in a lifetime. Out of about three hundred million sperm cells ejaculated during coitus,

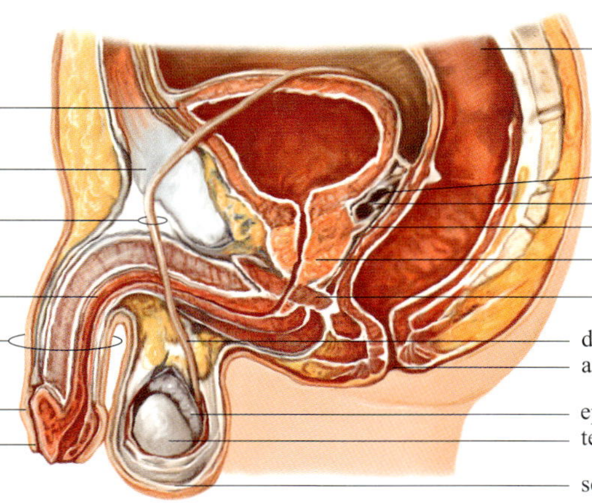

Figure 17-1 Sagittal cross-section of the male reproductive system

one sperm cell enters the ovum which constitutes fertilization. The male reproductive system secretes testosterone that induces secondary male characteristics, such as beard, pubic hair and masculine voice.

Anatomical Terms

Testis (testicle; plural: testes, testicles)

Testes are a pair of organs that produce sperm and male hormone testosterone, enclosed in the scrotum. Spermatogenesis occurs in the seminiferous tubules of the testis. Testosterone, which induces secondary male characteristics like beard and masculine voice, is produced by the interstitial cells in the testis.

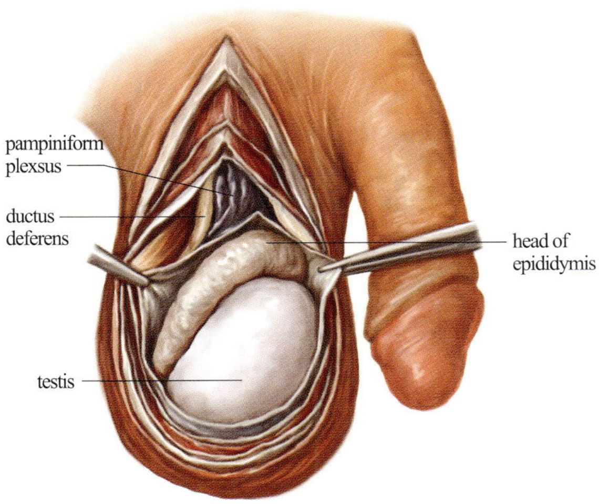

Figure 17-2 Testis

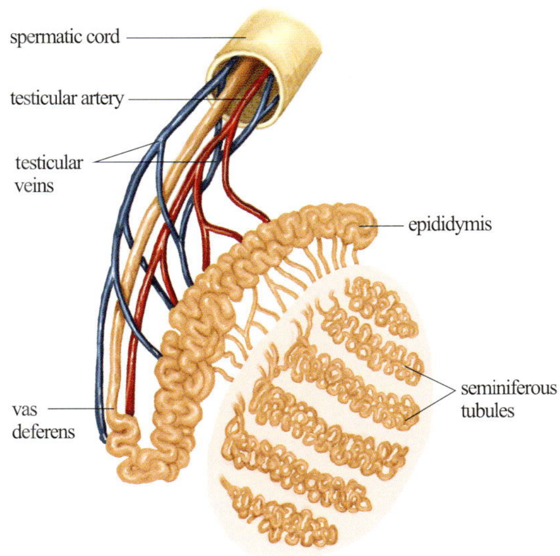

Figure 17-3 Internal structure of the testis and epididymis

Scrotum

A sac posterior to and on both sides of the penis that encloses testes and epididymides, formed as a small protuberance from the abdominal wall.

Perineum

The region between the anus and the scrotum.

Seminiferous tubules

The threadlike thin tubules in the testis where spermatogenesis occurs.

Epididymis (pl. : epididymides)

Tightly coiled tube superior to the testis, divided into three parts - head, body and tail. It stores sperm produced in the testis or carries them to the vas deferens. The sperm mature and acquire motility during their transit in the epididymis.

Vas deferens, ductus deferens

The sperm-carrying duct of about 45 cm long, connecting the epididymis and the urethra, passing through the pelvic cavity around the urinary bladder. When male sterilization is desired, the procedure called vasectomy is performed, where vas deference is disconnected or ligated.

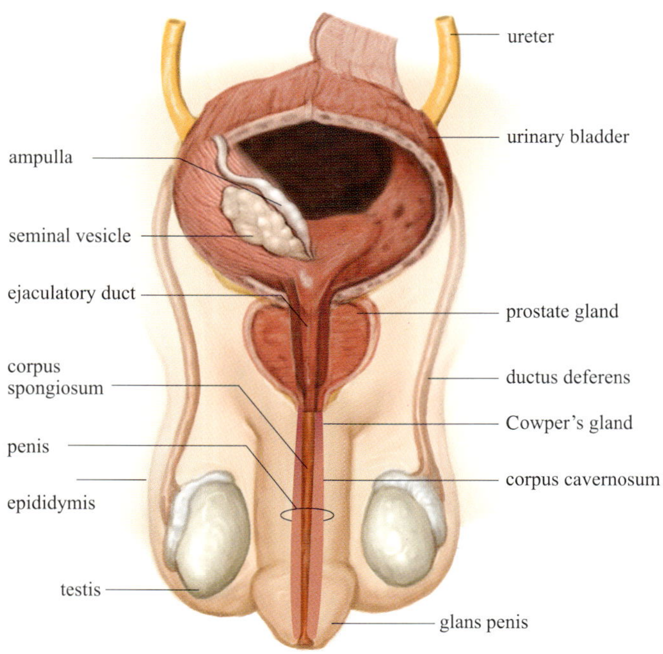

Figure 17-4 Male reproductive system and organs in the vicinity

Seminal vesicles

Located posterior to the urinary bladder, seminal vesicles store secretion from the testes and releases yellow fluid containing sperm's nutrients, which is a component of the semen.

Urethra

As a tube connected to the vas deferens, unlike females, it is a genital orifice for ejaculation of sperm as well as urinary opening.

Prostate gland

A gland surrounding the urethra inferior to the urinary bladder. It produces an alkaline secretion that is a component of the semen. The secretion neutralizes and maintains the acidity in the urethra and the vagina to protect the sperm and support their motility.

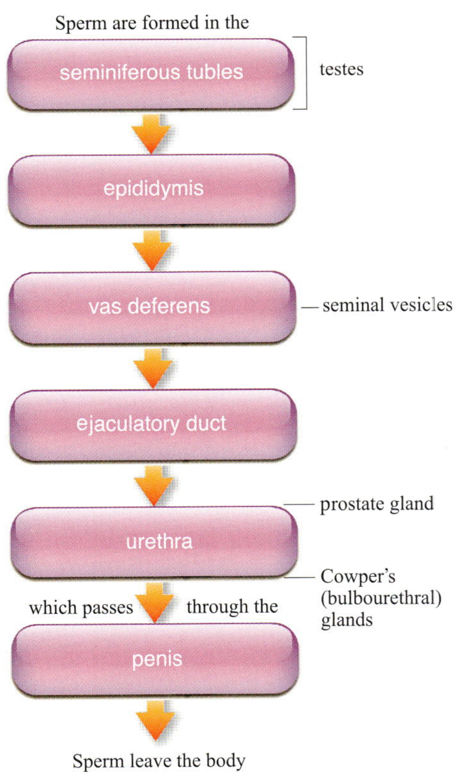

Figure 17-5 Path of travel for sperm

Cowper's glands, bulbourethral glands

Located inferior to the prostate gland, they secrete a mucus fluid upon sexual arousal in order to lubricate the glans penis.

Penis

The external male sexual organ that contains a pair of corpora cavernosa penis and a corpus cavernosum urethrae under the skin and the subcutaneous tissue. The urethra runs at the center axis of the penis, at the tip of which the foreskin covers the glans penis at birth.

Glans penis

The bulbous head portion at the distal end of the penis, at the tip of which the urethral orifice is located.

Prepuce

The foreskin that covers the glans penis of the male who hasn't had circumcision (surgical excision of the prepuce).

Semen

The fluid to be ejaculated, composed of the fluid released from the seminal vesicles and the sperm.

Ejaculation

Ejection of semen out from the male urethra.

Memory key

- Reproductive duct starts at the epididymis, runs through the vas deferens and ejaculatory duct, then passes the prostate gland to reach the urethra.

Terms for Symptoms and Diseases

Azoospermia

Lack of sperm in the semen.

Oligospermia

Abnormally low number of sperm in the semen.

Chancre

Hard skin ulceration, associated with certain infections such as syphilis.

Chancroid

Painful soft skin ulceration, caused by nonsyphilitic infection.

Balanitis

Inflammation of the glans penis.

Epididymitis

Inflammation of the epididymis.

Prostatitis

Inflammation of the prostate gland.

Orchitis

Inflammation of the testis.

Phimosis

The condition in which the opening of the foreskin is too small or the prepuce (foreskin) is fused to the glans penis, rendering prepuce retraction difficult or impossible. Circumcision can correct this condition.

Anorchism, anorchia

A congenital condition in which one or both testes are absent.

Cryptorchidism, cryptorchism

A congenital condition where one or both testes fail to descend into the scrotal sac and stay in the abdominal cavity or the inguinal canal. Orchiopexy can be performed to correct this condition.

Benign prostatic hyperplasia, benign prostatic hypertrophy (BPH)

A common condition for men of 60 years or older. Normal urination becomes difficult because of urethral constriction due to enlargement of the glandular tissue of the prostate. The patient can experience urinary stasis, urethral infection or hydronephrosis. Treatments include prostatectomy, especially TUR (or TURP, transurethral resection of prostate) in which case a part of the prostate is removed through the urethra.

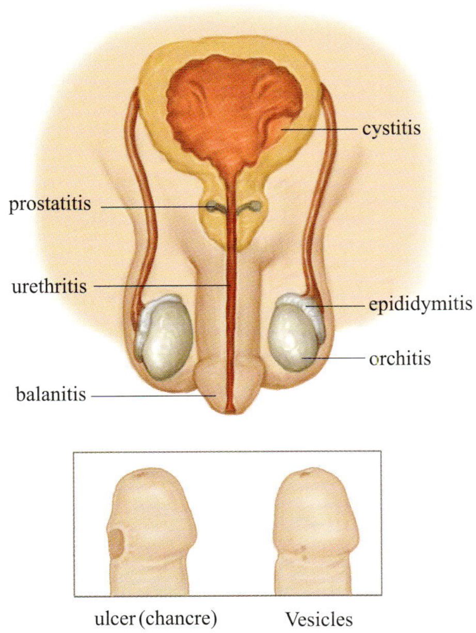

Figure 17-7 Inflammation of the male reproductive organs

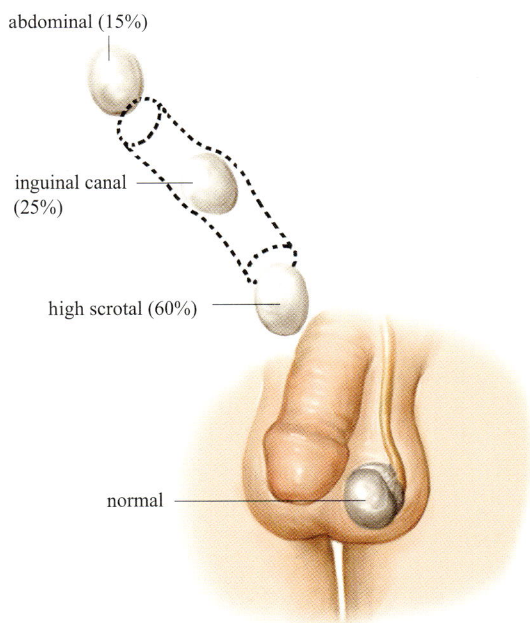

Figure 17-8 Cryptorchidism

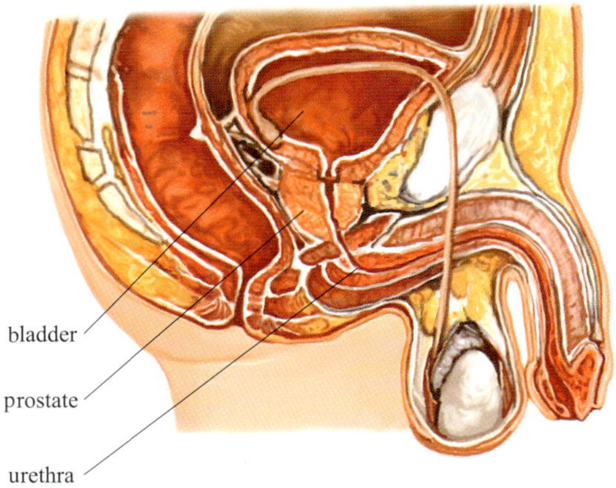

Figure 17-9 Normal prostate

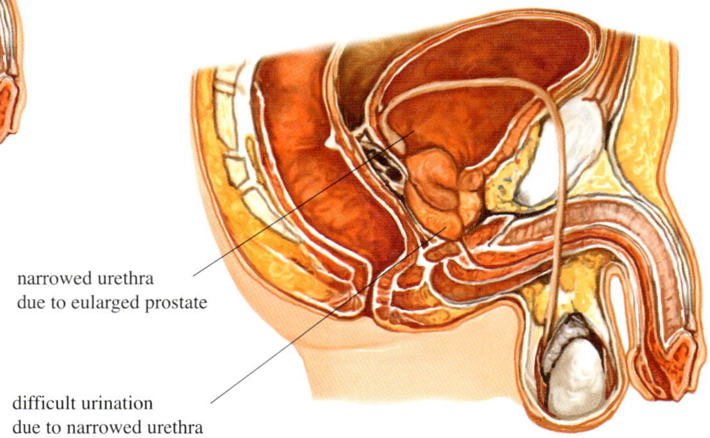

Figure 17-10 Hypertrophic prostate

Hydrocele

Abnormal buildup of serous fluid around the testis and perhaps along the vas deferens. In extreme cases the penis can be buried in the scrotum. Hydrocelectomy may be necessary to treat this condition.

Varicocele

Varicose veins (enlargement of the veins) in the area near the testis. This condition may induce oligospermia that leads to male infertility. Varicocelectomy can relieve this contition.

Hypospadias, hypospadia

A birth defect of the penis, where the urethral external orifice is placed under the penis instead of at the tip.

Epispadias, epispadia

A birth defect of the penis, where the urethral external orifice is at the dorsal part of the penis instead of at the tip. Urethroplasty is needed to correct this condition.

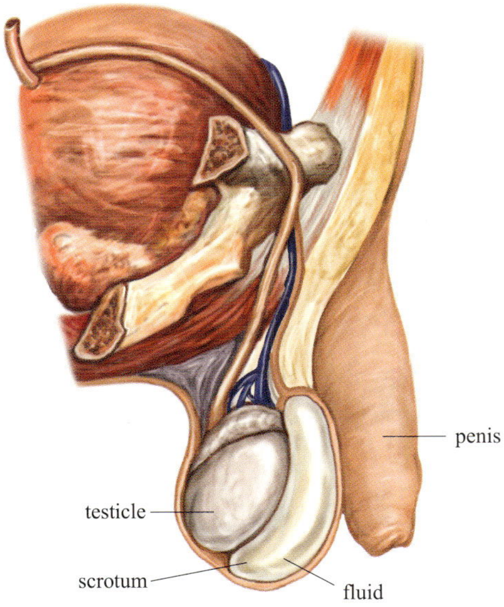

Figure 17-11 Hydrocele

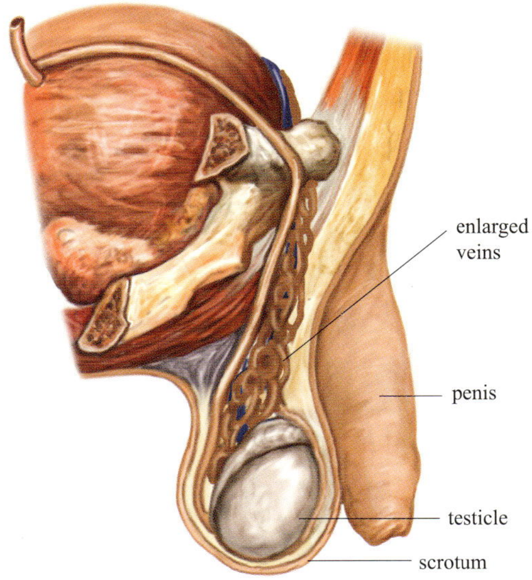

Figure 17-12 Varicocele

Adenocarcinoma of prostate

Cancer of the prostate gland, usually adenocarcinoma of epithelial tissue. Available treatments are prostatectomy, radiotherapy, chemotherapy and hormone therapy, etc.

Testicular carcinoma

Malignant tumor of the testis. The testis swells and becomes firm without pain but the tumor may spread to other organs if left untreated. Depending on the origin, this cancer can be classified as choriocarcinoma, embryonal carcinoma, seminoma, teratocarcinoma, etc. Available treatments are radiotherapy, chemotherapy, orchiectomy, etc.

Memory key

- Commonly occurring in men of 60 years or older, benign prostatic hyperplasia constricts the urethra that makes normal urination difficult.

Sexually Transmitted Infections, STI

Sexually transmitted infections are the diseases transmitted through sexual contact, and in the past were called venereal diseases or sexually transmitted diseases.

Gonorrhea

STI caused by the gonococcus bacteria, that affects the mucous membrane of the genital and urinary tracts. Symptoms are dysuria and yellow mucous pyogenic discharge.

Syphilis

STI caused by Treponema pallidum, a spirochete bacterium. In the initial stage, several weeks after the exposure, painless and round chancres will appear. In the second stage, about six weeks after the initial infection, skin rash, lymphadenopathy, etc. will occur and papules called condylomata lata will arise at the genital, anus, oral cavity, etc., and it becomes very infectious. In the third stage, the symptoms become dormant temporarily, however, the pathogens will invade the central nervous system, cardiovascular system, the eyes, etc. and cause gumma involving necrosis and fibrosis of tissues. A pregnant woman with untreated syphilis can have miscarriage or deliver a deformed baby. Treatment is with antibiotics including penicillin.

Trichomoniasis

A genital infection by trichomonas, a parasitic pathogen, occurring primarily on women. Treatment with metronidazole (Flagyl) is usually effective against this inflammation.

Chlamydial infection

Infection in the reproductive system by Chlamydia trachomatis bacteria. Males suffer anuresis, and can discharge white or transparent excretions. It can be treated with tetracycline, an antibiotic.

Terms for Surgery and Treatment

Castration

Surgical removal of the testis or the ovary.

Circumcision

Surgical excision of the prepuce in the case of phimosis, so that the glans penis is always exposed.

Epididymectomy

Surgical excision of the epididymis.

Orchiectomy, orchidectomy, orchectomy

Surgical excision of the testis.

Orchiopexy, orchidopexy

Surgical procedure to move and fixate the testis in the scrotum in the case of cryptorchidism.

Hydrocelectomy

Surgical procedure to correct the condition of hydrocele.

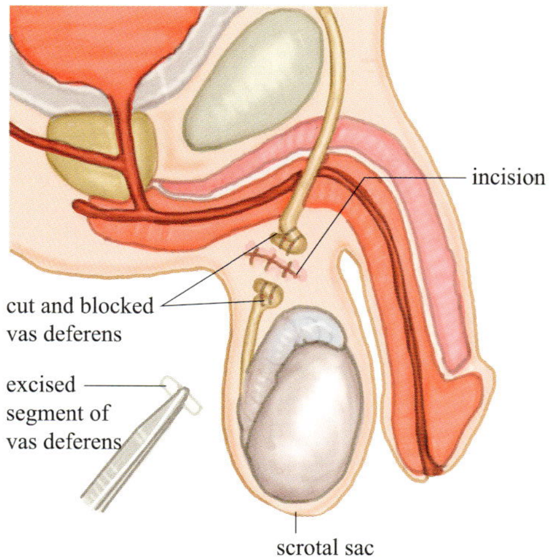

Figure 17-13 Vasectomy

Prostatectomy

Surgical excision of the prostate. Several methods exist for benign prostatic hyperplasia (BPH), such as transurethral prostatectomy, suprapubic prostatectomy, retropubic prostatectomy, perineal prostatectomy, etc.

Vasectomy

Surgical procedure for permanent male contraception, by cutting the vas deferens and sealing both cut ends so that the sperm can't join the semen in ejaculation.

Vasoligation

Surgical procedure in which the vas deferens is ligated, for male contraception or prevention of epididymitis.

Vasovasostomy

Surgical procedure to restore fertility for males who previous had the vas deference disconnected.

Terms for Test and Intervention

VDRL (Venereal Disease Research Laboratory) test

Blood serum screening test to detect syphilis.

FTA-ABS (fluorescent treponemal antibody absorption test)

This test is useful for confirmation, early detection, judgment of prognosis or cure of syphilis. Other syphilis tests include STS (serological test for syphilis), Wasserman test, TPHA, etc.

Semen analysis

Microscopic examination of the semen for sperm count and their motility. Sterility is usually defined as fewer than 10 million sperm cells in 1 mL of semen.

Transurethral resection of the prostate (TURP)

Surgical removal of a part of the prostate, using a resectoscope inserted into the urethra, for treatment of benign prostatic hyperplasia.

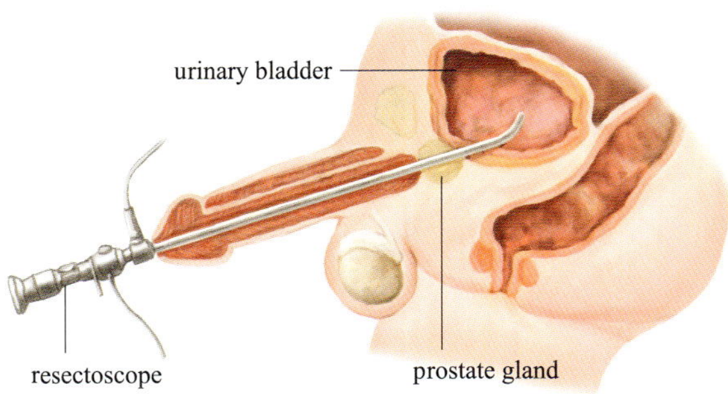

Figure 17-14 Thransurethral resection of the prostate

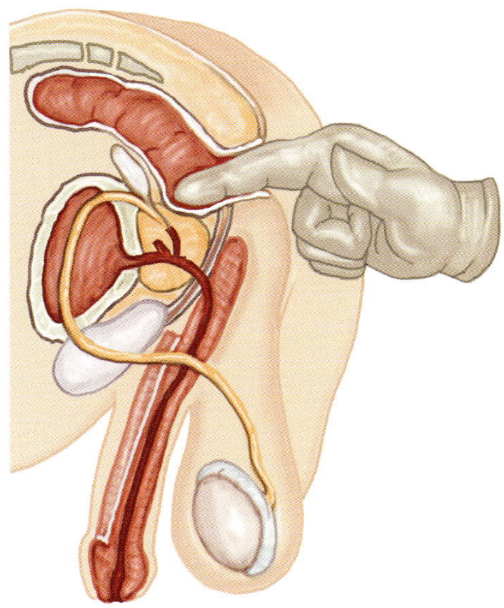

Figure 17-15 Digital rectal examination (DRE)

Digital rectal examination (DRE)

Physical examination of the rectum by inserting a finger through the anus, for diagnosis of prostatic disorder.

Analysis and Meaning of Key Terms

Term	Term Analysis	Meaning
orch/o, orchi/o, orchid/o, test/o :		**testicle, testis**
orchitis [ɔ́:rkáitis]	-itis = inflammation	inflammation of the testis
cryptorchidism [kriptɔ́:rkizəm]	-ism = process crypt/o = hidden	congenitally hidden testis in the abdominal cavity
orchidopexy [ɔ́:rkidoupeksi]	-pexy = surgical fixation	surgical fixation of the testis in the scrotum for a patient with cryptorchidism
balan/o :		**glans penis**
balanitis [bæ̀lənáitis]	-itis = inflammation	inflammation of the glans penis
balanorrhea	-rrhea = flow, discharge	a discharge from the glans penis
epididym/o :		**epididymis**
epididymitis [èpədídəmatis]	-itis = inflammation	inflammation of the epididymis
epididymotomy [èpədídəmɑtəmi]	-tomy = cutting	surgical removal of the epididymis
prostat/o :		**prostate**
prostatitis [prɑ̀stətáitis]	-itis = inflammation	inflammation of the prostate
prostatectomy [prɑ̀stətéktəmi]	-ectomy = excision	surgical excision of the prostate
testicul/o :		**testicle, testis**
testicular [testíkjulər]	-ar = pertaining to	pertaining to the testis

Term	Term Analysis	Meaning
sperm/o, spermat/o :		**sperm**
oligospermia [àligouspə́:rmiə]	oligo = scanty, deficient	abnormally low number of sperm in the semen
vas/o :		**vas deference**
vasectomy [væséktəmi]	-ectomy = excision	surgical cutoff of the vas deferens
-cele :		**hernia**
hydrocele [háidrousì:l]	hydr/o = water	abnormal accumulation of serous fluid around the testis
varicocele [vǽrəkousì:l]	varic/o = varicose vein, dilated vein	dilation of the veins in the scrotum
-trophy :		**nourishment, development**
benign prostatic hypertrophy [bináin pràstətátic haípɜ:trəfi]	hyper- = excessive	benign expansion of the prostate that constricts the urethra causing dysuria
circum- :		**around**
circumcision [sə̀:rkəmsíʒən]	cis/o = cutting; -ion = process	surgical excision of the prepuce

Abbreviations

Abbreviation	Full Term	Meaning
BPH	benign prostatic hyperplasia	benign expansion of the prostate that constricts the urethra causing dysuria
GU	genitourinary	pertaining to the genital and urinary system
TUR	transurethral resection	surgical removal (of a part of the prostate) through the urethra
TURP	transurethral resection of the prostate	surgical removal of a part of the prostate, using a resectoscope inserted into the urethra
STI	sexually transmitted infections	infections caused by pathogens transmitted through sexual contact

Exercises

1. Analyze the following medical terms into prefix, root, suffix and write the meaning.

① orchidopexy　orchid/o (testis) + -pexy (fixation)

surgical fixation of the undescended testis in the scrotum

② prostatitis　prostat/o (prostate) + -itis (inflammation)

inflammation of the prostate

2. Write the meaning of the following medical terms.

① benign prostatic hypertrophy

excessive benign growth of the prostate that constricts the urethra and causes dysuria

② cryptorchism

congenital condition in which the testis has not descended into the scrotum

③ epididymitis

inflammation of the epididymis

④ epispadias

congenital condition in which the external urethral orifice is on the dorsal part of the penis instead of at the tip

⑤ syphilis

an STI caused by a spirochete bacterium

3. Write the medical terms that mean the following.

① surgical excision of the prepuce — circumcision

② an STI caused by gonococcus bacteriaum — gonorrhea

③ external urethral orifice being underside of the penis — hypospadias, hypospadia

④ inflammation of the testis — orchitis

⑤ surgical resection of the prostate — prostatectomy

4. Write the medical terms that mean the following.

① accumulation of fluid around the testicles — hydrocele

② scanty production and expulsion of spermatozoa — oligospermia

③ inflammation of glans penis — balanitis

④ failure of one or both of the testes to descend into the scrotum — cryptorchism

5. Write full terms for the following abbreviations.

① STI sexually transmitted infection

② BPH benign prostatic hyperplasia

③ TURP transurethral resection of the prostate

6. Write the medical term for each item in the figure.

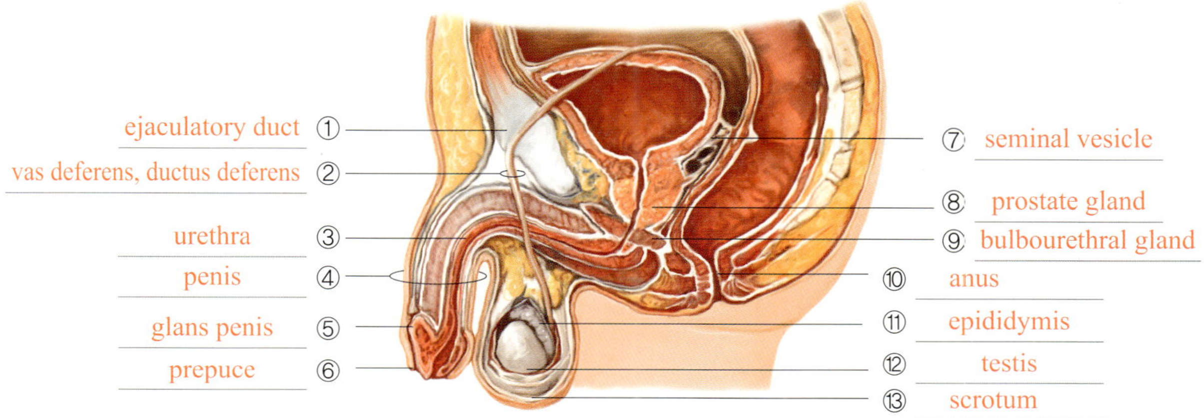

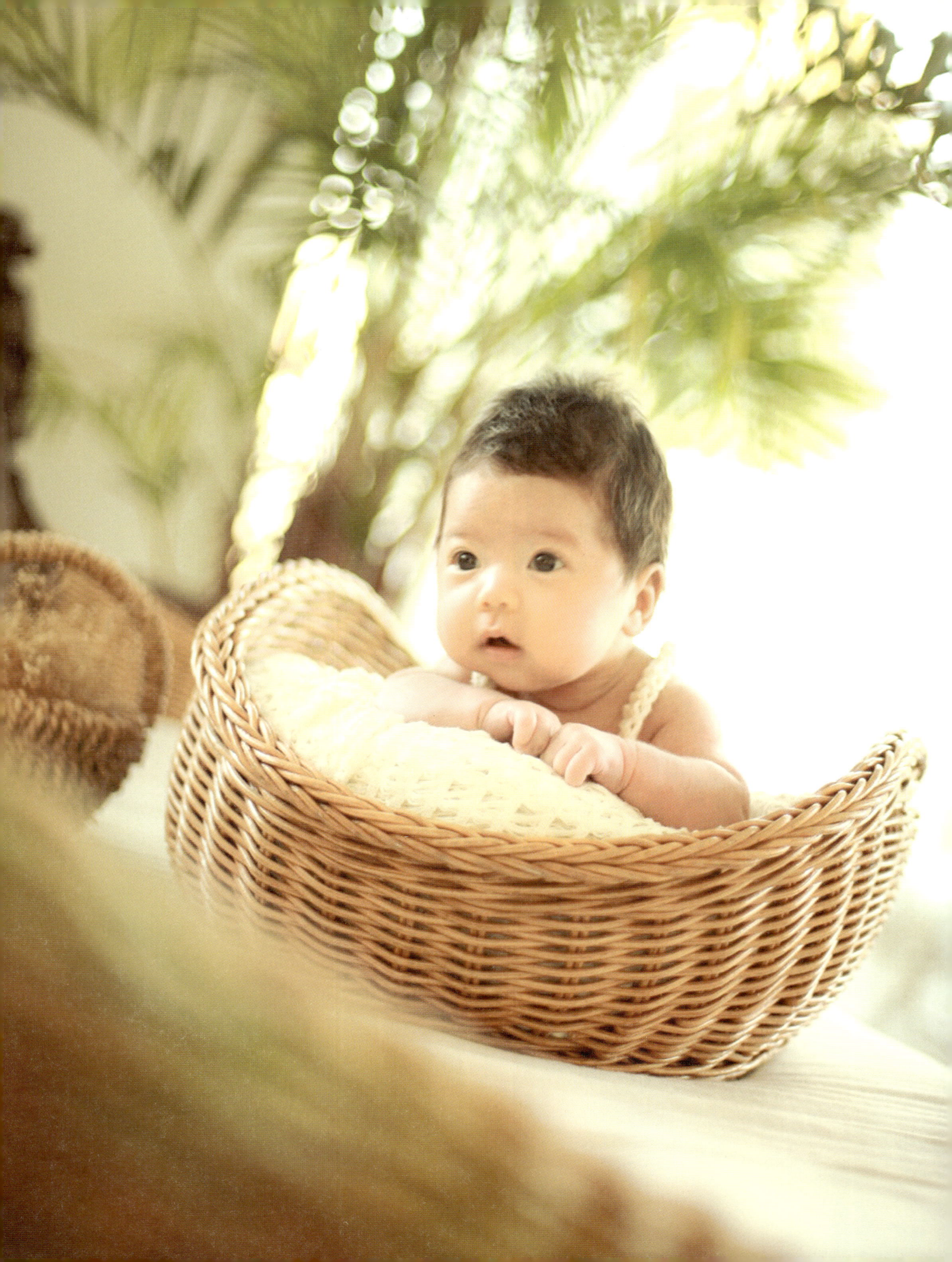

Chapter 18

Female Reproductive System and Obstetrics

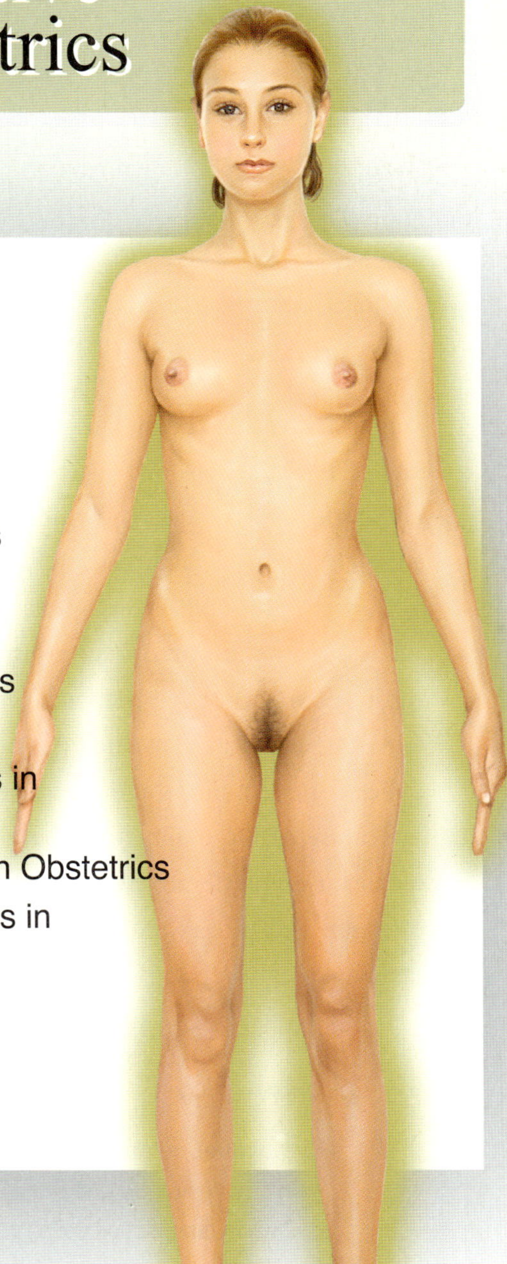

Chapter Contents

- Prolog
- Anatomical Terms
- Terms for Symptoms and Diseases
- Terms for Surgery and Treatment
- Terms for Test and Intervention
- Analysis and Meaning of Key Terms
- Anatomical Terms in Obstetrics
- Terms for Symptoms and Diseases in Obstetrics
- Terms for Surgery and Treatment in Obstetrics
- Analysis and Meaning of Key Terms in Obstetrics
- Abbreviations
- Exercises

Learning Objectives

- Understand anatomical structures and functions of the female reproductive system.
- Understand menstruation, ovulation, pregnancy and related hormones.
- Understand diseases and treatments of the female reproductive system.
- Pronounce and define medical terms relating to the female reproductive system.
- Learn abbreviations relating to the female reproductive system.
- Understand terms in obstetrics including pregnancy and parturition.

Prolog

The female reproductive system consists of the internal and external reproductive organs including the uterus, ovaries, uterine tubes (fallopian tubes), vagina and vulva. The ovaries produce ovum, and the uterus provides itself as the site of implantation for the fertilized ovum and allows the fetus to grow until childbirth. The important sex hormone produced by the ovaries helps form the secondary female characteristics.

Upon fertilization of the ovum, progesterone stimulates growth of the blood vessels of the uterus to supply blood and thicken the uterine walls. If no fertilization occurs, the endometrium (uterine lining) sheds and bleeding occurs, which is called menstruation. Ovum production by the ovaries commences at puberty and terminates at menopause.

Release of the ovum from the ovaries starts at puberty and continues until menopause. The fertilized egg grows and develops in the uterus. Sex hormones estrogen and progesterone secreted by the ovaries control menstrual cycles, maintain pregnancy and induce secondary female characteristics.

Memory key

- The ovaries release ovum, which is called ovulation, and secretes sex hormones estrogen and progesterone that control menstrual cycles, maintain pregnancy and induce secondary female characteristics.

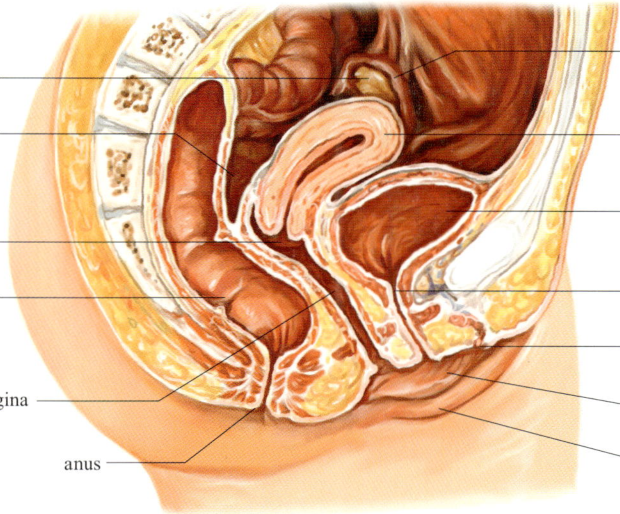

Figure 18-1 Sagittal cross-section of the female reproductive organs

Anatomical Terms

Vulva and Vagina

Vulva

This is a general term for the female external reproductive organ.

- **Clitoris :** The organ with abundance of blood vessels and nerves with erectile tissue, homologous with the male penis.
- **Hymen :** A mucous membrane that partially or completely covers the vaginal opening.
- **Labia majora :** Two prominent longitudinal left and right cutaneous folds (lips) of the vulva that cover the labia minora and clitoris. Opening of the labia minora exposes the vaginal entrance.
- **Labia minora :** The lip-shaped inner parts near the vaginal opening covered by the labia majora.
- **Bartholin's glands, greater vestibular glands, vulvovaginal glands :** A pair of glands on the sides of the vaginal opening that secrete viscous fluid

for lubrication during sexual arousal. These glands are homologous with the male bulbourethral glands.

- **Vestibule :** The recessed area of the vulva formed by the clitoris and the open labia minora, where the vagina and the urethral orifice open, and where the Skenes ducts and Bartholin's glands locate.
- **Mons pubis :** The mound of fatty tissue covering the symphysis pubis and superior to the vulva, normally covered with pubic hair in adult females.

Perineum

The region between the anus and the vagina, where the labia majora and labia minora link.

Vagina

This female internal reproductive organ is the canal lined with mucous membrane, posterior to the urethra and anterior to the rectum. It is the passage for uterine excretions from menstruation as well as the organ for sexual intercourse and the canal for childbirth.

Skene's glands, paraurethral ducts

The glands on both sides of the female urethra.

Memory key

- The female external reproductive organs include the clitoris, labia majora, labia minora, Bartholin's glands, mons pubis, etc. The perineum is the region between the vulva and the anus.

Uterus and Pelvic Supporting Structure

Uterus

The uterus (womb) is a major female reproductive organ, located between the urinary bladder and the rectum, where the fertilized ovum implants, receives nutrients and develops into a fetus. Depending on the region, the uterus is divided into fundus (superior section), corpus (middle section), and cervix (inferior section). The lowest recessed space or pouch of the peritoneal cavity between the rectum and the uterus is called Douglas' pouch or cul-de-sac. The uterine wall consists of three layers : endometrium, myometrium and perimetrium.

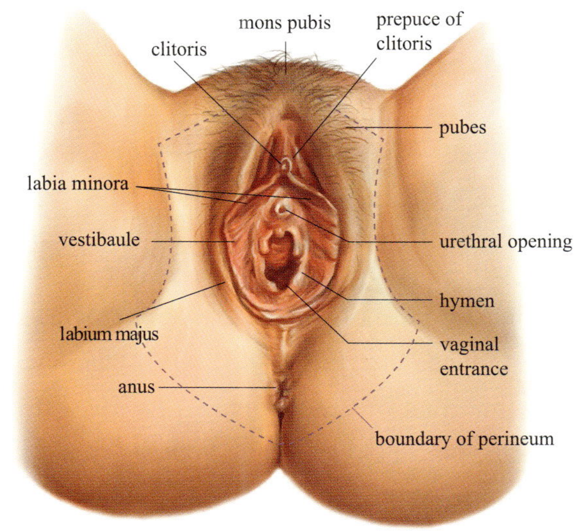

Figure 18-2 External female reproductive organs

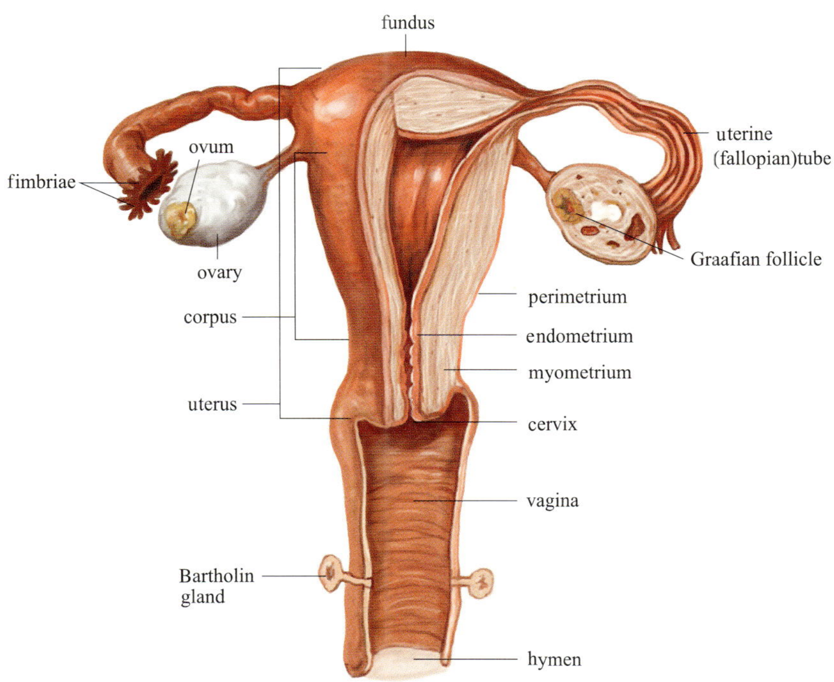

Figure 18-3 Frontal view of the female reproductive organs

Ovaries and Fallopian Tubes

Adnexa uteri

Adnexa uteri are the organ appendages to the uterus, namely ovaries, uterine (fallopian) tubes and ligaments.

Ovaries (singular : ovary)

A pair of organs that produce, develop and release the ovum as well as secrete hormones after puberty.

Estrogen

Estrogen is the female hormone produced in the ovaries, adrenal cortex, placenta, etc., that induces the secondary female characteristics, stimulates buildup of the endometrium of the uterus and prepares the environment for fertilization, implantation and nutrient supply to the early stage embryo.

Progesterone

The hormone produced in the corpus luteum, adrenal cortex and placenta, which stimulates secretion from the endometrium for preparation as a good environment for maintaining pregnancy, and development of the mammary gland.

Ova (singular : ovum)

The reproductive cells produced in the ovary.

Fimbriae

The fimbriae are fringes of tissues around the ovary, connected to the fallopian tube for the ovum to be carried to the uterus, so that fertilization of the ovum with the spermatozoa can occur. The fallopian tube can be divided into four sections, namely ampulla, isthmus, interstitial (intramural) and infundibulum.

Memory key

- The ovary produces the ovum and sex hormones. Ovulation is the process of releasing the ovum.

Breast

The breast is an organ that produces milk for feeding the infant after birth, and consists of the mammary gland, nipple, areola, lactiferous sinuses and lactiferous ducts. The areola is the round dark part of the skin that surrounds the nipple.

The most important function of the mammary gland is lactation. Milk produced in the alveolus tissues is stored in the lactiferous sinuses, and discharged from the nipple via lactiferous ducts. Lactation is the process of milk production stimulated by prolactin secreted by the pituitary gland after childbirth.

Menstrual Cycle

A female's first menstrual cycle occurs at puberty, which is called menarche. The cycle continues until menopause. Menstruation is a periodic bleeding from the endometrium, a natural physiological phenomenon occurring approximately every four weeks. The decrease of estrogen and progesterone hormones, when fertilization of the ovum fails, induces local anemia and involution of the uterus, causing the endometrium to shed and bleed through the vaginal canal.

The menstrual cycle includes menstrual period (days 1 ~ 5), proliferative period (days 5 ~14), ovulatory period (day 14) and secretory period (day 15 ~28).

The period of ovulation starts around the 14th day of the start of menstruation, when the graafian follicle bursts and the ovum is released in the process of ovulation to enter the uterine tube.

Terms for Symptoms and Diseases

Amenorrhea

Absence or abnormal discontinuity of menstrual discharge.

Dysmenorrhea

Menstruation accompanied by excessive pain in the uterine region.

Menorrhagia, hypermenorrhea

Excessive uterine hemorrhage during regular menstruation cycle, in which case the menstrual period is longer than normal.

Metrorrhagia

Uterine bleeding at a time other than during regular menstrual period.

Oligomenorrhea

Menstruation occurring less frequently than normal, or being too light.

Polymenorrhea

Menstruation occurring more often than normal.

Dyspareunia

Painful, difficult or unpleasant sexual intercourse, especially in women.

Leukorrhea

White, viscous excretion from the uterus or uterine cavity.

Pruritus vulvae

Pruritus of the vulva; severe itching sensation of the vulva.

Menarche

The first menstrual period in a female's life, starting at puberty.

Menopause

The ending of menstruation in a woman's life.

Infertility

The inability for a woman to reproduce by natural means. This term does not exactly mean sterility, where she can't possibly bear children. In primary infertility the woman is infertile and has never been pregnant, whereas in secondary infertility she has experienced pregnancy.

Sterility

The condition of not being able to bear children (female sterility). Male sterility is the inability for a man to fertilize.

Gynecomastia

Excessive development of breasts in males, resembling the female's.

Mastalgia, mastodynia

Pain or tenderness in the mammary gland.

Vulva and Vagina

Atresia of vulva

Congenital occlusion of the vagina or adhesion of the vaginal walls.

Condyloma acuminatum, genital warts

A sexually transmitted disease with a verrucous lesion in the vulva or perineum, with warts of various sizes.

Colpitis, vaginitis

Inflammation of the vagina.

Vulvitis

Inflammation of the vulva.

Rectovaginal fistula

An abnormal connection (hole) between the rectum and the vagina.

Vesicovaginal fistula

An abnormal connection (hole) between the bladder and the vagina.

Uterus and Pelvic Supporting Structure

Cervicitis

Inflammation of the cervix. Absence of immediate treatment of the acute condition will lead to chronic cervicitis. Causes are infection by streptococcus, staphylococcus or gonococcus. Leukorrhea is a conspicuous symptom. Treatments include administration of antibiotics, or depending on the inflamed region, electrocauterization, cryotherapy or conization can be performed.

Carcinoma of the cervix

Malignant tumor in the cervix.

Endometriosis

Growth of tissues histologically and functionally similar to the endometrium outside the uterine cavity. The tissues may bleed during menstruation, just like the normal endometrium.

Endometritis

Inflammation of the endometrium, that causes increased excretions, pain in the lower abdomen, irregular menstruation, etc.

Parametritis, pelvic cellulitis

Inflammation of the cellular connective tissues in the vicinity of the uterus caused by bacterial infection.

Displacement of uterus

- **anteflexion :** state of the uterus being bent forward
- **retroflexion :** state of the uterus being bent backward
- **anteroversion :** state of the uterus being tilted forward
- **retroversion :** state of the uterus being tilted backward

Dysfunctional uterine bleeding (DUB)

Abnormal or irregular menstrual uterine bleeding due to hormonal disturbances including that of estrogen and progesterone production.

Myoma of uterus (uterine fibroid)

Benign tumor of the smooth muscle tissue of the uterus, the myometrium. Symptoms include irregular uterine bleeding, dysmenorrhea, leukorrhea, anemia, infertility, etc.

Endometrial carcinoma

Malignant tumor of the uterus arising from the endometrium.

Pelvic inflammatory disease (PID)

Inflammation of the pelvic region with accompanying salpingitis, endoparametritis, oophoritis, etc. typically caused by STIs such as gonorrhea and chlamydia.

Ovaries and Uterine Tubes

Oophoritis

Inflammation of the ovary.

Salpingitis

Inflammation of the fallopian tube.

Oophorosalpingitis

Inflammation of the ovary and the fallopian tube.

Hydrosalpinx

Swelling of the fallopian tube due to accumulation of the serous fluid.

Pyosalpinx

Fallopian tube being filled with pus.

Ovarian cyst

Collection of fluid in cysts in the ovary. Out of several types of cysts, serous or follicular cysts arise most often.

Ovarian carcinoma

Malignant tumor of the ovary, with higher mortality than that of the uterus or the cervix. Because there are no symptoms in the initial stage, in many cases the cancer is spread to the neighboring region of the pelvis before being diagnosed.

Memory key

- Pelvic inflammatory disease is inflammation of the organs in the pelvic region other than the uterus, including salpingitis, endoparametritis, oophoritis, etc,

Breasts

Mastadenitis

Inflammation of the mammary gland.

Thelitis

Inflammation of the nipple.

Amastia

Absence of the breast tissue, nipple and areola.

Breast carcinoma

Malignant tumor in the mammary gland or the lactiferous duct.

Terms for Surgery and Treatment

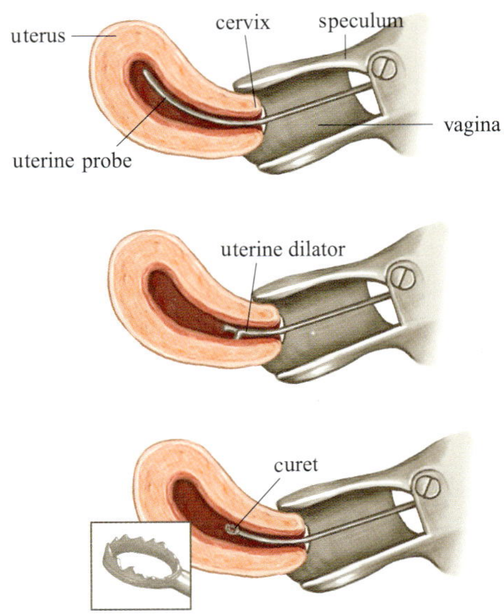

Figure 18-4 Dilatation & curettage

Dilation (or dilatation) and curettage (D&C)

Surgical procedure in which the cervix is dilated and the lining of the uterus is cleaned up by scraping the remaining placenta, myoma, polyp, etc. after abortion or biopsy of the endometrium or cervix, using a tool called curette.

Hysterectomy

Surgical extraction of the uterus, by laparotomy (abdominal incision) or using a laparoscope.

Hysteropexy

Surgical procedure to restore the uterus to its original position, with surgical fixation of the ovaries to the abdominal wall.

Cryotherapy

Medical therapy using low temperatures.

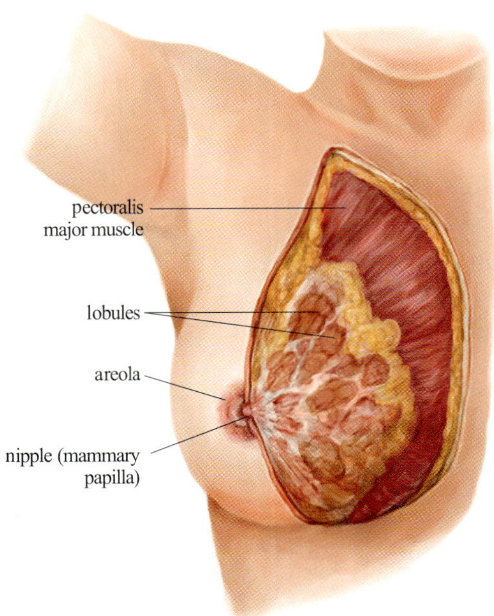

Figure 18-5 Breast of the female

Cauterization

Medical technique of promoting growth of granulation tissues by searing inflamed tissues with heat, electricity or chemical means.

Oophorectomy, ovariectomy

Surgical excision of an ovary or both.

Salpingectomy

Surgical excision of the fallopian tube.

Salpingo-oophorectomy

Surgical excision of the fallopian tube and the ovary.

Tubal ligation

Surgical procedure for contraception by disconnecting and ligating (both) fallopian tubes.

Tuboplasty, salpingoplasty

Surgical reconstruction of the fallopian tubes, in order to achieve fertility.

Mastectomy

Surgical excision of part or all of the breast. Choices are simple mastectomy, partial mastectomy and radical mastectomy.

Terms for Test and Intervention

Pap test (Papanicolou smear)

A screening test to detect cancerous cells by taking a sample (smear) of cells from the cervix and the vagina.

Conization

Surgical excision of a cone-shaped tissue from the cervix as a treatment or biopsy.

Culdocentesis

A diagnostic procedure in which serous fluid from the Douglas' pouch at the lowest part of the abdominal cavity is taken using a needle, in order to detect ectopic pregnancy, acute pyogenic salpingitis or cancer cells.

Mammography

X-ray examination of the breasts for diagnosing abnormalities, especially tumors.

Pelvimetry

Examination of the pelvis, for its shape and size relating to the birth canal, in the assessment for safe natural delivery.

Amniocentesis

A procedure used in prenatal diagnosis, by draining a sample of amniotic fluid using a needle into the amniotic sac.

Analysis and Meaning of Key Terms

Term	Term Analysis	Meaning
ovari/o, oophor/o :		ovary
oophorectomy [òuəfəréktəmi]	-ectomy = excision	surgical excision of the ovary
salping/o :		fallopian tube, oviduct
salpingectomy [sæ̀lpəndʒéktəmi]	-ectomy = excision	surgical excision of the fallopian tube
hysterosalpingec-tomy [hístərousælpiŋzek-təmi]	hyster/o = uterus, -ectomy = excision	surgical excision of the uterus and the fallopian tube
dysmenorrhea [dìsmenərì:ə]	dys- = bad, painful, abnormal	pain during menstruation
men/o :		menses, menstruation
menorrhea [mènərí:ə]	-rrhea = discharge, flow	blood discharge during menstruation
menorrhagia [menəréidʒiə]	-rrhagia = rapid blood flow	excessive blood discharge during menstruation

Term	Term Analysis	Meaning
hyster/o, uter/o, metr/o :		uterus
hysterectomy [histərektəmi]	-ectomy = excision	surgical extraction of the uterus
cervic/o :		cervix, neck of uterus, cervix uteri
cervicitis [sə́:rvəsátis]	-itis = inflammation	inflammation of the cervix
vagin/o, colp/o :		vagina
vaginitis [vӕ̀dʒənáitis]	-itis = inflammation	inflammation of the vagina
colpectomy [kɑlpectomi]	-ectomy = excision	vaginectomy, surgical removal of all or a part of the vagina
vulv/o :		vulva
vulvectomy [vʌlvəctomi]	-ectomy = excision	surgical removal of all or a part of the vulva
episi/o :		vulva, external genitalia, pudendum
episiotomy [ipi:silɑ:təmi]	-tomy = process of cutting	surgical incision of the vulva toward the perineum to enlarge the birth canal and assist childbirth
perine/o :		perineum
perineorrhaphy [periniɔ́:rəfi]	-orrhaphy = suture	surgical suture of the perineum
labi/o :		lips
labial [léibiəl]	-al = pertaining to	pertaining to the labia
lact/o :		milk
lactogenesis [latədʒénisis]	-genesis = production, formation	production of milk by the mammary gland
mast/o, mamm/o :		breast
mammogram [mǽməgrӕ̀m]	-gram = record, picture	X-ray image of the breast
mastectomy [mæstéktəmi:]	-ectomy = excision	surgical excision of all or a part of the breast
-salpinx :		fallopian tube, uterine tube
hematosalpinx [hí:mətsǽlpiŋs]	hemat/o = blood	accumulation of the blood in the fallopian tube

Term	Term Analysis	Meaning
-cele :		hernia
cystocele [sístousì:l]	cyst/o = bladder	hernia of the bladder through the vaginal wall
rectocele [rékəsí:l]	rect/o = rectum	hernia of the rectum through the vaginal wall
-arche :		beginning
menarche [mináːrki:]	men/o = menses	the first menstrual experience for a female
ante- :		before
anteflexion [æ̀ntiflékʃən]	flex/o = bending	state of the uterus being bent forward
retro- :		back, behind
retroflexion [rètrəflékʃən]	flex/o = bending	state of the uterus being bent backward

Anatomical Terms in Obstetrics

Pelvis

The pelvis consists of the hip bones, sacrum and coccyx.

Placenta

The vascular structure that supplies oxygen and nutrients to the fetus.

Amnion

The innermost membrane of the fetal membranes that contain the embryo and the amniotic fluid.

Chorion

The outermost membrane of the fetal membranes that contain the embryo and the amniotic fluid.

Amniotic fluid

The fluid contained in the amnion that surrounds and protects the fetus from physical impacts.

Memory key

- The placenta is a vascular structure that supplies oxygen and nutrients to the fetus. The chorion is the outer membrane of the sac that encloses the embryo, while the amnion is the inner membrane. The shape of the amnion in the amniotic cavity is maintained for the embryo to float within.

Umbilical cord

The flexible tube with two arteries and a vein, connecting the fetus with the placenta.

Contraception

The device or procedure intended to prevent conception (pregnancy).

Gestation

The period or process in which the embryo or fetus develops in the uterus.

Parturient

The woman giving birth.

Labor

Pain and effort borne by the parturient, accompanying the process of giving birth.

Quickening

The first noticeable movements of the fetus, typically during 16~18th weeks of pregnancy.

Embryo

The pre-fetal entity, during the two months after fertilization.

Fetus

The post-embryonic entity, from the third month through childbirth.

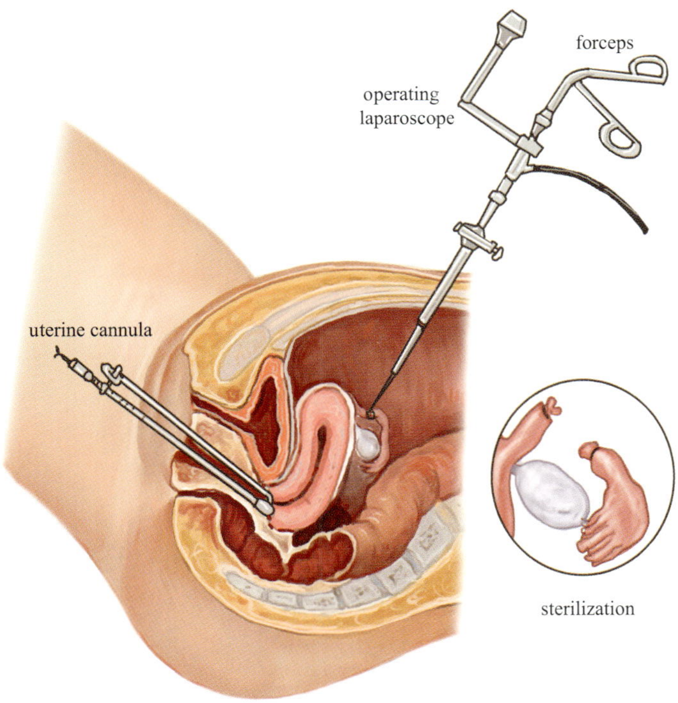

Figure 18-6 Laparoscopic tubal sterilization

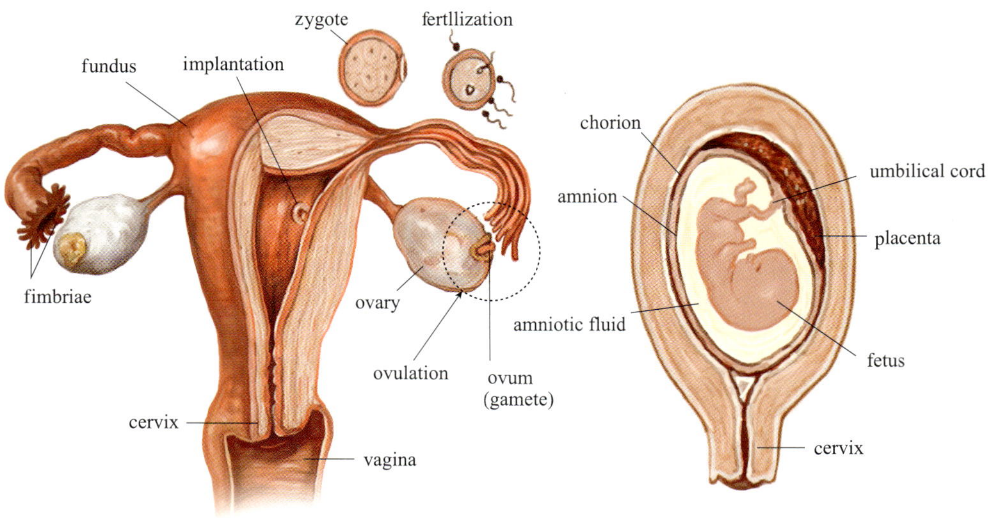

Figure 18-7 Process of ovulation, fertilization, implantation and fetal development

Apgar score

A zero to ten point score given to newborns, assessed at 1 minute and 5 minutes after birth. The assessment criteria are Appearance (complexion or skin color), Pulse (heart rate), Grimace (facial response to stimulation), Activity (muscle flexion or tone) and Respiration, each of which is given a score of 0, 1 or 2.

Meconium

The first discharge of feces by the infant.

Colostrum

The yellowish fluid secreted from the mammary gland on the first through third days after delivery.

Lochia

Uterine and vaginal discharge, during first and second weeks after delivery, in the order of lochia urbra, lochia serosa, lochia alba.

Delivery

The process of giving birth to a child.

Memory key

- Apgar scoring is the assessment of newborn's health by giving up to 2 points each on criteria including heart rate, respiration, complexion, muscle tone and response to stimuli, with a possible total score of 10.

Prenatal fetal position relative to the uterus and the pelvis

Lie

The relative alignment of the longitudinal axes of the fetus and the mother. In most cases the lie is roughly longitudinal.

Attitude

The relationship of the fetal head vs. extremity. In most cases the attitude is in flexion.

Presentation

Fetal lie means the relationship of the presenting part vs. the birth canal, as well as the alignment of the longitudinal axes of the fetus and the mother. The presenting part is the body part of the fetus that is headed toward the birth canal, which varies depending on the lie. The various presentations are cephalic presentation (head first, the most desirable and common), breech presentation (buttocks or feet first) and shoulder presentation.

Terms for Symptoms and Diseases in Obstetrics

Stillbirth

Giving birth of a dead fetus.

Dystocia

Slow and difficult labor and delivery.

Uterine inertia

Weak or absence of contraction of the uterus during labor.

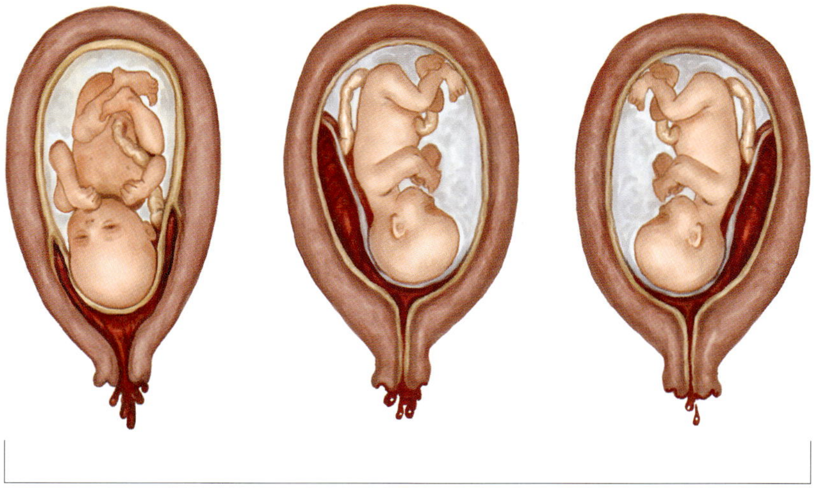

Figure 18-8 Placenta previa

Atony of the uterus

Inability of the uterus to contract following delivery after long labor, the leading cause of postpartum hemorrhage.

Abortion

Unintended or intended cessation of pregnancy with miscarriage or extraction of the embryo or fetus that cannot be kept alive. It can be classified as habitual abortion, threatened abortion, incomplete abortion, induced abortion, missed abortion, etc.

Ectopic pregnancy

Implantation of the fertilized ovum in the region other than the uterine cavity, i.e. fallopian tube, ovary, abdomen, etc. About 90% of the cases are tubal pregnancies.

Hyperemesis gravidarum

Abnormally severe vomiting during pregnancy.

Preeclampsia

A complication of pregnancy, characterized by hypertension, weight gain due to edema, proteinuria, or albuminuria.

Eclampsia

A complication of pregnancy, characterized by hypertension, edema, proteinuria, convulsion and, in extreme cases, coma.

Placenta abruptio, placental abruption

Separation of the placenta from the uterine wall before delivery.

Hydatidiform mole

An abnormal initial period of pregnancy with implantation of non-viable fertilized ovum and the swelling of chorionic villi, resulting in colporrhagia and no fetal quickening. The villi resembles grapes (hydatidiform) and starts as a benign lesion, however, the lesion may develop into malignant choriocarcinoma.

Placenta previa

An obstetric complication in which the placenta is attached to the lower uterine (opening) segment of the uterus. As a major cause for parturient mortality before giving birth, the placenta enters the birth canal before the fetus. The patient often experiences colporrhagia without pain in late stage of pregnancy, especially in the 8th month. Depending on the configuration, the condition can be graded as complete (complete blockage of the opening), marginal (blockage of the periphery of the opening) or partial (partial blockage of the opening).

Involution of uterus

The uterus returning to its pre-pregnancy size.

Prolapse of cord

The condition in which the umbilical cord descends prematurely or precedes the fetus into the birth canal, a cause of fetal death.

Physiologic jaundice

Yellowing of the skin and other tissues of the infant for the first several days after birth.

Kernicterus, nuclear jaundice

The condition of the infant with severe neurological disorder relating to abnormally high level of bilirubin.

Nuchal cord

The status of the fetus's neck wrapped with the umbilical cord.

Terms for Surgery and Treatment in Obstetrics

Forceps delivery

Surgical assisting of child delivery by grabbing and pulling the head of the fetus out with the forceps.

Vacuum extraction

Inducing the delivery of the fetus with a ventouse (vacuum device). The process can occasionally leave a lump (swelling) or cephalohematoma on the fetus's head.

Version (external cephalic version)

This is a process in which a breech position of the fetus can be turned around from buttocks or feet first to head first, for normal delivery.

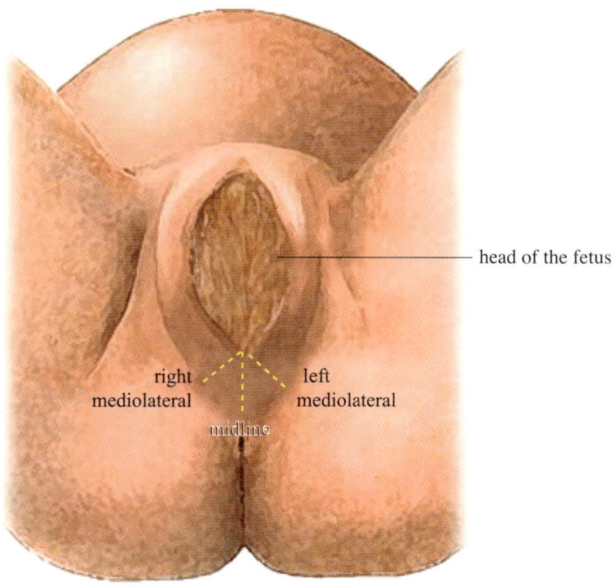

Figure 18-9 Episiotomy

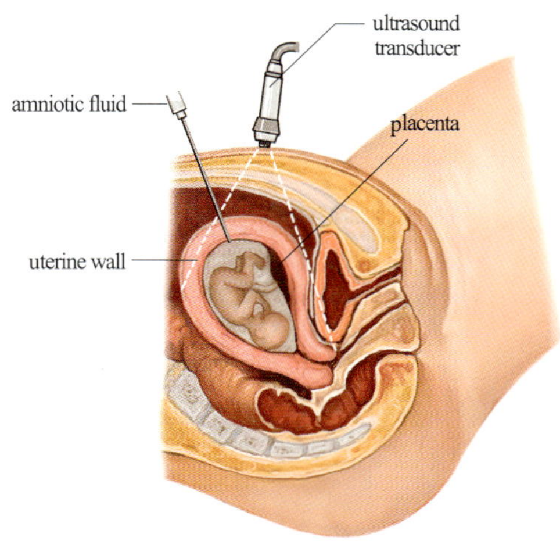

Figure 18-10 Amniocentesis

Cesarean section

Delivery of a baby through incisions into the abdomen and the uterus. Cervical cesarean section, classical cesarean section, etc. can be performed.

Episiotomy

Surgical incision of the vulva toward the perineum to enlarge the birth canal makes delivery easier and prevents laceration. It is widely practiced for women's first delivery.

Amniotomy

Artificial rupture of the amnion, in order to induce labor and subsequent delivery of the fetus.

Analysis and Meaning of Key Terms in Obstetrics

Term	Term Analysis	Meaning
amni/o :		amnion
amniocentesis [æ̀mniousentì:sis]	-centesis = surgical puncture	draining a sample of amniotic fluid using a needle into the amniotic sac, for prenatal diagnosis
oligohydramnios [ɑ́ligouhai-drouǽmni:ɔ̀us]	olig/o = scanty, poor; hydr/o = water	too little amniotic fluid
polyhydramnios [pa:lihaidrouǽm-ni:ɔ̀us]	poly- = many, much; hydr/o = water	too much amniotic fluid
nat/o :		birth
antenatal [æ̀ntinéitl]	-al = pertaining to; ante- = before	occurring before birth
postnatal [pòustnéitl]	-al = pertaining to; post- = after	occurring after birth

Term	Term Analysis	Meaning
-gravida :		pregnancy
multigravida [mʌ́ltigrǽvidə]	multi- = multiple	a woman who has been pregnant twice or more
primigravida [prìːmigrǽvidə]	primi- = first	a woman who has been pregnant once
-para :		to bear, give birth
multipara [mʌltípərə]	multi- = multiple	a woman who has given birth to at least two children
nullipara [nʌlípərə]	nulli- = none	a woman who has given birth to no child
primipara [praimípərə]	primi- = once	a woman who has given birth to one child
-partum :		labor, delivery, childbirth
antepartum [æ̀ntipɑ́ːrtəm]	ante- = before	before giving birth
postpartum [póustpɑ́ːrtəm]	post- = after	after giving birth
-tocia :		labor
dystocia [distóuʃə, ʃiə]	dys- = painful	difficult labor and delivery
-emesis :		vomiting
hyperemesis [hàipərémәsis]	hyper- = excessive	abnormally severe nausea and vomiting during pregnancy
-cyesis :		pregnancy
pseudocyesis [sùːdousaiíːsis]	pseudo- = false	false pregnancy, with the appearance of signs and symptoms associated with pregancy

Memory key

- Gravida is the number of pregnancies for a woman, while para is the number of viable children she has given birth to.

Abbreviations

Female reproductive organs

Abbreviation	Full Term	Meaning
BSO	bilateral salpingo-oophorectomy	surgical removal of both fallopian tubes and both ovaries
BTL	bilateral tubal ligation	surgical procedure for contraception by disconnecting and ligating both fallopian tubes
CIS	carcinoma in situ	cancer cells that are limited in their place of origin and have not spread
D&C	dilatation and curettage	surgical procedure in which the cervix is dilated and the lining of the uterus is cleaned up by scraping
PID	pelvic inflammatory disease	inflammation of the pelvic region, involving ovaries, fallopian tubes or endometrium, etc.
IUD	intrauterine device	contraceptive device placed in the uterus to prevent implantation
OB	obstetrics	medical specialty in the care of women during and after pregnancy
GY	gynecology	medical specialty in the care of female, especially the reproductive organs
TAH	total abdominal hysterectomy	surgical removal of internal female reproductive organs including at least the uterus and cervix through the incision of the abdominal wall
UC	uterine contraction	contraction of the uterine smooth muscle
STD	sexually transmitted disease	diseases caused by infections by pathogens mostly transmitted through sexual behavior
VD	venereal disease	sexually transmitted disease
HRT	hormone replacement therapy	medical treatment by administration of hormone (usually sex hormone such as estrogen and androgen) to supplement or substitute for naturally occurring hormone

Obstetrics

Abbreviation	Full Term	Meaning
C/S	cesarean section, C-section	delivery of a baby through incisions into the abdomen and the uterus
DOB	date of birth	
EDC	estimated day of confinement	expected date of delivery
LMP	last menstrual period	
AB	abortion	termination of pregnancy by miscarriage or intentional destruction of the embryo or fetus

Exercises

1. Analyze the following medical terms into prefix, combining form, suffix, and write the meaning.

① salpingectomy
salping/o = fallopian tube; -ectomy = excision
surgical excision of the fallopian tube

② vaginitis
vagin/o = vagina; -itis = inflammation
inflammation of the vagina

③ cervicitis
cervic/o =cervix; -itis = inflammation
inflammation of the cervix

④ primigravida
primi- = first, -gravida = pregnancy
woman who has been pregnant only once

⑤ nullipara
nulli- = none; -para = to bear, give birth
woman who has never given birth to a viable child

2. Write the meaning of the following medical terms.

① amenorrhea

absence or abnormal discontinuity of menstrual discharge

② menarche

first menstrual period in a female's life, starting at puberty

③ endometriosis

growth of tissues histologically and functionally similar
to the endometrium outside the uterine cavity

④ oophorosalpingitis

inflammation of the ovary and the fallopian tube

⑤ stillbirth

giving birth of a dead fetus

3. Write the medical term that means the following.

① surgical extraction of the uterus — hysterectomy

② surgical incision of the vulva toward the perineum to enlarge the birth canal — episiotomy

③ collection of fluid in cysts in the ovary — ovarian cysts

④ separation of the placenta from the uterine wall before delivery — placenta abruptio, placental abruption

⑤ placenta being attached to the lower uterine (opening) segment of the uterus — placenta previa

4. Write the medical term that means the following.

① painful menstruation — dysmenorrhea

② cessation of menstruation — menopause

③ fertilized ovum implanted outside of uterine cavity : in tube, ovary, or free in abdomen attached to a viscus ectopic pregnancy

④ mucous membrane partially or completely covering the vaginal orifice hymen

5. Write full terms for the following abbreviations.

① PID pelvic inflammatory disease

② D&C dilatation and curettage

③ TAH total abdominal hysterectomy

④ C/S cesarean section, C-section

6. Write the medical terms for the parts shown in the figure.

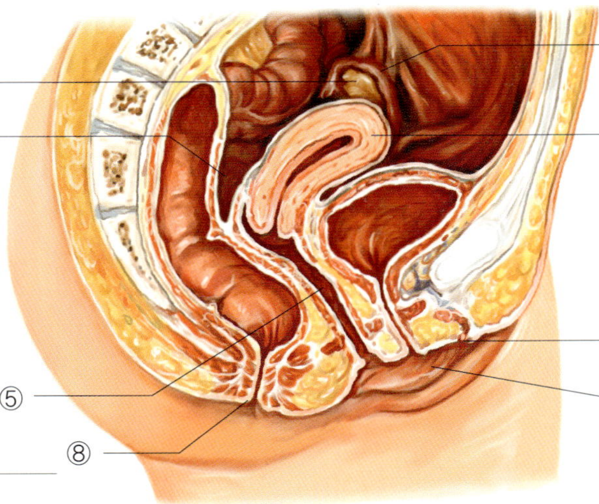

INDEX

A

abdominal cavity 76
abdominocentesis, paracentesis 338
abdominopelvic cavity 75
abducens nerve 171
abduction 82
abortion 410
abrasion 96
accessory digestive system 306
acholia 330
acidosis 356
acne 98
acoustic neuroma 197
acromegaly 219
adduction 82
adenocarcinoma of prostate 381
adenoid 276
adenoidectomy 289
adenoiditis 282
adenoiditis 294
adenoma 102
adenotonsilitis 323
adenotonsillectomy 332
adjectival Suffixes 48
adnexa uteri 396
adrenal gland 211
adrenalectomy 217
agglutination 258
agranulocyte 260
albinism 100
albumins 256
albuminuria 355
alimentary canal 306
alopecia 97
alveolar ducts 279
alveolar sac 280
alveoli 280
alveolitis 294
Alzheimer's disease 159
amastia 401
amblyopia 176
amenorrhea 397
amniocentesis 404
amniocentesis 413
amnion 406
amniotic fluid 406
amniotomy 413
ampulla of Vater 320
anal fissure 329
anal fistula 329
analgesia 159
anastomosis 333
anatomical position 74
anatomy 30
anesthesia 160
angina pectoris 237
angiography 242
angioplasty 241
angiospasm 237
anhidrosis 97
aniridia 176
anisocoria 186
anorchism 379
anorexia 323
anorexia 342
anotia 196
anoxia 282, 295
ANS function test 161
anteflexion 400
anterior chamber 174
anteroversion 400
antidiuretic hormone 221
antigen-antibody reaction 258
anuresis 354
anuria 355
anus 317
aorta 235
aortic insufficiency 237
aortic stenosis 237
aortic valve 230
aortogram 242
apex of lung 280
apgar score 408
aphagia 320
aphakia 176
aphasia 159
aphonia 282, 297
aphthous stomatitis 321
apnea 282, 297
apocrine glands 93
aponeurosis 140
appendectomy 334
appendectomy 339
appendicitis 327
aqueous humour 175
arcus senilis 176
arrhythmia 237
arterial blood gas analysis 265, 292
arteries 234
arteriography 243
arterioles 235
arteriosclerosis 237
arthritis 125
arthroplasty 127
arthroscopy 127
asbestosis 282
ascites 326
aspiration 283
asthma 283
astigmatism 181
atelectasis 283
atherectomy 241
atherosclerosis 237
atony of the uterus 410
atresia of vulva 399
atrial fibrillation ablation 241
atrioventricular bundle 233
atrioventricular node 233
atrioventricular valve 229
atrium 228
atrophy 95
attitude 409
audiometer 199
audiometry 199
auditory ossicle 192

auditory tube 193
auricle 191
autonomic nerves 155
autonomic nervous system 157
azoospermia 378
azotemia 356

B

Babinski's reflex 161
bacteriuria 356
balanitis 378, 385
Bartholin's glands 393
basal cell carcinoma 103
base of lung 281
basophil 260
basophils 257
benign prostatic hyperplasia 379
biliary stricture 331
bleb 101
blepharectomy 183
blepharitis 178, 186
blepharoplasty 183
blepharoptosis 179
blood formation 114
blood plasma 256
blood urea nitrogen 364
blood vessels 234
body Cavities 75
body 315
bone marrow transplantation 264
bone marrow 116
bone matrix 116
bone membrane 116
bony labyrinth 194
borborygmus 326
Bowman's capsule 349, 352
bradykinesia 146
bradypnea 283, 297
brain tumor 159
brain 155
breast carcinoma 401
Broca's aphasia 159
bromhidrosis 97
bronchiectasis 283, 294
bronchioles 279
bronchiolitis 283
bronchitis 283
bronchography 292
bronchoplasty 289
bronchoscopy 292
bronchospasm 283
bronchus 278
bubo 263
buccal cavity 309
bulimia 323
bulla 101
burn 98
bursitis 126
bypass surgery 241

C

caloric test 161
calyx 349
canthoplasty 183
canthus 172
capillaries 236
carcinoma of pancreases 332
carcinoma of the cervix 399
cardiac arrest 237
cardiac catheterization 243
cardiac muscles 141
cardiac region, cardia 315
cardiac scan 243
cardiac tamponade 237
cardiac valve 229
cardiomegaly 238
cardiomyopathy 238
cardioversion 243
carina 278
castration 383
cataract surgery 183
cataract 180
cauterization 103, 403
cecectomy 334
cecopexy 335, 339
cecum 317
celiotomy 334
cells 31
cementum 312
central nervous system 155
cerebral hemorrhage 160
cerebral infarction 159
cerebrospinal fluid 161
cerumen 191
ceruminous glands 93
cervicitis 399, 405
cesarean section 413
chambers 229
chancre 378
chancroid 378
cheek 309
cheilitis 321
cheiloplasty 332
chest computed tomography 292
chest pain 238
Cheyne-Stokes respiration 283
chiroplasty 128
chlamydial infection 382
chloasma 97
cholangioma 332
cholangitis 331
cholecystectomy 336
cholecystitis 331
cholecystogastrostomy 336
cholecystostomy 336
cholecystotomy 336
choledochoduodenostomy 336
choledocholithiasis 330
choledocholithotomy 336
choledocholithotripsy 337
choledochotomy 336
cholelithiasis 330
cholestasis 330
cholesteatoma 196
cholesterol 257
choriocarcinoma 381
chorion 406
choroid 173
choroiditis 178
choroidocyclitis 186
chronic obstructive pulmonary disease 283
cilia 275
ciliary body 174
circumcision 383
circumduction 83
cleft lip 322
cleft palate 322
clitoris 393
coarctation of aorta 238
cochlea 194
cochlear duct 195
colectomy 334
colic 326
colitis 327
colon 317
colonoscopy 338
colorectal cancer 329
colostomy 335
colostrum 408
colpitis 399

combining vowel 19
comedo 98
common bile duct 319
compact bone 116
complete blood count 265
computed tomography 162
condylectomy 128
condyloma acuminatum 399
cone cells 172
congenital hip dislocation 125
congenital word deafness 197
congestion 263
congestive heart faillure 238
conization 403
conjunctiva 173
conjunctival sac 186
conjunctivitis 178
constipation 326
continuous Positive Airway Pressure 292
contraception 407
cornea 171, 173
corneal abrasion 186
corneal transplant 184
coronary artery bypass graft 241
coronary artery 232
cortex 348
cough 284
Cowper's glands 377
crackles 284
cranial cavity 75
cranial nerve 158
C-reactive protein test 265
creatinine clearance test 364
cricoid cartilage 277
cricothyreotomy 289
cross-matching 258
crust 95
cryosurgery 103
cryotherapy 402
cryptorchidism 379
crystalline lens 174
culdocentesis 403
cyanosis 284
cyclitis 186
cyclodialysis 184
cyst 94
cystic fibrosis 284
cystitis 356, 365
cystocele 357
cystoscopy 362

D

dacryoadenectomy 184
dacryoadenitis 179
dacryocystectomy 184
dacryocystitis 179
dacryocystostomy 184
dactylitis 126
dactylospasm 127
deafness 197
debridement 104
deciduous teeth 312
decortication 289
decubitus, Bedsore 99
deep tendon reflex 161
defibrillation 238
delivery 408
dental calculus 321
dental caries 322
dental plaque 321
dental pulp 312
dentin 311
depression 83
dermabrasion 104
dermatitis 99, 145
dermatoplasty 104
dermis 90
diabetes mellitus 331
diabetic retinopathy 180
dialysis 360
diaphragm 75, 281
diaphysis 118
diarrhea 326
diastole 238
digestive organs 306
digital rectal examination 385
diopter 185
diplopia 181
dislocation 125
diuresis 354
diverticulectomy 334
diverticulitis 328
diverticulum 327
dizziness 195
doppler ultrasound 243
dorsal cavity 75
duodenal ulcer 325
duodenitis 327
duodenoscopy 338
duodenum 316
dwarfism 215
dysfunctional uterine bleeding 400
dyskinesia 149
dysmenorrhea 397, 404
dyspareunia 398
dyspepsia 323
dysphagia 320
dysphonia 284
dyspnea 284, 297
dystocia 409, 414
dystonia 146
dysuria 354

E

ecchymosis 97
eccrine sweat glands 93
echocardiogram 243
eclampsia 411
ectopic pregnancy 410
ectropion 181
eczema 98
edema 263
edentulous 340
ejaculation 378
electrocardiogram 234, 243
electrocochleography 200
electrodesiccation 104
electroencephalography 161
electromyography 147
electronystagmography 161
electrophoresis 269
electrophysiology study 243
elevation 83
embolectomy 241
embolus 246
embryo 407
embryonal carcinoma 381
emesis 323
emmetropia 182, 189
emphysema 284
empyema of gallbladder 331
empyema 284
enamel 311
endocarditis 238
endocardium 231
endocrine system 208
endometrial carcinoma 400
endometriosis 399
endometritis 400
endometrium 397

endoscopic ultrasonography 338
endoscopy 338
enteritis 327
enterocolitis 327
enterogastritis 327
enterolith 328
enterolysis 335
enterorrhaphy 335
enterostomy 335
entropion 180
enucleation 184
enuresis 354
eosinophil 260
eosinophils 257
epicardium 231
epidemic parotitis 322
epidermis 89
epididymectomy 383
epididymis 376
epididymitis 378
epidural block 160
epiglottis 277
epinephrine 211
epiphora 176
epiphysis 116
episiotomy 413
epispadias 380
epulis 322
erosion 95
eructation 323
eruption 94
erysipelas 99
erythema 94
erythrocyte sedimentation rate 265
erythrocyte 259
erythrocytes 257
erythrocytopenia 269
esophageal ring 324
esophageal spasm 324
esophageal varices 324
esophagectomy 333
esophagitis 324
esophagoplasty 333
esophagoscopy 338
esophagostomy 333
esophagotracheal fistula 324
esophagus 314
esotropia 183, 189
estradiol 213
estrogen 211, 396
ethmoidal sinus 275
eupnea 284
eversion 83
exercise stress test 243
exocrine system 208
exophthalmos 176, 215
exotropia 183, 189
extension 82
extracorporeal shock wave lithotripsy 364
extraocular muscles 171
eyeball 172
eyebrow 172
eyelash 173
eyelid 172

F

fasciectomy 147
fasciitis 145
fasciorrhaphy 147
fasting blood sugar 218
fatty liver 330
fetus 407
fibrillation 238
fibrinogen 256
fibrous Joint 123
fimbriae 396
fissure 96
flat bone 114
flatus, flatulence 326
flexion 82
flutter 238
folliculitis 99
forceps delivery 412
fracture 125
frenulum lingua 309
frequent urination 354
frontal plane 78
frontal sinus 275
frostbite 98
FTA-ABS 384
fundus 315
funduscopy 185

G

gallbladder 319
ganglion 163
gangrene 99
gastrectomy 333
gastric gavage 334
gastric lavage 334
gastric ulcer 325
gastritis 324
gastroduodenitis 324
gastroenteritis 324
gastroesophageal reflux disease 324
gastroesophageal 340
gastrointestinal series 339
gastropexy 333
gastroplasty 333
gastroptosis 325
gastroscopy 338
gastrostomy 333
gastrotomy 333
general suffixes 48
gestation 407
gigantism 215
gingiva 310
glans penis 377
glaucoma 180
globulins 256
glomerulonephritis 356, 365
glomerulus 349
glossitis 321
glossodynia 320
glossoplasty 332
glottis 277
glucagon 211
glycosuria 330, 355
goblet cells 279
goiter 215
gonad 209
gonorrhea 382
granulocyte 260
graves' disease 215
greater curvature 315
gynecomastia 398

H

hair bulb 91
hair follicle 91
hair root 91
hair shaft 91
halitosis 321
hard palate 309
harversian system 116
heart murmur 239
heart wall 230
hemangioma 103
hematemesis 323
hematochezia 327

hematopoiesis 257
hematosalpinx 405
hematuria 355
hemianopsia 182
hemocytoblast 268
hemocytoblasts 257
hemodialysis 360
hemolysis 262
hemolytic anemia 262
hemoperitoneum 327
hemophilia 262
hemoptysis 284
hemorrhage 263
hemorrhoid 329
hemorrhoidectomy 334
hemostasis 263, 269
hemothorax 284
hepatectomy 336
hepatic duct 319
hepatitis 331
hepatoma 332
hepatomalacia 330
hepatomegaly 330
hepatorrhaphy 336
hepatotomy 336
hernia 329
herniorrhaphy 335
herpes simplex 100
herpes zoster 100
hiatal hernia 329
hiccup 285
hilum 349
holter monitoring 243
homeostasis 208
hordeolum 180
hydatidiform mole 411
hydrocele 380
hydrocelectomy 383
hydronephrosis 358
hydrops of gallbladder 331
hydrosalpinx 401
hydrothorax 285
hymen 393
hyperacusis 200
hyperbilirubinemia 268, 330
hypercapnia 285, 296
hypercholesterolemia 239, 331
hyperemesis gravidarum 410
hyperemia 263
hyperglycemia 330
hypergonadism 219
hyperhidrosis 97
hyperkalemia 356
hyperkeratosis 95
hyperlipidemia 239
hypernephroma 359
hyperopia 182
hyperparathyroidism 215, 219
hyperpnea 285
hyperresonance 285
hypertension 239
hypertensive heart disease 239
hyperthyroidism 215
hypertriglyceridemia 239
hypertropia 183
hyperventilation 285
hypocapnia 285, 296
hypocholesterolemia 330
hypoglycemia 330
hypoparathyroidism 216
hypophysectomy 217
hypophysis 209, 210
hypopnea 285
hypopyon 177
hypospadias, hypospadia 380
hypotension 239
hypothalamus 209, 210
hypothyroidism 216
hypotropia 183
hypoventilation 285
hypoxemia 285
hypoxia 285, 295
hysterectomy 402
hysteropexy 402

I

ileitis 327
ileocolitis 327
ileostomy 335
ileum 317
immunosuppression 264
impetigo 100
implantable cardiac defibrillator 241
incus 192
inferior vena cavae 235
infertility 398
inguinal hernia 329
inner Ear 193
insertions 140
insulin 211
insulin-dependent diabetes 214
internal fixation 127
intervertebral discs 120
intestinal obstruction 328
intradermal test 105
intravenous pyelography 362
intussusception 328
inversion 83
involuntary muscles 141
involution of uterus 411
iridectomy 184
iris 174
iritis 179
irregular bone 115
irritable bowel syndrome 328
ischemic heart disease 239
itch 96

J

jaundice 330
jejunum 317
joint 123

K

Kaposi's sarcoma 102
keloid 96
keratitis 178
keratocentesis 184
keratomycosis 187
keratoplasty 184
kernicterus, nuclear jaundice 411
ketonuria 355
kidney transplantation 359
kidney 348
KUB 362

L

labia majora 393
labia minora 393
labor 407
labyrinth 190, 194
labyrinthitis 197
lacrimal apparatus 171
lacrimal duct 175
lacrimal gland 175
lacrimal sac 175
lactose intolerance 328
laparoscopy 338
large intestine 317
laryngeal cartilage 277

laryngectomy 290
laryngitis 286
laryngopharynx 276, 314
laryngoplasty 290
laryngoscopy 292
laryngostomy 290
larynx 277
left atrium 229
left coronary artery 233
left ventricle 229
leiomyosarcoma 148
lentigo 101
leprosy 100
lesser curvature 316
leucocytes 257
leukocyte 259
leukocytopenia 269
leukoderma 97
leukoplakia 321
leukorrhea 398
lichenification 96
lie 409
ligament 146
lingual tonsil 277
lips 309
lithotripsy 341, 366
liver biopsy 336
liver function test 339
liver 318
lobectomy 290
lochia 408
long bone 114
lower respiratory tract 274
lumbar puncture 161
lumpectomy 103
lung 280
lung abscess 286
lung biopsy 292
lung cancer 286
lymph node biopsy 264
lymph node 261
lymph 261
lymphadenitis 267
lymphangiography 265
lymphatic capillaries 258
lymphatic tissue 261
lymphatic vessel 261
lymphedema 267
lymphocyte 261
lymphocytopenia 264
lymphocytosis 264
lymphoma 264

M

macrotia 196
macula 174
macule 101
magnetic resonance imaging 161
malleus 192
mammography 404
mantoux test 105
mastadenitis 401
mastalgia 398
mastectomy 403, 405
mastoidectomy 198
mastoiditis 196
maxillary sinus 275
meconium 408
mediastinoscopy 292
mediastinum 281
medulla 349
melanocyte 90
melanoderma 97
melanoma 102
melatonin 210
melena 326
membranous labyrinth 194
menarche 397, 398
menopause 397, 398
menorrhagia 397
menstrual cycle 397
menstrual period 397
mesentery 318
mesocolon 318
metabolic acidosis 286
metabolic alkalosis 286
metaphysis 117
metrorrhagia 398
microtia 196
micturition 354
middle Ear 191
mineral storage 114
miosis 177
mitral commissurotomy 241
mitral insufficiency 239
mitral stenosis 239
mitral valve 230
monocyte 260
mons pubis 394
multigravida 414
muscle attachment 114
muscular dystrophy 146
myalgia 145
myasthenia 164
mydriasis 177
myelography 160
myocardial infarction 240
myocarditis 240
myocardium 231
myofibrosis 145
myofilaments 140
myoma of uterus 400
myoma 145
myopathy 145
myopia 182
myorrhaphy 147
myotonia 145
myringitis 196
myringoplasty 198
myringotomy 198
myxedema 216

N

nasal cavity 275
nasal septum 275
nasopharynx 276, 314
nausea 323
negative prefixes 60
nephrectomy 359
nephritis 356
nephrolithiasis 358, 365
nephrolithotomy 359
nephron 349
nephropexy 359
nephroptosis 357
nephrotic syndrome 357
neuron 162
neutrophil 260
neutrophils 257
nevus 102
nocturia 355
nodule 94
non-insulin-dependent diabetes 214
norepinephrine 211
nuchal cord 412
nyctalopia 177
nystagmus 177

O

obesity 216

obstructive sleep apnea 286
oculomotor nerve 171
oligomenorrhea 398
oligospermia 378
oligospermia 386
oliguria 355
omentum 318
onychia 99
oophorectomy 217, 403, 404
oophoritis 400
oophorosalpingitis 401
open heart surgery 242
optic nerve 170, 175
optic neuritis 179
optic tract 170, 175
oral cavity 307
orbit 172
orbital cavity 171
orchiectomy 217, 383
orchiopexy 383
orchitis 378, 385
origins 140
oropharynx 276, 314
orthopnea 286, 297
ossiculectomy 198
osteoarthropathy 126
osteoblast 116
osteochondritis 126
osteoclast 116
osteoid 116
osteoma 126
osteomalacia 125
osteomyelitis 125
osteoporosis 125
osteosarcoma 126
otalgia 195
otitis externa 196
otitis media 196
otomycosis 197
otoplasty 198
otorrhea 195
otosclerosis 197
otoscopy 199
outer Ear 191
ova 396
oval window 193
ovarian carcinoma 401
ovarian cyst 401
ovaries 396
ovary 211
ovulatory period 397
oxytocin 222

P

P wave 234
palate 309
palatine tonsils 276
palatoplasty 332
palpitation 240
pancarditis 246
pancreas 209, 211, 320
pancreatectomy 337
pancreaticoduodenectomy 337
pancreatitis 331
pansinusitis 286, 295
pap test 403
papilledema 178
papilloma 102
papule 94
paradoxical respiration 286
parametritis 400
paranasal sinuses 275
parasympathetic nervous system 157
parathyroid gland 210
parathyroid 209
Parathyroidectomy 217
paresthesia 164
parietal pericardium 231
parietal pleura 281
parotid gland 310
parotitis 322
paroxysmal nocturnal dyspnea 286
parturient 407
patch test 105
pathology 30
pelvic cavity 76
pelvic Girdle 122
pelvic inflammatory disease 400
pelvimetry 129, 404
pelvis 349, 406
pemphigus 100
penis 377
peptic ulcer 325
pericardial effusion 240
pericardial fluid 232
pericardiectomy 242
pericardiocentesis 241
pericarditis 240
pericardium 231
perineal prostatectomy 383
perineum 376, 394
periodontal disease 321
peripheral nervous system 155
peritoneal abscess 329
peritoneal dialysis 360
peritoneocentesis 338
peritoneum 318
peritonitis 328
permanent teeth 312
pernicious anemia 262
petechia 96
pharyngeal tonsil 276
pharyngitis 286, 323
pharynx 276, 313
pheochromocytoma 216
phimosis 379
phospholipid 257
photoallergy 189
photophobia 178
physiologic jaundice 411
physiology 30
pineal body 209, 210
pinealectomy 217
pitting edema 356
placenta abruptio 411
placenta previa 411
placenta 406
platelet 260
pleura 281
pleural cavity 281
pleural effusion 287
pleural fluid 281
pleural friction rub 287
pleurectomy 290
pleurisy 287
pleurodesis 290
pneumatic bone 115
pneumoconiosis 287, 294
pneumonectomy 290
pneumonia 287, 294
pneumothorax 287, 298
podalgia 127
poikilocytosis 268
polyarthritis 126
polycystic kidney disease 358
polydipsia 222
polymenorrhea 398
polyp 95, 328
polypectomy 335
polyphagia 323

polysomnography 292
polyuria 355
positron Emission Tomography 293
preeclampsia 410
prefix 17
prepuce 377
presbycusis 197, 200
presbyopia 182, 189
presentation 409
primigravida 414
proctectomy 335
proctitis 328
proctoplasty 335
progesterone 211, 396
prolapse of cord 411
proliferative period 397
pronation 83
prostate gland 377
prostatectomy 383
prostatitis 378, 385
protection 114
protraction 83
pruritus ani 327
pruritus vulvae 398
pruritus 97
pseudocyesis 414
pterygium 181
pulmonary abscess 287
pulmonary angiography 293
pulmonary edema 287
pulmonary Embolectomy 290
pulmonary embolism 287
pulmonary function test 293
pulmonary valve 230
pulpitis 321
pupil 174
purified Protein Derivative test 293
purkinje fibers 233
purpura 96
pursed lip breathing 287
pustule 94
pyelitis 356
pyelolithotomy 359
pyelonephritis 357
pyelotomy 359
pyloric stenosis 325
pyloroplasty 334
pylorospasm 325, 342
pylorus 315
pyosalpinx 401
pyothorax 287
pyuria 355

Q

QRS wave 234
quadrants 77
quickening 407

R

rachiometer 129
radical pancreatoduodenectomy 337
radioactive iodine uptake 218
radioimmunoassay 221
rales 288
rectocele 329
rectostenosis 342
rectovaginal fistula 399
rectum 317
reduction 127
reflux 340
regional anesthesia 160
regurgitation 323
renal angiography 363
renal biopsy 363
renal failure 357
renal hypertension 357
respiratory acidosis 288
respiratory alkalosis 288
reticulocytes 257
retina 174
retinal detachment 181
retinitis 179
retinoblastoma 181
retraction 83
retroflexion 400
retrograde pyelography 363
retropubic prostatectomy 383
retroversion 400
rh antigen 258
rhabdomyosarcoma 147
rhinoplasty 290
rhinorrhea 288
rhonchi 288
right atrium 228
right bundle branches 233
right coronary artery 233
right ventricle 229
rod cells 172
root 17
rosacea 98
rotation 82
round window 193
rugae 314

S

sagittal plane 79
salivary glands 310
salpingectomy 403, 404
salpingitis 401
salpingo-oophorectomy 403
scabies 101
scale 95
sclera 171, 173
sclerectomy 184
scleritis 179
scleroderma 95
sclerotherapy 247
scotoma 178
scratch test 105
scrotum 376
sebaceous glands 92
sebum 92
secretory period 397
segmental resection 290
semen 377
semen analysis 384
semicircular canal 194
semilunar valve 230
seminal vesicles 377
seminiferous tubules 375, 376
seminoma 381
sepsis 263
septoplasty 290
septotomy 290
short bone 114
shoulder girdle 121
shunt surgery 242
sialadenitis 322
sickle cell anemia 262
sigmoidoscopy 339
silicosis 288
Simmonds' disease 216
sinoatrial node 233
sinusitis 288
skeletal muscles 141
Skene's glands 394
skin biopsy 105
skin graft 104
small intestine 316
smooth muscles 141

sneezing 288
SOAP 16
soft palate 309
somatic nervous system 157
sphenoidal sinus 275
sphincter of Oddi 320
sphincteroplasty 337
spinal block 160
spinal cavity 75
spinal cord injury 160
spinal cord 75, 156
spinal nerve 158
spleen 261
splenorrhaphy 267
spondylitis 126
spongy bone 116
sprain 146
sputum 288
squamous cell carcinoma 102
stapedectomy 198
stapes 192
steatorrhea 326
sterility 398
stillbirth 409
stomach cancer 325
stomach 314
stomatitis 321
stomatitis 343
stomatoplasty 332
strabismus 182
strain 146
stratum basale 90
stratum corneum 89
stratum granulosum 89
stratum lucidum 89
stratum papillarosum 90
stratum reticularosum 90
stratum spinosum 90
stridor 289
sublingual gland 310
submandibular gland 310
suffix 17
supination 83
support 114
suprapubic prostatectomy 383
suprarenal gland 209
sweat glands 93
syllables 20
sympathetic nervous system 157
synchondrosis 124
synovial joint 124
syphilis 382
syringitis 197
systemic lupus erythematosus 101
systole 240

T

T wave 234
tachycardia 247
tachypnea 289
tactile fremitus 289
tarsus 172
teeth, tooth 311
tendinitis 126, 145
tendon 140
tenesmus 326
tenodesis 147
tenosynovitis 126
tenotomy 127, 147
teratocarcinoma 381
testicular carcinoma 381
testis 211, 375
testosterone 211
tetany 217
tetraplegia 165
thallium test 244
thelitis 401
thoracentesis 293
thoracic cage 120
thoracic cavity 76
thoracic duct 261
thoracoplasty 291
thoracoscopy 293
thoracotomy 290
thrombocytes 257
thrombocytopenia 269
thrombus 246
thymopoietin 210
thymosin 210
thymus 261
thymus gland 210
thymus 209
thyroid cartilage 277
thyroid function test 218
thyroid gland 210
thyroid scan 218
thyroid 209
thyroidectomy 217
thyroidotomy 217
thyroxine 210
tinnitus 195
tissues 31
tongue cancer 322
tongue 313
tonometer 189
tonometry 185
tonsil 261, 276
tonsillectomy 291
tonsillitis 289, 295, 324
trachea 277
tracheal cartilage 277
tracheoplasty 291
tracheostomy 291
tracheotomy 291
trachoma 181
transesophageal echocardiogram 244
transfusion 264
transurethral prostatectomy 383
transverse plane 79
trichiasis 180
trichomoniasis 382
tricuspid atresia 240
tricuspid valve 230
triglycerides 256
trigone 351
trochlear nerve 171
tubal ligation 403
tuboplasty 403
tubule 349
tuning fork test 199
TUR 379
TURP 384
tympanic cavity 192
tympanic membrane 192
tympanites 326
tympanometry 199
tympanoplasty 198
tympanotomy 198

U

ulcer 96
ulcerative colitis 327
umbilical cord 407
umbilical hernia 329
upper respiratory infection 289
upper respiratory tract 274
urea 348
uremia 356, 366
ureter 351
ureterectasis 357

ureterectomy 359
ureteritis 356
ureterolithiasis 358
ureterostenosis 359
urethra 352, 377
urethritis 356
urethroscopy 362
uric acid 348
urinalysis 364
urinary bladder 351
urinary catheterization 364
urinary incontinence 354
urinary meatus 352
urinary retention 355
urinary stasis 354
urinary tract infection 357
urinary urgency 354
urine 348, 352
uterine inertia 409
uterus 394
utricle 195
uvea 171, 173
uveitis 179
uvula 309
uvulectomy 291
uvulitis 322
uvulopalatopharyngoplasty 291

V

vacuum extraction 412
vagina 394
vagotomy 334
valve replacement 242
valvotomy 242
valvuloplasty 242
varicocele 380
vas deferens 376
vasectomy 383
vasoconstriction 240
vasodilator 240
vasoligation 383
vasovasostomy 384
VDRL test 384
veins 235
vena cavae 235
venography 244
ventilation / perfusion scan 293
ventral cavity 75
ventricle 229
ventriculography 244
ventriculostomy 163
venules 235
vermiform appendix 317
version 412
vertebral column 119
vertigo 195
vesical tenesmus 355
vesicle 95
vesicovaginal fistula 399
vestibule 193, 394
video-assisted thoracic surgery 291
viral hepatitis 331
virillism 217
visceral muscles 141
visceral pericardium 232
visceral pleura 281
visual acuity test 185
visual acuity 185
visual field test 185
visual field 185
vitiligo 101
vitrectomy 184
vitreous humour 175
vitreous 175
vocal cords 277
voiding cystourethrogram 363
voluntary muscles 141
volvulus 328
vowel 17
vulva 393
vulvitis 399

W

wart 102
wedge resection 291
Wernicke's aphasia 159
wheal 95
wheeze 289
Whipple's operation 337
Wilms' tumor 359

X

xenograft 103
xerophthalmia 178
xerostomia 321

Z

Zollinger-Ellison syndrome 325